Palit K. Kataki, PhD
Suresh Chandra Babu, PhD
Editors

T0252813

Food Systems for Improved Human Nutrition: Linking Agriculture, Nutrition, and Productivity

Food Systems for Improved Human Nutrition: Linking Agriculture, Nutrition, and Productivity has been co-published simultaneously as *Journal of Crop Production*, Volume 6, Numbers 1/2 (#11/12) 2002.

Pre-publication REVIEWS, COMMENTARIES, EVALUATIONS . . .

"The subject matter addresses a very important nexus: agriculture, nutrition and productivity. Hitherto, these topics have been treated singly and in isolation. Researchers and development experts of late have attempted to link these issues, but oftentimes only in a conceptual way. I can see an attempt in this manuscript to link them in a real practical way. Further, I can see what often is the real situation on the ground being documented.

. . . It will form a most valuable resource for professionals across the fields of agriculture, nutrition and production economics."

Ruth K. Oniang'o, PhD
Professor
Food Science and Nutrition
Executive Director
Rural Outreach Program
and Editor-in-Chief
African Journal of Food and
Nutritional Sciences (AJFNS)

"This book endeavors to provide linkages between agricultural production and nutritional quality using an umbrella food systems perspective. The chapters bridge a broad range covering vegetable, animal and fish production and their potential for addressing global food security and health issues. . . . Readers interested in food security issues from various disciplines will benefit from the cross-cutting concerns expressed in the various chapters.

Several chapters deal with economic issues, food consumption elasticities and use of model approaches to predict future needs, as well as health consequences. Case studies in Bangladesh illustrate the importance of fish and, in China, how rapidly changing consumption and activity patterns are shifting concerns from undernutrition to overnutrition and chronic diseases. The historical account of the development of Quality Protein Maize (QPM) is especially interesting as it illustrates how barriers initially thought to be insurmountable were overcome. The nutritional and economic benefits of enhanced vegetable production and consumption are put in perspective, identifying barriers and risks to farmers and providing suggestions for government and trade policies to stabilize production in light of increased consumer demand. And, the chapter on fisheries in Bangladesh has implications for meeting micronutrient needs in other countries."

Barbara A. Underwood, PhD
Chair
Food and Nutrition Board
Scholar-in-Residence
Institute of Medicine
The National Academies

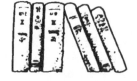

Food Systems
for Improved
Human Nutrition:
Linking Agriculture,
Nutrition, and Productivity

Food Systems for Improved Human Nutrition: Linking Agriculture, Nutrition, and Productivity has been co-published simultaneously as *Journal of Crop Production*, Volume 6, Numbers 1/2 (#11/12) 2002.

The *Journal of Crop Production* Monographic "Separates"

Below is a list of "separates," which in serials librarianship means a special issue simultaneously published as a special journal issue or double-issue *and* as a "separate" hardbound monograph. (This is a format which we also call a "DocuSerial.")

"Separates" are published because specialized libraries or professionals may wish to purchase a specific thematic issue by itself in a format which can be separately cataloged and shelved, as opposed to purchasing the journal on an on-going basis. Faculty members may also more easily consider a "separate" for classroom adoption.

"Separates" are carefully classified separately with the major book jobbers so that the journal tie-in can be noted on new book order slips to avoid duplicate purchasing.

You may wish to visit Haworth's website at . . .

http://www.HaworthPress.com

. . . to search our online catalog for complete tables of contents of these separates and related publications.

You may also call 1-800-HAWORTH (outside US/Canada: 607-722-5857), or Fax 1-800-895-0582 (outside US/Canada: 607-771-0012), or e-mail at:

getinfo@haworthpressinc.com

Food Systems for Improved Human Nutrition: Linking Agriculture, Nutrition, and Productivity, edited by Palit K. Kataki, PhD and Suresh Chandra Babu, PhD (Vol. 6, No. 1/2 #11/12, 2002). *Discusses the concepts and analyzes the results of food based approaches designed to reduce malnutrition and to improve human nutrition.*

Quality Improvement in Field Crops, edited by A. S. Basra, PhD, and L. S. Randhawa, PhD (Vol. 5, No. 1/2 #9/10, 2002). *Examines ways to increase nutritional quality as well as volume in field crops.*

Allelopathy in Agroecosystems, edited by Ravinder K. Kohli, PhD, Harminder Pal Singh, PhD, and Daizy R. Batish, PhD (Vol. 4, No. 2 #8, 2001). *Explains how the natural biochemical interactions among plants and microbes can be used as an environmentally safe method of weed and pest management.*

The Rice-Wheat Cropping System of South Asia: Efficient Production Management, edited by Palit K. Kataki, PhD (Vol. 4, No. 1 #7, 2001). *This book critically analyzes and discusses production issues for the rice-wheat cropping system of South Asia, focusing on the questions of soil depletion, pest control, and irrigation. It compiles information gathered from research institutions, government organizations, and farmer surveys to analyze the condition of this regional system, suggest policy changes, and predict directions for future growth.*

The Rice-Wheat Cropping System of South Asia: Trends, Constraints, Productivity and Policy, edited by Palit K. Kataki, PhD (Vol. 3, No. 2 #6, 2001). *This book critically analyzes and discusses available options for all aspects of the rice-wheat cropping system of South Asia, addressing the question, "Are the sustainability and productivity of this system in a state of decline/stagnation?" This volume compiles information gathered from research institutions, government organizations, and farmer surveys to analyze the impact of this regional system.*

Nature Farming and Microbial Applications, edited by Hui-lian Xu, PhD, James F. Parr, PhD, and Hiroshi Umemura, PhD (Vol. 3, No. 1 #5, 2000). *"Of great interest to agriculture specialists, plant physiologists, microbiologists, and entomologists as well as soil scientists and evnironmentalists. . . . very original and innovative data on organic farming." (Dr. André Gosselin, Professor, Department of Phytology, Center for Research in Horticulture, Université Laval, Quebec, Canada)*

Water Use in Crop Production, edited by M.B. Kirkham, BA, MS, PhD (Vol. 2, No. 2 #4, 1999). *Provides scientists and graduate students with an understanding of the advancements in the understanding of water use in crop production around the world. You will discover that by utilizing good management, such as avoiding excessive deep percolation or reducing runoff by increased infiltration, that even under dryland or irrigated conditions you can achieve improved use of water for greater crop production. Through this informative book, you will discover how to make the most efficient use of water for crops to help feed the earth's expanding population.*

Expanding the Context of Weed Management, edited by Douglas D. Buhler, PhD (Vol. 2, No. 1 #3, 1999). *Presents innovative approaches to weeds and weed management.*

Nutrient Use in Crop Production, edited by Zdenko Rengel, PhD (Vol. 1, No. 2 #2, 1998). *"Raises immensely important issues and makes sensible suggestions about where research and agricultural extension work needs to be focused." (Professor David Clarkson, Department of Agricultural Sciences, AFRC Institute Arable Crops Research, University of Bristol, United Kingdom)*

Crop Sciences: Recent Advances, Amarjit S. Basra, PhD (Vol. 1, No. 1 #1, 1997). *Presents relevant research findings and practical guidance to help improve crop yield and stability, product quality, and environmental sustainability.*

Food Systems for Improved Human Nutrition: Linking Agriculture, Nutrition, and Productivity

Palit K. Kataki, PhD
Suresh Chandra Babu, PhD
Editors

Food Systems for Improved Human Nutrition: Linking Agriculture, Nutrition, and Productivity has been co-published simultaneously as *Journal of Crop Production*, Volume 6, Numbers 1/2 (#11/12) 2002.

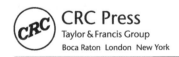

CRC Press
Taylor & Francis Group
Boca Raton London New York

CRC Press is an imprint of the
Taylor & Francis Group, an **informa** business

Published by

The Food Products Press®, 10 Alice Street, Binghamton, NY 13904-1580 USA

The Food Products Press® is an imprint of The Haworth Press, Inc., 10 Alice Street, Binghamton, NY 13904-1580 USA.

Food Systems for Improved Human Nutrition: Linking Agriculture, Nutrition, and Productivity has been co-published simultaneously as *Journal of Crop Production*, Volume 6, Numbers 1/2 (#11/12) 2002.

The development, preparation, and publication of this work has been undertaken with great care. However, the publisher, employees, editors, and agents of The Haworth Press and all imprints of The Haworth Press, Inc., including The Haworth Medical Press® and Pharmaceutical Products Press®, are not responsible for any errors contained herein or for consequences that may ensue from use of materials or information contained in this work. Opinions expressed by the author(s) are not necessarily those of The Haworth Press, Inc. With regard to case studies, identities and circumstances of individuals discussed herein have been changed to protect confidentiality. Any resemblance to actual persons, living or dead, is entirely coincidental.

Cover design by Jennifer Gaska

Library of Congress Cataloging-in-Publication Data

Food systems for improved human nutrition: linking agriculture, nutrition, and productivity / Palit K. Kataki, Suresh Chandra Babu, editors.
    p. cm.
    "Co-published simultaneously as Journal of crop production, volume 6, numbers 1/2(#11/12)".
    Includes bibliographical references and index.
    ISBN 1-56022-102-X (hard: alk. paper)–ISBN 1-56022-103-8 (pbk: alk. paper)
    1. Malnutrition–Prevention. 2. Nutrition policy. 3. Sustainable agriculture. I. Kataki, Palit K.
II. Babu, Suresh Chandra. III. Journal of crop production.
RA645.N87 F684 2002
363.8–dc21

2002010069

Indexing, Abstracting & Website/Internet Coverage

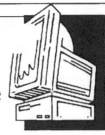

This section provides you with a list of major indexing & abstracting services. That is to say, each service began covering this periodical during the year noted in the right column. Most Websites which are listed below have indicated that they will either post, disseminate, compile, archive, cite or alert their own Website users with research-based content from this work. (This list is as current as the copyright date of this publication.)

Abstracting, Website/Indexing Coverage . . . . Year When Coverage Began

- *AGRICOLA Database <www.natl.usda.gov/ag98>* 1998

- *BIOBASE (Current Awareness in Biological Science)*
  <URL: http://www.elsevier.nl> 1998

- *Cambridge Scientific Abstracts (Water Resources*
  Abstracts/Agricultural & Environmental Biotechnology
  Abstracts) <www.csa.com> 2001

- *Chemical Abstracts Services <www.cas.org>* 1998

- *CNPIEC Reference Guide: Chinese National Directory*
  of Foreign Periodicals 1998

- *Derwent Crop Production File* 1998

- *Environment Abstracts. Available in print–CD-ROM–*
  on Magnetic Tape. For more information check:
  <www.cispubs.com> 1998

- *Field Crop Abstracts (c/o CAB Intl/CAB ACCESS)*
  <www.cabi.org/> 1998

(continued)

Special Bibliographic Notes related to special journal issues (separates) and indexing/abstracting:

- indexing/abstracting services in this list will also cover material in any "separate" that is co-published simultaneously with Haworth's special thematic journal issue or DocuSerial. Indexing/abstracting usually covers material at the article/chapter level.
- monographic co-editions are intended for either non-subscribers or libraries which intend to purchase a second copy for their circulating collections.
- monographic co-editions are reported to all jobbers/wholesalers/approval plans. The source journal is listed as the "series" to assist the prevention of duplicate purchasing in the same manner utilized for books-in-series.
- to facilitate user/access services all indexing/abstracting services are encouraged to utilize the co-indexing entry note indicated at the bottom of the first page of each article/chapter/contribution.
- this is intended to assist a library user of any reference tool (whether print, electronic, online, or CD-ROM) to locate the monographic version if the library has purchased this version but not a subscription to the source journal.
- individual articles/chapters in any Haworth publication are also available through the Haworth Document Delivery Service (HDDS).

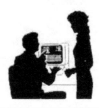

Food Systems for Improved Human Nutrition: Linking Agriculture, Nutrition, and Productivity

CONTENTS

ABOUT THE EDITORS

Palit K. Kataki, PhD, received his doctorate at Cornell University, USA. He is currently CIMMYT Adjunct Scientist and Research Assistant at University of Guelph, Ontario, Canada. His research activities include: tillage and crop establishment, carbon sequestration under conservation and conventional tillage systems, development of Ontario wheat database research information system for crop modelling. His earlier work experience includes: GIS Assistant, Corporation of Halton Hills, Canada; Coordinator, Cornell University, USA; Assistant Professor, Assam Agriculture University, India; Research Associate, Indian Council of Agriculture Research, Barapani; Assistant Manager, Namroop Tea Estate, Tata Tea Ltd., India. His past research and academic activities included research on micronutrients, crop sterility, tillage and crop establishment, and legume establishment in the rice-wheat cropping system of South Asia (Bangladesh, India, Nepal and Pakistan) for several years, seed physiology, weed management in rice-rice cropping system , tea production, and teaching undergraduate courses. Dr. Kataki has been the recipient of several awards and scholarships, has authored or co-authored several scientific papers, and has edited a two-volume book on the Rice-Wheat cropping system of South Asia.

Suresh Chandra Babu, PhD, is Senior Research Fellow and Senior Training Advisor at the International Food Policy Research Institute in Washington, DC. He joined IFPRI in 1992 as a research fellow and currently head IFPRI's Training and Capacity Strengthening Program, conducting research on issues related to food security, rural poverty, and natural resource sustainability. He has been a senior advisor to the government of Malawi on food and nutrition policy issues. He has taught at Iowa State University, Tamil Nadu Agricultural University, and Bunda College of Agriculture in Malawi.

Preface

Nutritional status of humans is determined by the chain of events from food production to consumption, and against the backdrop of cultures and nations, it is a complex relationship. Despite an increase in staple food grain production and consumption during the last few decades, malnutrition in humans is still alarming, and is the primary reason for reduced human productivity. This publication brings together information on various aspects of a food systems strategy from different regions of the world. The information presented in this publication is in three forms–first: analysis, interpretation and discussions of data from different research programs, second: econometric models supported by field data, where applicable, and third: discussion of concepts and approaches that can be taken to address issues of malnutrition.

All the articles are woven around the central concept of Food Systems, elaborated in Table 1 of the Article 1. The science of food production and human nutrition are specialist subjects, that have been mutually exclusive primarily at the policy and institutional level in general, have has perhaps been one of many reasons why malnutrition amongst humans is still alarming. It is therefore fitting that this compilation is being published as a journal-cum-book issue in the *Journal of Crop Production*, a small step towards bridging the gap between the activities of agriculture and human nutrition.

Our invitation to all the experts to share their data, analysis and discussion for this publication has been overwhelming, for which we are grateful. We are honored to have Dr. Per Pinstrup-Andersen, Director General, IFPRI, and recipient of 2001 World Food Prize, for sharing his views (Foreword), on this publication. Finally, we will value any comments and suggestions from the readers of this publication.

Palit K. Kataki
Suresh Chandra Babu

[Haworth co-indexing entry note]: "Preface." Kataki, Palit K., and Suresh Chandra Babu. Co-published simultaneously in *Journal of Crop Production* (Food Products Press, an imprint of The Haworth Press, Inc.) Vol. 6, No. 1/2 (#11/12), 2002, pp. xxi; and: *Food Systems for Improved Human Nutrition: Linking Agriculture, Nutrition, and Productivity* (ed: Palit K. Kataki, and Suresh Chandra Babu) Food Products Press, an imprint of The Haworth Press, Inc., 2002, pp. xiii. Single or multiple copies of this article are available for a fee from The Haworth Document Delivery Service [1-800-HAWORTH, 9:00 a.m. - 5:00 p.m. (EST). E-mail address: getinfo@haworthpressinc.com].

Foreword

It is increasingly being recognized that agricultural scientists and human nutritionists should jointly explore options to solve the problem of malnutrition. International agricultural research has made significant contributions towards increasing the food supplies in developing countries, which has lowered food prices and has improved access to food staples for the poor and malnourished. In spite of the successes, high levels of micronutrient malnutrition remain a major public health concern. The crucial role of poor dietary quality has been recognized as a major contributing cause for increasing the level of micronutrient malnutrition. Therefore, what role can agriculture and food-based interventions play in addressing micronutrient malnutrition? What strategies are needed to simultaneously address both low levels of energy and micronutrient intake? How do we bring together a multidisciplinary team of agricultural researchers, planners, and policymakers to design and implement holistic food and nutrition strategies?

The editors of this volume have attempted to provide answers for the above questions by compiling a set of papers written by a multidisciplinary group of researchers. Termed as "food systems approach," the issues and strategies addressed by the papers of this volume range from crop diversification to fortification through plant breeding and planning, monitoring and evaluation of food and nutrition interventions. Several food-based strategies have been reviewed for their impact on the nutritional well being of the population. Several ideas for designing nutritional intervention programs have been identified by the papers of this volume. The recommendations made by the authors for furthering the goals of improving human nutrition are worth emulating in various settings.

It is my hope that this book will stimulate debate and further research on this

[Haworth co-indexing entry note]: "Foreword." Pinstrup-Andersen, Per. Co-published simultaneously in *Journal of Crop Production* (Food Products Press, an imprint of The Haworth Press, Inc.) Vol. 6, No. 1/2 (#11/12), 2002, pp. xxiii-xxiv; and: *Food Systems for Improved Human Nutrition: Linking Agriculture, Nutrition, and Productivity* (ed: Palit K. Kataki, and Suresh Chandra Babu) Food Products Press, an imprint of The Haworth Press, Inc., 2002, pp. xv-xvi. Single or multiple copies of this article are available for a fee from The Haworth Document Delivery Service [1-800-HAWORTH, 9:00 a.m. - 5:00 p.m. (EST). E-mail address: getinfo@ haworthpressinc.com].

xv

important topic of addressing malnutrition through food systems and that it will lead to improved programs and policies for addressing food insecurity and malnutrition in the future.

Per Pinstrup-Andersen
Director General
International Food Policy Research Institute
Washington, DC, USA

Food Systems
for Improved Human Nutrition:
An Introduction

P. K. Kataki

S. C. Babu

SUMMARY. Food insecurity and malnutrition continue to be the major developmental challenge at the beginning of the 21st century. An estimated 11 percent of children are born with low birth weight, 165 million pre-school children are stunted, an estimated 2 billion people suffer from anemia, 74 million from iodine deficiency, and one-quarter of a billion children are deficient in vitamin A in developing countries. Despite an overall decrease in the levels of malnutrition over the past 30 years, food and nutrition insecurity, particularly among women and children, the two most vulnerable population groups, is still very high. Since malnutrition manifests itself throughout the life cycle, it has serious repercussions on the quality of human capital, productivity, and economic development of nations. In addition, malnutrition in the form of obesity is also increasing in several developing and developed countries. This introductory chapter describes the background, structure, and topics covered in this publication on "Food Systems for Improved Human Nutrition" as key components of a food systems strategy. *[Article copies available for a fee from The Haworth Document Delivery Service: 1-800-HAWORTH. E-mail address: <getinfo@haworthpressinc.com> Website: <http://www.HaworthPress.com> © 2002 by The Haworth Press, Inc. All rights reserved.]*

P. K. Kataki is currently at the Department of Plant Agiculture, Crop Science Building, University of Guelph, Guelph, Ontario, Canada N1G 2W1 (E-mail: pkataki@uoguelph.ca).

S. C. Babu is Senior Research Fellow and Senior Training Advisor, IFPRI, 2033 K Street, N.W., Washington, DC 20006 USA (E-mail: s.babu@cgiar.org).

[Haworth co-indexing entry note]: "Food Systems for Improved Human Nutrition: An Introduction." Kataki. P. K., and S. C. Babu. Co-published simultaneously in *Journal of Crop Production* (Food Products Press, an imprint of The Haworth Press, Inc.) Vol. 6, No. 1/2 (#11/12), 2002, pp. 1-5; and: *Food Systems for Improved Human Nutrition: Linking Agriculture, Nutrition, and Productivity* (ed: Palit K. Kataki, and Suresh Chandra Babu) Food Products Press, an imprint of The Haworth Press, Inc., 2002, pp. 1-5. Single or multiple copies of this article are available for a fee from The Haworth Document Delivery Service [1-800-HAWORTH. 9:00 a.m. - 5:00 p.m. (EST). E-mail address: getinfo@haworthpressinc.com].

KEYWORDS. Food systems, micronutrients, malnutrition, nutrition

FOOD SYSTEMS: AN INTRODUCTION

Efforts to tackle protein-energy malnutrition have been fairly successful, primarily through increased cereal production and government food distribution programs, including subsidies and safety net programs of various kinds. Increased cereal production, especially of rice and wheat, has been achieved primarily through green-revolution technologies. More recently, the progress made with Quality Protein Maize (QPM) and promises of nutritious rice should add to the success stories of the cereal revolution of the 1970s. Such production-oriented efforts need to continue to receive support through appropriate policies and institutions in order for it to build on the progress made over the past 30 years. However, despite the progress made, there are an estimated 4.5 billion people to feed in developing countries and 800 million of them are food insecure (Pinstrup-Andersen, 1999).

Recently, micronutrient malnutrition has been recognized as a major problem in developing countries where staple foods make up a large percentage of the diet. Micronutrient deficiency related malnutrition in humans has largely been addressed through supplementation and fortification of foods. Supplementation can dramatically and relatively quickly overcome micronutrient deficiency problems in population groups, but such programs are not always sustainable on a long-term basis for developing countries. For example, Bangladesh has made significant progress towards controlling vitamin A deficiencies by increasing the coverage of vitamin A capsules amongst its population, largely through foreign aid. However, there are concerns that if foreign assistance were to stop due to reduced flow or lack of funds (which did for a brief period in 1996), the vitamin A program in Bangladesh may lapse and its deficiency amongst its population would increase. It is in this backdrop that sustainable strategies to link agriculture and nutrition, which were largely exclusive until recently, have gained momentum in recent years. For example, "Food Systems Approach," "Food-Based Strategies" and "Field Fortification Methods" are approaches that make the foods that people already eat more nutritious.

The chain of events, from production to consumption of foods, determines the nutritional status of various population groups in different regions. Therefore, the "Food Systems" strategies seek to address problems of food insecurity and malnutrition by understanding the production requirements for diverse foods (cereals, legumes, vegetables, and fruits), to increase their supply, affordability and their consumption. This approach argues that addressing nutrition-related health problems associated with micro- and macronutrient deficiencies exclusively through capsules and fortification of foods is not cost-effective and is unsustainable, especially for developing and least-developed countries, and therefore should be inclusive of a larger "Food Systems" strategy. Such an approach has two advantages–it avoids repeated high annual costs for research and development and once the system is developed in one country, it can be adapted so the benefits could be spread to the rest of the world avoiding cost of supplementation in each country. Furthermore, many of the traditional management skills, knowledge, and preservation of indigenous foods are slowly eroding; therefore, there is an increasing need to identify and enhance the food production systems that could contribute to increasing the macronutrient and micronutrient content of the local food supply.

This publication, therefore, brings together biological and social scientists from renowned research and policy institutions and non-governmental organizations to discuss multidisciplinary "Food Systems" strategies. As shown by the empirical evidence and discussions presented in the articles of this publication, purposeful linking of agriculture and human nutrition is unavoidable and necessary.

The first article of this publication by P. K. Kataki, introduces the concept of "Food Systems." "Food Systems" encompasses activities related to production, acquisition, and utilization of foods that affect human nutrition and health. This article introduces several key anthropometrical terms as indicators of human well being that are often used by nutritionists and economists. These indicators should serve to link agricultural scientists to nutrition issues better. This article also seeks to lay the background for the subsequent articles.

The article by M. Ruel and C. E. Levin gives an overview of food-based approaches for micronutrient malnutrition, with examples from three deficiencies: vitamin A, iron, and iodine. They also discuss the importance of investing in education for a food-based systems strategy to be successful. Micronutrient deficiencies result in serious sub-clinical and clinical health problems and appropriate government support for nutrition programs are essential to reduce its severity. The article by T. Schaetzel and R. Shankar, with data from South Asia illustrates this point. They argue that in addition to food systems strategies, micronutrient supplementation and fortification will continue to be major interventions for some time to come.

As economies of nations grow, diets change. Changes in diets have both positive and negative impacts on the nutritional status of various population groups as shown in the article by B. M. Popkin, L. Bing, and X. Guo with illustrations from China. Similarly, technologies change cropping systems. Green Revolution catalyzed the adoption of high-yielding rice-wheat cropping systems in South Asia that impacted the nutritional status in this region as demonstrated in the article by P. K. Kataki. Crop diversification is important to produce sufficient quantities of diverse foods, to increase farm incomes, and to increase diversity in diets. Vegetables, like pulses and oilseeds, are important components of crop diversification strategies and can positively contribute to human health. The article by M. Ali and Abedullah with data from South and South-East Asia illustrate the role of enhanced vegetable production and consumption on nutritional and economic benefits. Introduction of tree crops along with field crops in the form of agroforestry could bring substantial benefits to farm income, food, and nutrition security. While empirical evidence on the contribution of agroforestry to nutritional status continue to be scarce, the article by S. C. Babu and V. Rhoe develops a theoretical model that could form a basis for empirical investigations.

Though the Green Revolution technologies, with an emphasis on cereal production, largely succeeded in addressing the problem of hunger-related malnutrition, its impact on micronutrient-related malnutrition has been limited. To address this concern, breeding for nutritious cereals has been a more recent area of research thrust. This strategy is becoming attractive since the delivery of nutrients through staple grains can reach large populations, and therefore is viewed to be a sustainable tactic to address micronutrient deficiencies. In this context, Quality Protein Maize (QPM) research described in the article by S. K. Vasal has made tremendous progress in recent years and the prospects of growing QPM in the Americas, Africa, and Asia is highly promising. Similarly, efforts to enrich the rice grain with micronutrients are gaining momentum and there is hope for nutritious rice (in combination with other desirable agronomic traits) to be part of the solution to malnutrition in the developing world as shown in the article by S. K. Datta and G. S. Khush.

A "Food Systems" strategy also includes programs to enhance production and consumption of smaller animals, poultry, and fish. Every year, monsoon rains inundate large areas with water in the coastal country of Bangladesh. As shown in the article by P. Thompson, N. Roos, P. Sultana, and S. H. Thilsted, fish farming has tremendous potential to improve the quality of the diets for people in Bangladesh. Similarly, adoption of cross-bred cow technologies can increase food and nutrition security for small dairy farmers in the eastern African highlands (article by M. Ahmed, S. Ehui, and M. Saleem).

Fortification of foods, which has been successful in developed countries, has had a limited impact in developing countries due to the decentralized, localized (and therefore problems with quality control), and unorganized food production and distribution systems. However, fortification holds promise for developing countries if strategies to overcome these constraints are formulated. The article by M. G. Venkatesh Mannar outlines some of these strategies.

Planning, communication, monitoring, and evaluation are essential for the adoption and implementation of all nutrition interventions. S. C. Babu and V. Rhoe discuss the basic processes needed for carrying out these functions. Furthermore, they review the challenges and constraints that are faced by the implementers of these activities.

"Food Systems" strategies will, therefore, be region specific (summary article by S. C. Babu and P. K. Kataki). This publication not only introduces the concept and strategies of "Food Systems," but also supports the concept with data and analysis from different countries for an understanding of the options available for addressing issues related to human nutrition. The discussions presented in this publication will be of interest not only to researchers in the field of agriculture, economics, and nutrition, but will also be useful as study materials for students in these areas.

Good nutrition is both a developmental and ethical imperative. Reducing food insecurity and malnutrition is the first and most important step towards increasing the quality of life of millions in the developing world. As demonstrated by the articles of this volume, the role of a "Food Systems" approach in achieving this goal could hardly be overemphasized.

REFERENCES

Pinstrup-Andersen, P. 1999. The Developing World Simply Can't Afford to Do Without Agricultural Biotechnology. *International Herald Tribune*. October 28th.

Food Systems and Malnutrition: Linking Agriculture, Nutrition and Productivity

P. K. Kataki

SUMMARY. The strategic linkages between agriculture and nutrition to combat malnutrition have been described as "Food systems," "Field fortification," and "Food based" strategies. These new strategies have evolved due to the realization of the limitations of supplementation and food fortification programs in developing countries. The measures, extent and causes of malnutrition and the components of the "Food systems" strategies to combat malnutrition in humans, will be dependent on the target population group of a region. The framework for this linkage encompasses several components, and "Food systems" strategies employed will be specific to a region. Traditionally, linkages between the management and production of crops, especially staple crops, and human nutrition were not strong, and research in these two areas was mutually exclusive. This article discusses the concepts behind the linkages between agriculture and human nutrition and the strategies to combat human malnutrition. *[Article copies available for a fee from The Haworth Document Delivery Service: 1-800-HAWORTH. E-mail address: <getinfo@ haworthpressinc.com> Website: <http://www.HaworthPress.com> © 2002 by The Haworth Press, Inc. All rights reserved.]*

P. K. Kataki is currently at the Department of Plant Agiculture, Crop Science Building, University of Guelph, Guelph, Ontario, Canada N1G 2W1 (E-mail: pkataki@ uoguelph.ca).

[Haworth co-indexing entry note]: "Food Systems and Malnutrition: Linking Agriculture, Nutrition and Productivity." Kataki, P. K. Co-published simultaneously in *Journal of Crop Production* (Food Products Press, an imprint of The Haworth Press, Inc.) Vol. 6, No. 1/2 (#11/12), 2002, pp. 7-29; and: *Food Systems for Improved Human Nutrition: Linking Agriculture, Nutrition, and Productivity* (ed: Palit K. Kataki, and Suresh Chandra Babu) Food Products Press, an imprint of The Haworth Press, Inc., 2002, pp. 7-29. Single or multiple copies of this article are available for a fee from The Haworth Document Delivery Service [1-800-HAWORTH, 9:00 a.m. - 5:00 p.m. (EST). E-mail address: getinfo@haworthpressinc.com].

KEYWORDS. Agriculture, body mass index, fortification, food based, food systems, human nutrition, malnutrition, stunting, underweight, wasting

INTRODUCTION

In recent years, various terms have been used to describe strategies to link food production (agriculture) to human nutrition and overall human productivity. These terms include: "Food Systems," "Food-Based Strategies," and "Field Fortification" (Bouis, Graham, and Welch, 1999; Combs, Duxbury, and Welch, 1997; Combs et al., 1996; Duxbury and Welch, 1999; FAO, 1997; Gibson 1996; Graham et al., 1996; Lupien 1996b). This is in addition to the already familiar terms and strategies of "Food Fortification" and "Supplementation" to improve human nutrition (Lachance, 1996; Lofti et al., 1996; MI, 1998; SUSTAIN, 1997, 1998, and 1999). Will these newer approaches remain "conceptual" to be described or defined by various "terms"? Can practical steps be taken at a community, country, or regional level to meet the goals of a "Food Systems" strategy? Is a definition of "Food Systems" really necessary and should this concept be used in different ways for different contexts? This chapter discusses the measures and extent of malnutrition, similarities between the causes of malnutrition and "Food systems" model, and the "Food Systems" concepts for alleviating malnutrition. Moreover, this chapter aims to introduce agricultural researchers to terms and anthropometrical measures used frequently by human nutritionists, and to lay the background for the subsequent chapters.

The basis for the above strategies is to reduce human malnutrition and improve human productivity. Several definitions of malnutrition exist and all of these definitions highlight the physical and/or mental impairment, and associated infections of individuals that occur due to nutritional inadequacies. The result of macronutrient malnutrition is from an imbalanced consumption of energy providing foods, and includes under- and over-nutrition. Macronutrient or energy intake and utilization by humans is achieved by the adequate consumption of carbohydrates, fats and proteins. Under-nutrition, due to insufficient calorie (energy) intake is prevalent in many countries and is a major health-related problem. Over-nutrition, due to excess calorie intake leading to obesity is not as severe as under-nutrition, but is showing an increasing trend both in developed and developing countries.

Coupled with macronutrient malnutrition is the problem of micronutrient malnutrition. Micronutrients refer to vitamins and minerals required in very small quantities relative to the macronutrients, for optimum (adequate) human health and productivity. For example, only a teaspoonful consumption of the micronutrient iodine is required in a lifetime by humans to avoid the adverse effects of iodine deficiency disorders or IDD (MI, 1997; UNICEF, Kiwani, and MI, 1999). Hence micronutrients are absolutely essential towards fulfilling human physiological needs and its deficiencies cause serious ailments (Alnwick, 1996; ACC and SCN, 2000; Calloway, 1995; HMG/N et al., 1998; Narasinga Rao, 1997; deOnis, Frongillo, and Blössner, 2000; Ross and Horton, 1998; Underwood, 1999; UNICEF, 1998; UNICEF et al., 1998; UNICEF and WHO, 1999). Both these forms of malnutrition can be closely related when food deficit is acute, depth of hunger is high, and diets are deficient in calories, minerals, and vitamins. The depth of hunger is a measure (in kilocalories) of the "per person" food deficit of the undernourished population within each country (FAO, 2000). In a second scenario, calorie production, its availability, and consumption may be sufficient, but communities may still suffer from micronutrient malnutrition resulting in a "hidden hunger." The consequences of both forms of malnutrition are severe and long lasting.

Variety is the key to solving macro and micronutrient malnutrition. One end of this "variety" spectrum is the variety of crop (e.g., cereals, legumes, vegetables, fruits, etc.) and non-crop (e.g., meat, milk, eggs, etc.) food sources grown, produced, distributed, and made available. At the opposite end of this spectrum is the variety of food consumed by various groups (communities of different cultures and countries) and categories (adults, adolescents, children) of people. In between the two ends of this spectrum are issues related to sustainable food production, marketing, government policies, economic status, status of women in society, culture, health, hygiene, education, and political stability in a region or country (Allaway, 1984; Andrews, 1997; Banda, 1996; Bargriansky et al., 1996; Bhalla, Hazel, and Kerr, 1999; Bouis, Graham, and Welch, 1999; Bouis and Slack, 1996; Brown, 1996; DeWalt, 1996; Evans, 1998; Evenson, Pray, and Rosegrant, 1999; Harison, 1996; Johnson-Welch, 1999; Lupien, 1996a; Narasinga Rao, 1997; Ronk, 1996; Shapiro, 1996; Tsou, 1996; Underwood, 1996).

The concept of "Food Systems" therefore seeks to encompass all activities related to production, acquisition, and utilization of food (Combs et al., 1996; Combs, Duxbury, and Welch, 1997; Duxbury and Welch, 1999; FAO, 1997) that affect human nutrition and health, thereby, forming the basis for a "Food-Based Strategy" towards preventing malnutrition, specifically micronutrient malnutrition. In the past, when the requirements in this variety spectrum did not fulfill the nutritional needs of population groups, deficiencies, e.g., micronutrient deficiencies, arose. Exclusively supplementation and food fortification programs were adopted in the past to tackle these deficiencies.

MEASURES OF MALNUTRITION

The combination of inadequate dietary intake of protein energy and micronutrients, and infection leads to malnourishments (UNICEF, 1998). Undernourishment and its associated growth failure are more prevalent, especially amongst children in many developing countries. For adults, Body Mass Index (BMI) is used as a crude measure of body composition (FAO, 2000) and is calculated as:

$$BMI = Body\ weight\ (in\ kgs)/(height\ in\ meters)^2$$

A healthy BMI is considered to be in the range of 18.5 to 25. A BMI above or below this range indicates obesity and underweight, respectively, and the severity of malnourishment increases the further apart the BMI of an individual is from this normal or healthy range. The mild (BMI = 17.00 to 18.49 kg/m^2), moderate (BMI = 16.00 to 16.99 kg/m^2), and severe (BMI = < 16.00 kg/m^2), underweight categories of people are considered to be chronologically energy deficient (CED). Similarly, the overweight categories of people are grouped into three grades: Grade 1, 2, and 3 with BMI of (25.00 to 29.99), (30.00 to 39.99), and (> 40.00) kg/m^2), respectively. During the last few decades, the ratio of CED:obesity, which is an indicator of undernutrition to overnutrition for a population group, has been decreasing due to the gradual increase in the numbers of obese people in population groups. Another measure of malnourishment in adults is the mid-upper-arm circumference (MUAC) (ACC and SCN, 2000). The healthy macronutrient intake as a percent of total energy can be 50-75%, 15-35%, and 10-15%, for carbohydrates, fats, and proteins, respectively.

For infants and young children, the extent of malnourishment is quantified by recording the weight, height, and age of this population group compared to a "reference population" known to have grown well (UNICEF, 1998; ACC and SCN, 2000; HMG/N et al., 1998). The measures of weight, height, and age are used to obtain indices on the percent of this population group that are underweight, wasted, or stunted. *Underweight* is the *low weight for age* in children occurring from the inadequate food intake, past episodes of under nutrition, and (or) poor health environment. *Wasting* is the *low weight for height* occurring due to recent period of starvation or disease. Stunting is a good indicator of *long-term cumulative effects* of low height for age due to past episode(s) of under nutrition. These three measures of malnutrition are considered to be moderate or severe when the data for the percent population under study is minus two or three standard deviations, respectively, from the median weight for age (underweight), weight for height (wasting), and height for age (stunting) of the reference population (UNICEF, 1998; ACC and SCN, 2000; HMG/N et al., 1998).

Growth failure can be due to Protein-Energy Malnutrition or PEM, or due to micronutrient malnutrition (UNICEF, 1998; ACC and SCN, 2000; HMG/N et al., 1998). Dietary energy deficits determine the type of severe PEM produced.

A diet that is deficient in total proteins and essential amino acids but is excessive in nonprotein calories from starch or sugar, results in kwashiorkor. In young children, severe forms of inadequate energy and nutrients cause inanition and is called marasmus. The intermediate forms are called marasmic-kwashiorkor. Marasmus is the predominant form of PEM existing in most parts of the developing countries while kwashiorkor is less common, manifesting itself in its intermediate state. Kwashiorkor is more common in regions where the staple food is comprised of yam, cassava, sweet potatoes, green banana, etc., leading to the diets being excessively starchy and deficient in proteins, e.g., in rural Africa, Caribbean, and Pacific islands.

Though growth failure is often associated with PEM, it is also caused by micronutrient deficiencies (UNICEF, 1998; ACC and SCN, 2000; HMG/N et al., 1998). There are dozens of these micronutrients, of which the deficiency of iron, vitamin A, and iodine is most widespread (Alnwick, 1996; ACC and SCN, 2000; Calloway, 1995; HMG/N et al., 1998; Narasinga Rao, 1997; deOnis, Frongillo and Blössner, 2000; Ross and Horton, 1998; Underwood 1999; UNICEF, 1998; UNICEF et al., 1998; UNICEF and WHO, 1999). The fat-soluble vitamins (A, D, E, and K) and minerals are stored in the body and therefore take time for deficiency diseases to develop. However, the water-soluble vitamins (B group and C) are not stored in the body and their deficiency symptoms develop quickly. The major reasons for micronutrient deficiencies are: uneven distribution in foods, environmental deficiency, and low bio-availability (Beebee, Gonzalez, and Rengifo, 1999; Bouis, Graham, and Welch, 1999; Calloway, 1995; Cardwell, 1999; Gopalan, Sastri, and Balasubramanian, 1995; Graham and Welch, 1994; Graham et al., 1996; Gruhn, Goletti, and Yudelman, 2000; House and Welch, 1984; Rendig, 1984; VanCampen, 1996; Welch, 1996; Welch et al., 1999; Welch and House, 1984). In addition, the crop species grown and consumed, economic status, and culture, influences the degree of micronutrient malnutrition.

EXTENT OF MALNUTRITION

Quantitative estimation of malnutrition is dependent on the quality and the extent of data available for a population group in a region. Information on the BMI and MUAC for adults, and stunting, wasting, and underweight for children, severity of anemia, iron deficiency, IDD, and other micronutrient deficiencies for different age groups, is generally collected through structured surveys using questionnaires, sample collections (blood, urine, etc.) and analysis. The quality of the data is a concern, and often time course data is not available as it is expensive, time-consuming, logistically tedious, and requires careful planning.

Deficiencies of iron, iodine, and vitamin A are considered most severe micronutrient deficiencies in many countries, and these are being discussed in subsequent articles of this publication. For children under age five, stunting, underweight, and wasting are good anthropometrical indices of malnutrition. The extent of stunting and underweight incidences for children under age five is lower for Latin America and the Caribbean (LA&C) compared to Africa and Asia (Figure 1). The present percentage points of under five children's population that are stunted and underweight for the year 2000 and the forecasting for the year 2005 is similar for Africa and Asia (Figures 1 A and C), but the numbers for Asia are double that of Africa (Figures 1 B and D) due to its higher population base. However, unlike Africa, data show an overall decreasing stunting and underweight trends for Asia and for LA&C (Figure 1 and 2). Of the 31 countries in Africa that were analyzed for trends in stunting (< −2 SD stunting), the number of countries showing an increasing (12) and decreasing (10) trend were quite similar with 9 countries remaining unchanged (Figure 2). On the contrary, of the 19 Asian and 20 LA&C countries, 15 countries each for both regions showed a decreasing trend in stunting amongst children (Figure

FIGURE 1. Trends in the percent and total numbers of children stunted and underweight in Asia, Africa, and Latin America and the Caribbean (adapted from deOnis, Frongillo, and Blössner, 2000).

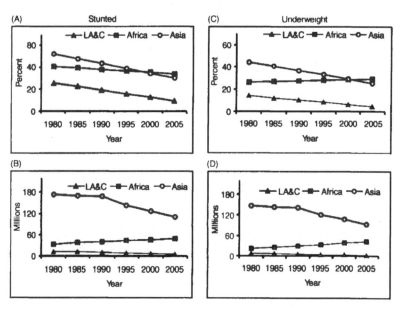

FIGURE 2. Number of countries showing increasing, decreasing, or static trends in Asia, Africa, and Latin America and the Caribbean (adapted from deOnis, Frongillo, and Blössner, 2000).

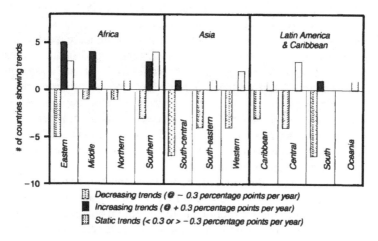

2). Details of these analysis and trends are discussed in deOnis, Frongillo, and Blössner (2000) and ACC and SCN (2000).

Nutritional status can manifest itself as a life cycle: a malnourished child is likely to be a malnourished adult and children of malnourished adults are likely to get caught in this malnourishment cycle (ACC and SCN, 2000). Since the health status of children is a good indicator of a nation or community's health services and care abilities (and also due to the availability of this form of data), especially for the vulnerable groups of women and children, it is often a favored measure of malnourishment for a region. Data on other measures of malnutrition have been scattered and scarce.

NUTRIENTS FOR CROPS AND HUMANS

Nutrient requirements for both plants and humans are categorized as the macro- and micronutrients, based on their total amounts needed. Macronutrients are required in large quantities (kilograms) while micronutrients are required in smaller quantities (in milligrams or even in lesser units). If one or more of these nutrients are deficient and do not satisfy physiological needs of either plants or humans, its deficiency results in adverse growth effects. Deficiency of macronutrients in plants (e.g., nitrogen) and in humans (e.g., lack of energy from carbohydrates, proteins or fat) is visible and striking. It leads to yellowing, stunting, and significantly low grain yield in plants and stunting, underweight, wasting, starvation, and possibly death in humans.

Deficiency symptoms of micronutrients for both plants (B, Cu, Fe, Mn, Zn, etc.) and humans (iodine, zinc, vitamins, etc.) are not always visible and are therefore hidden, except under extreme cases of its deficiencies, additionally influenced by climatic conditions for plants. Macronutrient are mostly supplied to plants through fertilizers and native soil (nitrogenous, phosphatic or potassic) and to humans through consumption of staple foods that contain high quantities of carbohydrates and proteins, derived from plants. Micronutrients are supplied to plants either from the native micronutrients present in the soil, or from soil microbes, organic fertilizers (e.g., cattle manure, other crop or plant residues), or from inorganic micronutrient fertilizers. Micronutrient requirements for humans are often met through the variety of foods consumed (in addition to the staples) and from sunlight.

Most of the nutrients identified for both plants and humans are termed "essential." They are "essential" because deficiency of any one of these nutrients even when other nutrients are supplied in the optimum quantities leads to a decreased expression of the genetic potential for disease resistance and yield in plants or cognitive, development, work capacity, productivity, and immunity to infections in humans. Many of the nutrients needed for plants and humans are similar, therefore strategic linkages (i.e., Food Systems) between agriculture and human nutrition is a very attractive and long-term sustainable approach to reduce and contain the extent of malnutrition amongst humans.

CAUSES OF MALNUTRITION

The "Food Systems" approach seeks to tackle not only the present malnutrition problems, particularly micronutrient malnutrition, but also to have a long-term sustainable impact on the productivity and well being of human populations and its generation. Understanding the causes of malnutrition is therefore a key towards tackling malnutrition. Recent analysis by Smith and Haddad (2000 a and b; for detailed analysis and discussion, refer to these publications) on the causes of child malnutrition is being discussed briefly in this section.

Evaluation of the health and nutritional status of children is considered to be an excellent measure of inequalities in human development faced by populations (deOnis, Frongillo, and Blössner, 2000). The conceptual framework for empirical analysis of children's nutritional status (Figure 3) has been built on three nutritional status determinants, i.e., immediate, underlying, and basic (Smith and Haddad, 2000a and b). The immediate determinant includes the interacting factors of dietary intake and health status that governs a child's nutri-

FIGURE 3. A comparison between models of the "Determinants of Nutritional Status" (or malnutrition model) and "Food Systems." Similarly shaded areas depict commonalities between the two models (adapted from Smith and Haddad, 2000a and b; Combs Jr., Duxbury, and Welch, 1997).

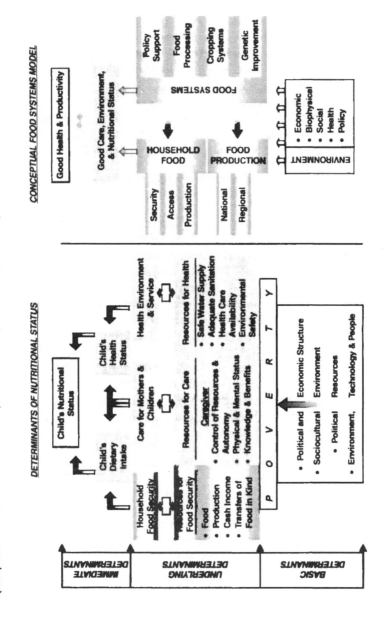

tional status, which is at the level of an individual being. The underlying determinants (Figure 3) of household food security, care for mothers and children, and the health environment and services influences the immediate determinant. Each of the underlying determinants is dependent on a set of resources (Figure 3). These resources, i.e., of food security, care and health, are influenced by the extent of poverty in the region (Figure 3). The underlying determinant is further influenced by the basic determinants of potential resources available in a country (natural resources, technology, people, etc.), socio-cultural, political, and economic environment (Figure 3).

Similarities Between the "Causes of Malnutrition" and "Food Systems" Model

The conceptual models proposed independently on the "causes of malnutrition" (henceforth referred to as the malnutrition model) by Smith and Haddad (2000a and b), and that of the "Food Systems" by Combs, Duxbury, and Welch (1997), and Combs et al. (1996), contain several key but common components. At the core of both of these models is the nutritional status of a population under study. The malnutrition model analyzes the determinants of a child nutritional status, which is a good indicator of the socio-economic and health status of a nation, region, or community. The "Food Systems" model aims to achieve adequate nutrient intake for improving human productivity, especially of women and children, the two most vulnerable groups to malnutrition. The similarities (Figure 3, shaded areas in this figure shows similarities between the two models) between these two models is in the three key areas of (a) environmental influence, (b) food production, security and intake, and (c) care and health, as described below.

> *Environmental influence:* The basic determinants of the causes of malnutrition are similar to the environments within which the food systems concept exists (similarly shaded boxes in Figure 3). These environments include the biophysical, political, economic, social and associated policies, which describes their complex and dynamic interactions. A favorable environment will facilitate the achievement of the common goals depicted in both these models.
>
> *Food production, security, and intake:* The dietary intake of a child in the malnutrition model is dependent on the household food security, which in turn, relies on the resources for food security, i.e., food production and income (Figure 3). Similarly, the "Food Systems" model emphasizes adequate nutrient intake for good health. Nutrient intake in the "Food Systems" model is dependent on food production and access at the household, regional, and national level. In addition, the "Food Sys-

tems" technologies of crop genetic improvement, cropping systems, etc., influence food production and access in the Food Systems model.
Care and health: Both these models emphasize the need for adequate care for mothers and children, and good health environment and services.

The malnutrition model was further tested empirically by a cross-country analysis of 63 developing countries between 1970 and 1996 (Smith and Haddad, 2000a and b). This broad-based analysis showed a statistically significant, but a negative correlation between child malnutrition (defined as underweight children, < 5 years of age) and the basic (per capita GDP, democracy) and underlying (access to safe water, female school enrolment, female-to-male life expectancy ration, and dietary energy supplies) determinants. Though the authors (Smith and Haddad, 2000a and b) emphasizes the need for careful diagnosis and analysis to understand the causes of child malnutrition for each subpopulation of developing countries, the components of the malnutrition and "Food Systems" models are strikingly similar.

The possibilities of a "Food Systems" approach towards reducing malnutrition and improving human productivity as a long-term sustainable strategy is therefore real. Both these models do not emphasize supplementation or food fortification as exclusive, but as inclusive means of reducing malnutrition. Given the enormity of the model components, food systems strategies will, therefore, have to be country and region specific.

FOOD SYSTEMS STRATEGY

Expanding on the conceptual "Food Systems" model of Figure 3, the strategies that can be employed to implement this concept would be many-fold. These strategies include food production, food fortification, communication, planning, and monitoring (surveillance and evaluation) strategies (Table 1). A summary of the goals and objectives for each of these strategies, and its associated constraints and requirements are shown in Table 1.

Food production strategies would include six major activities (Table 1): crop diversification; breeding for micronutrient enriched staple food grains; large-scale vegetable, fruit, and milk production and distribution; improved post-harvest storage; small-scale vegetable production; and, production of small animals, poultry, and fish. Within the last three decades, cereal grain production has increased in several countries but crop diversification has decreased tremendously. Breeding for cereal varieties has been with an emphasis on higher yield and disease resistance. Research on increasing micronutrient content of grain crops, e.g., rice, has tremendous long-term potential for delivering micronutrients to populations (Allaway, 1984; Abd El-Moneim et al.,

TABLE 1. The Strategies, Goals, Objectives, Constraints, and Requirements of a Food Systems Approach.

STRATEGIES	GOALS and OBJECTIVES	MAJOR CONSTRAINTS and REQUIREMENTS
A. FOOD–PRODUCTION STRATEGIES		
1. *Crop Diversification*	• Increased cultivation and production of *legumes* for fodder and grains, and **vegetables**. • *Oil seed* crop production for availability of low-cost dietary fat. • Increasing *diversity* in food consumption through production.	• Legumes and oil seed crops are generally grown in *harsher* environments. • Higher *risks* due to low yields (compared to cereals), *vulnerability* to insects, pests and diseases. • Requires appropriate *varieties* and *management skills* for stable yield. • Appropriate government *policies* to encourage diversification.
2. *Breeding for and production of micronutrient enriched staple food grains (e.g., wheat, rice, maize, potatoes, etc.)*	• Breed for one or multinutrient *varieties* of staple crops. • To improve *quality* of staple crops that are consumed. • Reach a *wider population* base for reducing micronutrient malnutrition.	• Tools exists (e.g., conventional plant breeding and selection, biotechnology) but is time *consuming* and *costly.* • *Bioavailability* studies need to be conducted. • *Varietal adaptation* to different agro-ecological zones, though enriched seeds (varieties) should have agronomic advantages in general.
3. *Large-scale (commercial) vegetable & fruit production, organized milk & milk product production & distribution (e.g., dairy co-operatives)*	• Supply of *micronutrient rich food* at reasonable prices. • Competitive *pricing* lowers prices for purchase by consumer.	• Need for improved *post-harvest storage* (see constraints for post-harvest strategy).
4. *Improved post-harvest storage*	• To prevent (reduce) *post-harvest losses* in quantity and quality of perishables. • Increased year-round *availability* of several micronutrient rich foods.	• At *commercial level:* Good marketing, grading, packaging, transport, and cold storage facilities needed. • At *household level:* Practical and simple food processing and preservation methods (e.g., solar drying) required.

5. Small-scale community vegetable and fruit gardening	• To increase micronutrient rich-foods at *local level*. • Indirectly, this should lead to *increased consumption* by increasing availability.	• Land and water *limitations*. • Good understanding of local conditions needed. • *Community* participation. • *Women's* involvement. • *Government* interventions & assistance.
6. Production of *small animals, poultry and fish*	• Increased *production* of micronutrient rich-foods. • Increased *bio-availability* of micronutrients in diet, especially of Fe and vitamin A.	• *Cost constraints* need to be addressed. • Need for *promoting* small livestock and fishery projects. • Need for *education* and *support* for producers.
B. FOOD FORTIFICATION STRATEGY	• To *deliver micronutrients* without a major change in taste and appearance of food.	• Careful *planning*. • Identify appropriate *food vehicles* and *fortificants*. • Adequate *consumption* of fortified foods. • *Enforcement* of regulation. • *Cost* consideration. • Consumer *education*. • Effective *quality* assurance.
C. COMMUNICATION STRATEGY	• To change *dietary practices* (especially of vulnerable groups, e.g., women and children) by changing eating habits and increasing intake. • To preserve *traditional nutritional* beneficial practices.	• *Plan* communication interventions. • *Strategies* should be based on information obtained from target groups.
D. PLANNING STRATEGY	• Conduct *situation analysis* to assess extent of micronutrient malnourishment problems, analyze causes, and review available sources.	• Involvement of *expert personnel* from health, agriculture, food industry, and education required. • National *policy formulation* and associated strategies essential.
E. MONITORING, SURVELLIANCE and EVALUATION STRATEGY	• To improve *implementation*. • To demonstrate comparative *effectiveness* of food-based approaches.	• Must be *simple*, of reasonable cost and easy to obtain. • Regular *data* updates, compilation, and processing.

1999; Beebee, Gonzalez, and Rengifo, 1999; Bouis, Graham, and Welch, 1999; Graham and Welch, 1994; Graham et al., 1996; Vasal, 1999; Welch et al., 1999). In many countries, post-harvest losses of perishables are high due to poor storage conditions coupled with an inadequate food distribution network. The components of food production strategies should be combined with appropriate food fortification, communication, planning, and monitoring strategies. In the past, strategies towards combating malnutrition have been mutually exclusive. Though single-approach strategies (e.g., food fortification, supplementation) have made impacts in combating malnutrition, their limitations especially in relation to long-term sustainability have been recognized. "Food Systems" approach, therefore, seeks to develop strategies specific to a region or a country that would have a long-term sustainable impact in combating malnutrition.

EXAMPLES OF FOOD SYSTEM STRATEGIES

Food systems strategies are multi-pronged and seem overwhelming, but with a good understanding of the requirements of population groups in a geographical region, these strategies can be narrowed to lay focus on a select few. This principal of selectivity will be advantageous because nutritional problems and its solutions vary between regions. Example strategies of "Food Systems" discussed in this publication are on the food production, food fortification, communication, and evaluation strategies.

With respect to Table 1, examples of food production strategies discussed in this publication are:

- The urgent need for shifting cereal-cereal cropping system for inclusion of legumes (including pulse crops) and vegetables with example from South Asia.
- Nutritional benefits of community and commercial vegetable production.
- Agroforestry systems in which trees, animals, and annual crops are strategically planted and grown to maximize output through various interactions of the system components.
- Breeding staple crops for improved nutritional quality of grains to reach a larger population in a region, with examples of Quality Protein Maize (QPM) and nutritious rice. This strategy is viewed to be a long-term approach to solving micronutrient malnutrition by combining the skills of conventional and modern (biotechnology) breeding tools.
- Changing significance of fisheries and the introduction of cross-bred cow technologies for livelihoods and nutrition with example from Bangladesh and Ethiopia, respectively.

The *food fortification* strategy of "Food Systems" has been very successful in many developed countries, and partially successful in developing countries due to inherent problems of decentralized food processing and lack of strict quality control. However, food fortification when properly implemented has had tremendous impacts in addressing micronutrient malnutrition.

"FOOD SYSTEMS" VERSUS "FOOD BASED STRATEGIES"

Two terms "Food Systems" and "Food Based Strategies" are often used interchangeably in the literature. "Food Systems" is a preferred term used by agricultural professionals, and is looked upon as part of a system. The emphasis has been for agriculture professionals to be aware, and knowledgeable in, and to incorporate issues of human nutrition where appropriate. For example, the crop diversification component of a food-production strategy (Table 1) is an important component of sustainable crop production in a cropping and farming systems perspective. Crop diversification is often emphasized as an agronomic strategy to control pests (weeds, insects, diseases) by breaking the cycle of an otherwise preferred cropping system (example: growing of rice and wheat on the same piece of land for several cycles in South Asia). Introduction of the "break crop" disrupts the pest cycle thereby bringing the pest problem, if any, within manageable levels. Often the preferred cropping system adopted by farmers is for economic reasons and in the process, "less profitable" and "risky" crops belonging to the legume and oil seed families are not cultivated. However, cultivation of legumes for fodder, grains, and vegetables, and of oil seeds as a micronutrient(s) and low-cost dietary fat source is a cheaper and long-lasting alternative to providing variety to a diet because of its higher production, availability, and lower pricing. This is in addition to the agronomic benefits of growing legumes and (or) oilseeds as part of the cropping system.

Nutritionists and economists often use the term "Food Based Strategies." Traditionally, "Food Based Strategies" included food fortification and supplementation as a means of delivering micronutrients to target groups and populations towards combating micronutrient malnutrition. However, with the linking of agriculture and human nutrition as a strategic concept, both these terms are often used to mean the same, i.e., to develop long-term strategies towards reducing malnutrition with the knowledge of appropriate foods that can be grown, produced, and consumed for meeting adequate human nutritional needs. However, the "set" of strategies will be different for countries and communities of people. In conclusion, "Food Systems" or "Food Based" (the terms being used interchangeably in this chapter) strategies seek to further strengthen the linkages between agriculture and human nutrition as a long-term sustainable process towards reducing malnutrition. Once malnutrition is reduced in many parts of the developing (and developed) countries, the knowledge gained through these strategies will help in increasing and sustaining productivity.

REFERENCES

Abd El-Moneim, A.M., B. van Dorrestein, M. Baum, and M. Mulugeta. 1999. Role of ICARDA in improving the nutritional quality and yield potential of grasspea (*Lathyrus sativus* L.) for subsistence farmers in developing countries. Workshop on improving human nutrition through agriculture: The role of International Agricultural Research, October 5-7, IRRI, Philippines.

ACC / SCN. 2000. Fourth report on the world nutrition situation. Geneva: ACC / SCN in collaboration with IFPRI. 75 p.

Allaway, W.H. 1984. Plants as sources of nutrients for people: An overview. Presented at the symposium on "Crops as sources of nutrients for humans." Annual meetings, American society of Agronomy, Special publication # 48, 2nd December 1982, CA, USA. 7 p.

Alnwick, D. 1996. Significance of micronutrient deficiencies in developing and industrialized countries. In *Food-based approaches to preventing micronutrient malnutrition: an International research agenda*. Eds. G.F. Combs Jr., R.M. Welch, J.M. Duxbury, M.C. Nesheim. Abstract from Summary report of an International Workshop, Salt Lake City, Utah, USA, November 6-9, 1995. Published by Cornell International Institute for Food, Agriculture and Development. 68 p.

Andrews, M.P. 1997. Women's involvement in agriculture and food production in India. Third Agricultural Science Congress, PAU, Ludhiana, India, March 12-15, 1997. pp. 37-46.

Banda, T.W. 1996. The role of government in dealing with micronutrient malnutrition. In *Food-based approaches to preventing micronutrient malnutrition: an International research agenda*. Eds. G.F. Combs Jr., R.M. Welch, J.M. Duxbury, M.C. Nesheim. Abstract from Summary report of an International Workshop, Salt Lake City, Utah, USA, November 6-9, 1995. Published by Cornell International Institute for Food, Agriculture and Development. 68 p.

Bargriansky, J., R. Nathan, G. Maberly, and D. Michalak. 1996. preparing for a policy dialogue between the public and policy sectors in support of eliminating micronutrient malnutrition. In *Food-based approaches to preventing micronutrient malnutrition: an International research agenda*. Eds. G.F. Combs Jr., R.M. Welch, J.M. Duxbury, M.C. Nesheim. Abstract from Summary report of an International Workshop, Salt Lake City, Utah, USA, November 6-9, 1995. Published by Cornell International Institute for Food, Agriculture and Development. 68 p.

Beebee, S., A.V. Gonzalez, and J. Rengifo. 1999. Research on trace minerals in common bean. Workshop on improving human nutrition through agriculture: The role of International Agricultural Research, October 5-7, IRRI, Philippines.

Bhalla, G.S., P. Hazell, and J. Kerr. 1999. Prospectus for India's cereal supply and demand to 2020. Food, Agriculture, and the Environment Discussion paper 29. Food,

Agriculture, and the Environment Discussion Paper 29, International Food Policy Research Institute, Washington, DC. 24 p.

Bouis, H.E., R.D. Graham, and R.M. Welch. 1999. The CGIAR micronutrient project: Justification, history, objectives, and summary of findings. Workshop on improving human nutrition through agriculture: The role of International Agricultural Research, October 5-7, IRRI, Philippines.

Bouis, H. and A. Slack. 1996. Food policy perspective in evaluating alternative interventions for reducing micronutrient malnutrition. In *Food-based approaches to preventing micronutrient malnutrition: an International research agenda*. Eds. G.F. Combs Jr., R.M. Welch, J.M. Duxbury, M.C. Nesheim. Abstract from Summary report of an International Workshop, Salt Lake City, Utah, USA, November 6-9, 1995. Published by Cornell International Institute for Food, Agriculture and Development. 68 p.

Brown, D.L. 1996. Opportunities for non-intensive small livestock production: Animals are critical to sustainable food-based micronutrient delivery. In *Food-based approaches to preventing micronutrient malnutrition: an International research agenda*. Eds. G.F. Combs Jr., R.M. Welch, J.M. Duxbury, M.C. Nesheim. Abstract from Summary report of an International Workshop, Salt Lake City, Utah, USA, November 6-9, 1995. Published by Cornell International Institute for Food, Agriculture and Development. 68 p.

Calloway, D.H. 1995. Human nutrition: Food and micronutrient relationships. Working papers on agricultural strategies for micronutrients, No. 1, International Food Policy Research Institute, Washington, DC. 23 p.

Cardwell, K.F. 1999. Mycotoxin contamination in foods–Anti-nutritional factors. Workshop on improving human nutrition through agriculture: The role of International Agricultural Research, October 5-7, IRRI, Philippines.

Cervinskas, J. 1996. Industry as a partner in food fortification programs to alleviate micronutrient malnutrition. In *Food-based approaches to preventing micronutrient malnutrition: an International research agenda*. Eds. G.F. Combs Jr., R.M. Welch, J.M. Duxbury, M.C. Nesheim. Abstract from Summary report of an International Workshop, Salt Lake City, Utah, USA, November 6-9, 1995. Published by Cornell International Institute for Food, Agriculture and Development. 68 p.

Cervinskas, J. and R. Houston, eds. 1998. *Monitoring vitamin A programs*. The Micronutrient Initiative, Ottawa, Canada.

Combs Jr., G.F., J.M. Duxbury, and R.M. Welch. 1997. Food systems for improved health: linking agricultural production and human nutrition. European Journal of Clinical Nutrition, 51. pp. S32-S33.

Combs Jr., G.F., R.M. Welch, J.M. Duxbury, N.T. Uphoff, and M.C. Nesheim. 1996. *Food-based approaches to preventing micronutrient malnutrition: an International research agenda*. Summary report of an International Workshop, Salt Lake City, Utah, USA, November 6-9, 1995. Published by Cornell International Institute for Food, Agriculture and Development. 68 p.

deOnis, M., E.A. Frongillo, and M. Blössner. 2000. Is malnutrition declining? An analysis of changes in levels of child malnutrition since 1980. Bulletin of the World Health Organization, 78(10). pp. 1222-1233.

DeWalt, B.R. 1996. Social constraints affecting acceptance of new food crop systems. In *Food-based approaches to preventing micronutrient malnutrition: an International research agenda*. Eds. G.F. Combs Jr., R.M. Welch, J.M. Duxbury, M.C. Nesheim. Abstract from Summary report of an International Workshop, Salt Lake City, Utah, USA, November 6-9, 1995. Published by Cornell International Institute for Food, Agriculture and Development. 68 p.

Dexter, P.B. 1998. Rice fortification for developing countries. Department of Food Science, University of Arkansas-Fayetteville. OMNI / USAID publication. 12 p.

Duxbury, J.M. 1996. Analyzing the micronutrient outputs of major agricultural systems. In *Food-based approaches to preventing micronutrient malnutrition: an International research agenda*. Eds. G.F. Combs Jr., R.M. Welch, J.M. Duxbury, M.C. Nesheim. Abstract from Summary report of an International Workshop, Salt Lake City, Utah, USA, November 6-9, 1995. Published by Cornell International Institute for Food, Agriculture and Development. 68 p.

Duxbury, J.M. and R.M. Welch. 1999. Agriculture and dietary guidelines. Food Policy, 24. pp. 197-209.

Evans, L.T. 1998. *Feeding the ten billion: Plants and population growth*. Cambridge University Press.

Evenson, R.E., C.E. Pray, and M.W. Rosegrant. 1999. Agricultural research and productivity growth in India. Research Report 109, international Food Policy Research Institute. 88 p.

FAO. 1997. *Preventing micronutrient malnutrition. A guide to food-based approaches– A manual for policy makers and programme planners*. Prepared by Food and Agriculture Organization of the United Nations and International Life Sciences Institute. ILSI Press.

FAO. 1998. FAO-Nutrition country profiles: Bangladesh. Food and Agricultural Organization of the United Nations, Rome. 30 p.

FAO. 1998. FAO-Nutrition country profiles: India. Food and Agricultural Organization of the United Nations, Rome. 33 p.

FAO. 1998. FAO-Nutrition country profiles: Nepal. Food and Agricultural Organization of the United Nations, Rome. 31 p.

FAO. 1998. FAO-Nutrition country profiles: Pakistan. Food and Agricultural Organization of the United Nations, Rome. 26 p.

FAO. 2000. Food insecurity: When people live with hunger and fear starvation. The state of food insecurity in the world. Food and Agricultural Organization of the United Nations, Rome. 31 p.

Gibson, R.S. 1996. Monitoring the progress and evaluating the impact of food-based strategies to combating micronutrient deficiencies. In *Food-based approaches to preventing micronutrient malnutrition: an International research agenda*. Eds. G.F. Combs Jr., R.M. Welch, J.M. Duxbury, M.C. Nesheim. Abstract from Summary report of an International Workshop, Salt Lake City, Utah, USA, November 6-9, 1995. Published by Cornell International Institute for Food, Agriculture and Development. 68 p.

Gopalan, C., B.V.R. Sastri, and S.C. Balasubramanian. 1995. Nutritive value of Indian foods. Revised and updated by B.S. Narasinga Rao, Y.G. Deosthale and K.C. Pant.

National Institute of Nutrition. Indian Council of Medical Research, Hyderabad, India. 156 p.

Graham, R.D. and R.M. Welch.1994. Breeding for staple-food crops with high micronutrient density: Long-term sustainable agricultural solutions to hidden hunger in developing countries. Paper presented at the "Food policy and agricultural technology to improve diet quality and nutrition," a collaborative project among CGIAR centers organized by IFPRI and funded by the office of nutrition of USAID, Annapolis, Maryland, January 10-12, 1994. 115 p.

Graham, R., I. Monasterio, S. Beebe, and C. Iglesias. 1996. Potential for breeding micronutrient-dense staple food crops: "Field Fortification." In *Food-based approaches to preventing micronutrient malnutrition: an International research agenda.* Eds. G.F. Combs Jr., R.M. Welch, J.M. Duxbury, M.C. Nesheim. Abstract from Summary report of an International Workshop, Salt Lake City, Utah, USA, November 6-9, 1995. Published by Cornell International Institute for Food, Agriculture and Development. 68 p.

Gruhn, P., F. Goletti, and M. Yudelman. 2000. Integrated nutrient management, soil fertility, and sustainable agriculture: Current issues and future challenges. Food, Agriculture, and Environment Discussion Paper 32, International Food Policy Research Institute, Washington, DC. 31 p.

Harison, G.G. 1996. Potential for changing food consumption patterns. In *Food-based approaches to preventing micronutrient malnutrition: an International research agenda.* Eds. G.F. Combs Jr., R.M. Welch, J.M. Duxbury, M.C. Nesheim. Abstract from Summary report of an International Workshop, Salt Lake City, Utah, USA, November 6-9, 1995. Published by Cornell International Institute for Food, Agriculture and Development. 68 p.

HMG/N, New Era, Micronutrient Initiative, UNICEF Nepal, and WHO. 1998. Nepal Micronutrient Status Survey 1998.Kathmandu, Nepal: Ministry of Health, Child Health Division, HMG/N, New Era, Micronutrient Initiative, UNICEF Nepal, and WHO. 131 p.

House, W.A. and R.M. Welch. 1984. Effects of naturally occurring antinutrients on the nutritive value of cereals grains, potato tubers, and legume seeds. Presented at the symposium on "Crops as sources of nutrients for humans." Annual meetings, American society of Agronomy, ASA special publication # 48, 2nd December 1982, CA, USA. pp. 9-35.

Johnson, V.A. 1984. Potential for improved crop nutritional quality in cereals through plant breeding. Presented at the symposium on "Crops as sources of nutrients for humans." Annual meetings, American society of Agronomy, ASA special publication # 48, 2nd December 1982, CA, USA. pp. 79-89.

Johnson-Welch, C. 1996. Using multi-sectoral, human-centered approaches to resolving micronutrient malnutrition. In *Food-based approaches to preventing micronutrient malnutrition: an International research agenda.* Eds. G.F. Combs Jr., R.M. Welch, J.M. Duxbury, M.C. Nesheim. Abstract from Summary report of an International Workshop, Salt Lake City, Utah, USA, November 6-9, 1995. Published by Cornell International Institute for Food, Agriculture and Development. 68 p.

Johnson-Welch, C. 1999. Focussing on women works: Research on improving micronutrient status through food based interventions. Synthesis paper. International center for Research on Women (ICRW), Washington, USA. 31 p.

Lachance, P.A. 1996. Integrating fortification and supplementation programs to develop sustainable food-based solutions to micronutrient malnutrition. In *Food-based approaches to preventing micronutrient malnutrition: an International research agenda*. Eds. G.F. Combs Jr., R.M. Welch, J.M. Duxbury, M.C. Nesheim. Abstract from Summary report of an International Workshop, Salt Lake City, Utah, USA, November 6-9, 1995. Published by Cornell International Institute for Food, Agriculture and Development. 68 p.

Lofti, M., M.G.V. Mannar, J.H.M.M. Richard, P.N. Havel. 1996. *Micronutrient fortification of foods. Current practices, research and opportunities*. The Micronutrient Initiative, IDRC/IAC, Ottawa. Canada K1G 3H9. 107 p.

Lorri, W. 1996. Potential for developing new home-based food processing and preparation techniques to improve micronutrient nutrition. In *Food-based approaches to preventing micronutrient malnutrition: an International research agenda*. Eds. G.F. Combs Jr., R.M. Welch, J.M. Duxbury, M.C. Nesheim. Abstract from Summary report of an International Workshop, Salt Lake City, Utah, USA, November 6-9, 1995. Published by Cornell International Institute for Food, Agriculture and Development. 68 p.

Lupien J.R. 1996. Implementing the ICN world plan of action for nutrition: Focus on food and agriculture-based approaches to improve nutrition and prevent micronutrient deficiencies. In *Food-based approaches to preventing micronutrient malnutrition: an International research agenda*. Eds. G.F. Combs Jr., R.M. Welch, J.M. Duxbury, M.C. Nesheim. Abstract from Summary report of an International Workshop, Salt Lake City, Utah, USA, November 6-9, 1995. Published by Cornell International Institute for Food, Agriculture and Development. 68 p.

Lupien, J.R. 1996. Needs and constraints of food-based approaches to control and prevent micronutrient malnutrition. In *Food-based approaches to preventing micronutrient malnutrition: an International research agenda*. Eds. G.F. Combs Jr., R.M. Welch, J.M. Duxbury, M.C. Nesheim. Abstract from Summary report of an International Workshop, Salt Lake City, Utah, USA, November 6-9, 1995. Published by Cornell International Institute for Food, Agriculture and Development. 68 p.

Mehta, S.L. and I.M. Santha. 1997. *Genetic engineering for nutritional quality upgradation*. Third Agricultural Science Congress, PAU, Ludhiana. India, 12-15 March. pp 193-199.

MI. 1995. Sharing risk and reward. Public-private collaboration to eliminate micronutrient malnutrition. Report of the "Forum on food fortification. International dialogue on micronutrient malnutrition." December 6-8, 1995, Ottawa, Canada. 57 p.

MI. 1997. *Joining hands to end hidden hunger–A call to action*. Second Edition, Micronutrient Initiative, Ottawa, Canada. 30 p.

MI. 1998. Food fortification to end micronutrient malnutrition. Symposium report, August 2, 1997, Ottawa, Canada.

Narasinga Rao, B.S. 1997. *Nutritional scenario in India after independence: Past achievements and future aspirations.* Third Agricultural Science Congress, PAU, Ludhiana, India, March 12-15, 1997. pp. 11-36.

Nesheim, R.O. 1984 The effects of processing and refining on nutritional value of crops. Presented at the symposium on "Crops as sources of nutrients for humans." Annual meetings, American society of Agronomy, ASA special publication # 48, 2nd December 1982, CA, USA. pp 55-59.

Pinstrup-Andersen, P. and M.J. Cohen. 2000. Biotechnology and the CGIAR. Presented at the international conference on "Sustainable agriculture in the next millennium–The impact of modern biotechnology on developing countries," sponsored by Friends of the Earth, Oxfam Solidarity, Belgium, and the Dag Hammarskjold Foundation, Brussels, Belgium, 28-31 May, 2000. 22 p.

Rao, K.D. and S.C. Kyle. 1997.Effective incentives and chickpea competitiveness in India. Working paper series WP 97-16, Department of Agricultural, Resource, and Managerial Economics, Cornell University, Ithaca, New York 14853-7801, USA. 85 p.

Pinstrup-Andersen, P., R. Pandya-Lorch, and M.W. Rosegrant. 1999. *World food prospects: Critical issues for the early twenty-first century.* A 2020 vision Food Policy Report, IFPRI, Washington, DC. 32 p.

Rendig, V.V. 1984. Soil fertility and plant nutrition effects on the nutritional quality of crops. Presented at the symposium on "Crops as sources of nutrients for humans." Annual meetings, American society of Agronomy, ASA special publication # 48, 2nd December 1982, CA, USA. pp 61-77.

Ronk, R.J. 1996. Food quality / safety needs and constraints of food-based approaches. In *Food-based approaches to preventing micronutrient malnutrition: an International research agenda.* Eds. G.F. Combs Jr., R.M. Welch, J.M. Duxbury, M.C. Nesheim. Abstract from Summary report of an International Workshop, Salt Lake City, Utah, USA, November 6-9, 1995. Published by Cornell International Institute for Food, Agriculture and Development. 68 p.

Ross, J. and S. Horton. 1998. *Economic consequences of iron deficiency.* The Micronutrient Initiative, Ottawa, Canada, K1G 3G9. 39 p.

Schneeman, B.O. 1996. Re-orienting production and processing for consumer health. In *Food-based approaches to preventing micronutrient malnutrition: an International research agenda.* Eds. G.F. Combs Jr., R.M. Welch, J.M. Duxbury, M.C. Nesheim. Abstract from Summary report of an International Workshop, Salt Lake City, Utah, USA, November 6-9, 1995. Published by Cornell International Institute for Food, Agriculture and Development. 68 p.

Scott, G.J., M.W. Rosegrant, and C. Ringler. 2000. Roots and Tubers for the 21st Century: Trends, projections, and Policy options. Food, Agriculture, and the Environment Discussion Paper 31. International Food Policy Research Institute, Washington, D.C. 64 p.

Shapiro, B. 1996. Some key socio-economic research issues for food-based approaches to preventing micronutrient malnutrition: The example of market-oriented dairying. In *Food-based approaches to preventing micronutrient malnutrition: an International research agenda.* Eds. G.F. Combs Jr., R.M. Welch, J.M. Duxbury, M.C. Nesheim. Abstract from Summary report of an International Workshop, Salt

Lake City, Utah, USA, November 6-9, 1995. Published by Cornell International Institute for Food, Agriculture and Development. 68 p.

Singh, R.B. and K.V. Prabhu. 1997. *Designer crops for future nutritional and industrial needs*. Third Agricultural Science Congress, PAU, Ludhiana, India, March 12-15, 1997. pp 279-289.

Slack, A.T. 1999. Food and nutrition security data on the World Wide Web. Technical Guide # 2, IFPRI, Washington, DC, USA. 32 p.

Smith, L.C. and L. Haddad. 2000a. *Explaining child malnutrition in developing countries*. IFPRI Research Report 111, Washington, DC, USA. International Food Policy Research Institute. 107 p.

Smith, L.C. and L. Haddad. 2000b. Overcoming child malnutrition in developing countries: Past achievements and future choices. Food, Agriculture, and the Environment Discussion Paper 30. International Food Policy Research Institute, Washington DC, USA. 53 p.

SUSTAIN. 1997. Results report on Vitamin C Pilot Program. Sharing United States Technology to Aid in the Improvement of Nutrition (SUSTAIN), Washington DC, USA. 44 p.

SUSTAIN. 1998. Forum on Iron Fortification. Forum proceedings, Institute of Food Technologists Annual Meeting, June 21, 1998, Atlanta, Georgia, USA. Sharing United States Technology to Aid in the Improvement of Nutrition (SUSTAIN), Washington, DC, USA. 44 p.

SUSTAIN. 1999. First report of the "Micronutrient Assessment Project." Sharing United States Technology to Aid in the Improvement of Nutrition (SUSTAIN), Washington, DC, USA. 44 p.

Tontisirin, K. 1996. Experiences with enrichment programs and other food-based approaches to preventing malnutrition in developing countries. In *Food-based approaches to preventing micronutrient malnutrition: an International research agenda*. Eds. G.F. Combs Jr., R.M. Welch, J.M. Duxbury, M.C. Nesheim. Abstract from Summary report of an International Workshop, Salt Lake City, Utah, USA, November 6-9, 1995. Published by Cornell International Institute for Food, Agriculture and Development. 68 p.

Tsou, S.C.B. 1996. Opportunities offered by small-scale vegetable production to improve micronutrient status. In *Food-based approaches to preventing micronutrient malnutrition: an International research agenda*. Eds. G.F. Combs Jr., R.M. Welch, J.M. Duxbury, M.C. Nesheim. Abstract from Summary report of an International Workshop, Salt Lake City, Utah, USA, November 6-9, 1995. Published by Cornell International Institute for Food, Agriculture and Development. 68 p.

Underwood, B.A. 1996. An analysis of integrated approaches to combating hidden hunger. In *Food-based approaches to preventing micronutrient malnutrition: an International research agenda*. Eds. G.F. Combs Jr., R.M. Welch, J.M. Duxbury, M.C. Nesheim. Abstract from Summary report of an International Workshop, Salt Lake City, Utah, USA, November 6-9, 1995. Published by Cornell International Institute for Food, Agriculture and Development. 68 p.

Underwood, B.A. 1999. Micronutrient deficiencies as a public health problem in developing countries and effectiveness of supplementation, fortification, and nutrition education programs: Is there a role for agriculture? Workshop on improving human nutrition through agriculture: The role of International Agricultural Research, October 5-7, IRRI, Philippines.

UNICEF. 1998. *The state of the world's children 1998.* United Nations Children's Fund, New York, Oxford University Press. 131 p.

UNICEF / Kiwani / MI. 1999. Salt iodization programmes: Strengthening, monitoring for success. Report of the workshop on "Strengthening monitoring for iodized salt programme management," Tagatay city, The Philippines, 21-23 April 1999. 87 p.

UNICEF, UNU, WHO, MI. 1998. Preventing iron deficiency in women and children: Background and consensus on key technical issues and resources for advocacy, planning and implementing national programmes. A UNICEF / UNU / WHO / MI technical workshop, UNICEF, New York, October 7-9, 1998. 60 p.

UNICEF, WHO. 1999. Prevention and control of iron deficiency anaemia in women and children. Report of the UNICEF / WHO regional consultation, February 3-5, 1999, Geneva, Switzerland. 110 p.

Vasal, S.K. 1999. Quality protein maize story. Workshop on improving human nutrition through agriculture: The role of International Agricultural Research, October 5-7, IRRI, Philippines.

VanCampen, D.R. 1996. Role of food and meal composition in determining bioavailabilities of micronutrients. In *Food-based approaches to preventing micronutrient malnutrition: an International research agenda.* Eds. G.F. Combs Jr., R.M. Welch, J.M. Duxbury, M.C. Nesheim. Abstract from Summary report of an International Workshop, Salt Lake City, Utah, USA, November 6-9, 1995. Published by Cornell International Institute for Food, Agriculture and Development. 68 p.

Wein, H.C. 1996. Limitations of home gardens and agricultural diversification. In *Food-based approaches to preventing micronutrient malnutrition: an International research agenda.* Eds. G.F. Combs Jr., R.M. Welch, J.M. Duxbury, M.C. Nesheim. Abstract from Summary report of an International Workshop, Salt Lake City, Utah, USA, November 6-9, 1995. Published by Cornell International Institute for Food, Agriculture and Development. 68 p.

Welch, R.M. 1996. Overcoming the limitations of mineral availabilities from soils to plants. In *Food-based approaches to preventing micronutrient malnutrition: an International research agenda.* Eds. G.F. Combs Jr., R.M. Welch, J.M. Duxbury, M.C. Nesheim. Abstract from Summary report of an International Workshop, Salt Lake City, Utah, USA, November 6-9, 1995. Published by Cornell International Institute for Food, Agriculture and Development. 68 p.

Welch, R.M., W.A. House, S. Beebe, D. Senadhira, G. Gregorio, and Z. Cheng. 1999. Testing iron and zinc bioavailability in genetically enriched bean (*Phaseolus vulgaris* L.) and rice (*Oryza sativa* L.) using a rat model. Workshop on improving human nutrition through agriculture: The role of International Agricultural Research, October 5-7, IRRI, Philippines.

Welch, R.M. and W.A. House. 1984. Factors affecting the bioavailability of mineral nutrients in plant foods. Presented at the symposium on "Crops as sources of nutrients for humans." Annual Meetings, American Society of Agronomy, ASA Special Publication # 48, 2nd December 1982, CA, USA. pp. 37-54.

Food-Based Approaches
for Alleviating Micronutrient Malnutrition:
An Overview

M. T. Ruel
C. E. Levin

SUMMARY. This chapter reviews current knowledge and experience with using food-based approaches in reducing vitamin A and iron deficiencies. It reviews recently published literature, highlights some lessons learned, and identifies knowledge gaps and research priorities. The main strategies reviewed are food-based interventions that aim at: (1) increasing the production, availability, and access to vitamin A and iron-rich foods through the promotion of home production and (2) plant breeding strategies that have the potential to increase the content of vitamin A and iron in diet as well as their bioavailability. The review highlights the fact that significant progress has been achieved in the past few decades in the design and implementation of food-based approaches. Evaluations however remain weak, and without rigorous, carefully conducted evaluations the real potential of food-based approaches in addressing micronutrient malnutrition cannot be fully understood. Plant breeding strategies, although they are at a much earlier stage of development, hold great promise

---

M. T. Ruel is affiliated with the International Food Policy Research Institute (IFPRI), 2033 K Street, N.W., Washington, DC 20006 (E-mail: m.ruel@cgiar.org).

C. E. Levin, previously at IFPRI, is currently affiliated with PATH, 4 Nickerson Street, Suite 300, Seattle, WA 98109-1699 (E-mail: clevin@path.org).

The authors would like to thank Anna Winoto for her excellent research assistance. Support for this review was made possible by MOST, the USAID micronutrient program and the International Food Policy Research Institute.

[Haworth co-indexing entry note]: "Food-Based Approaches for Alleviating Micronutrient Malnutrition: An Overview." Ruel, M. T., and C. E. Levin. Co-published simultaneously in *Journal of Crop Production* (Food Products Press, an imprint of The Haworth Press, Inc.) Vol. 6, No. 1/2 (#11/12), 2002, pp. 31-53; and: *Food Systems for Improved Human Nutrition: Linking Agriculture, Nutrition, and Productivity* (ed: Palit K. Kataki, and Suresh Chandra Babu) Food Products Press, an imprint of The Haworth Press, Inc., 2002, pp. 31-53. Single or multiple copies of this article are available for a fee from The Haworth Document Delivery Service [1-800-HAWORTH, 9:00 a.m. - 5:00 p.m. (EST). E-mail address: getinfo@haworthpressinc.com].

31

because of their enormous potential to improve the dietary quality of populations relying mainly on cereal staples. Studies on human bioavailability are the next crucial step to help understand the potential contribution of plant breeding towards alleviating micronutrient malnutrition. Our review suggests that food-based interventions could be an essential part of the long-term global strategy for the fight against micronutrient malnutrition, but their real potential is still to be explored. *[Article copies available for a fee from The Haworth Document Delivery Service: 1-800-HAWORTH. E-mail address: <getinfo@haworthpressinc.com> Website: <http://www. HaworthPress.com>*

KEYWORDS. Food-based strategy, iodine, iron, nutrition, plant breeding strategies, vitamin A

INTRODUCTION

Balanced diets are not accessible for a large proportion of the world's population, particularly those who live in developing countries. Many populations or subgroups of populations subsist on staple plant-based diets that often lack diversity, which may result in micronutrient deficiencies. Vitamin A and iron deficiencies are among the nutritional deficiencies of greatest public health significance in the world today. Almost one-third of children in developing countries are affected to some degree by vitamin A deficiency, which impairs their growth, development, vision and immune function, and in extreme cases leads to blindness and death (UN ACC/SCN 1997; WHO 1995; Sommer and West 1996). Iron deficiency, which leads to anemia, is well recognized as the most common dietary deficiency in the world (including developed countries), affecting mostly children and women of reproductive age (Gillespie, 1998). It is estimated that more than half of all pregnant women in the world and at least one-third of preschoolers suffer from anemia, and many more are iron deficient to some degree (UN ACC/SCN 1997). Iron deficiency is harmful at all ages. In young children it impairs physical growth, cognitive development, and immunity; at school age it affects school performance; at adulthood it causes fatigue and reduced work capacity; and among pregnant women, anemia may cause fetal growth retardation or low birth weight, and is responsible for a large proportion of maternal deaths (Gillespie 1998). Since iron and vitamin A deficiencies disproportionately affect children and women during their reproductive years, they hinder both the development of individual human potential and national, social, and economic development.

Short-term and long-term interventions do exist to effectively address vitamin A and iron deficiencies. The most popular approaches are supplement distribution, food fortification, nutrition education, and food-based strategies.

Food-based strategies–also referred to as dietary modifications–encompass a wide variety of interventions that aim at: (1) increasing the production, availability and access to micronutrient-rich foods (i.e., agricultural activities to increase the supply of and access to food by vulnerable groups); (2) increasing the consumption of foods rich in micronutrients (i.e., nutrition education and behavior change interventions); and/or (3) increasing the bioavailability of vitamin A and iron in the diet (i.e., improved home processing techniques, better selection of food and dietary combinations, or through plant breeding technologies.

The present chapter focuses on a subset of these food-based interventions,[1] namely agricultural approaches that increase home production of vitamin A and iron rich foods and plant breeding strategies that increase the concentration or bioavailability of these nutrients in plant crops. Current knowledge and experience with these approaches is reviewed, and lessons learned, knowledge gaps and research priorities are discussed. A brief summary of relevant issues related to intake and bioavailability of vitamin A and iron in developing countries is presented first.

VITAMIN A, IRON INTAKE, AND BIOAVAILABILITY IN DEVELOPING COUNTRIES

Vitamin A

Vitamin A is available from animal sources in the form of retinol or retinol esters, and plant sources, particularly fruits and vegetables, in the form of provitamin A carotenoids. There are approximately 50 known active provitamin A carotenoids, of which β-carotene makes the largest contribution to vitamin A activity in plant foods (McLaren and Frigg 1997). Until recently, it was assumed that the activity of β-carotene was 1/6 of that of retinol, and for other carotenoids, the activity was estimated to be 1/12 of retinol (FAO/WHO 1988). Recent findings suggest that the bioavailability of carotenoids in fruits and vegetables may be lower than previously estimated and research is currently under way to revise these previously established conversion factors (de Pee et al. 1995; de Pee and West 1996; de Pee et al. 1998; Jalal et al. 1998).

In developing countries, most of the vitamin A ingested is from fruits and vegetables. Estimates suggest that more than 80 percent of dietary intake of vitamin A in Africa and South East Asia, for example, is from provitamin A carotenoids (WHO 1995). The main sources of provitamin A are yellow and orange fruits, orange roots, i.e., carrots, and some sweet potato varieties, dark green leafy vegetables, and palm oil.

Because of the current controversy regarding the bioavailability of provitamin A carotenoids, the potential of plant sources to significantly improve or even maintain vitamin A status in deficient populations is being questioned. One of the purposes of the present review is to shed light on this question by reviewing the experience to date with the use of food-based approaches to control vitamin A deficiency. Interventions and programs promoting home production of fruits and vegetables, small livestock production and aquaculture are reviewed. The potential of plant breeding to contribute to increasing vitamin A intake is also summarized.

Iron

Iron is present in both heme (meat, fish, and poultry) and non-heme forms (dairy products eggs, and in plant foods such as beans, cereals, nuts, fruits, and vegetables of food). Heme iron is highly bioavailable (15 to 35 percent is absorbed), whereas non-heme iron is much less bioavailable, with absorption rates ranging from 2 to 20 percent (Allen and Ahluwalia 1997). The factors that influence the amount of iron absorbed from a meal include the individual's iron status and requirements, the sources and content of iron in the meal, and the other meal constituents. Absorption of both heme and non-heme iron is affected by the individual's characteristics, but non-heme iron is particularly sensitive to the presence of inhibitors of iron absorption such as phytic acid, tannins, and selected dietary fibers (Hallberg 1981). On the other hand, ascorbic acid and even small amounts of meat and fish are active promoters of non-heme iron absorption (Fairweather-Tait 1995).

Staple crops provide a large proportion of the total daily intake of energy and micronutrients among poor populations who have limited access to animal foods (Allen et al. 1992; Ferguson et al. 1989). The main sources of iron in these populations—staple cereals, starchy roots, tubers, and legumes—are in the non-heme iron form and have low bioavailability (Gibson 1994). The main problem with these diets is that they usually contain large amounts of phytic acid (Gibson 1994; Allen et al. 1992), the most potent inhibitor of non-heme iron absorption. Interventions to improve iron status must, therefore, include both strategies to increase the iron content of the diet and to reduce the phytic acid content. Plant breeding strategies are one type of interventions that can achieve this combination. In addition, the potential of interventions to increase home production and intake of animal products rich in heme iron is reviewed.

STRATEGIES TO INCREASE PRODUCTION AND INTAKE OF MICRONUTRIENT-RICH FOODS

Vitamin A

Home gardening has long been a popular food-based strategy for controlling vitamin A deficiency, and various reviews of their impact have been published over the past 10 to 20 years. The first series of reviews, which was supported by the VITAL Vitamin A Support Project (Peduzzi 1990; Soleri, Cleveland, and Wood 1991; Soleri, Cleveland, and Frankenberger 1991), which reviewed over 40 publications and looked at the impact of home gardens on consumption, nutritional status, and in some cases income. More recently, the ACC/SCN reviewed 13 dietary modification programs that aim to control vitamin A deficiency during the late 1980s and early 1990s (Gillespie and Mason 1994). This chapter updates this work by reviewing 8 new projects published between 1995 and 1999 (see Table 1 for references and summary of the studies reviewed). Below we summarize the evidence of the impact of these interventions on three main outcomes: (1) production and income; (2) knowledge, attitude and practices (KAP), and intake of micronutrient-rich foods; and (3) nutritional status.

Impact on Production and Income

The literature indicates that most home gardens are implemented to increase household production of fruits and vegetables to supplement the grain-based diets of rural agricultural households (Solon et al. 1979; CARE/Nepal 1995; Greiner and Mitra 1995; English et al. 1997, English and Badcock 1998; HKI/AVRDC 1993). Thus, their main objective is to improve both household food supply and dietary quality. There are also reports of home gardens that aim at increasing the total food supply to the household during certain lean seasons (Immink, Sanjur, and Colon 1981), or to increase the availability of micronutrient-rich vegetables and fruits throughout the year (Marsh 1998). Few home garden projects mention the objective of increasing household income through the sale of products or of increasing women's control over income even in cases where the intervention is mainly targeted to women.

Only a few projects looked at the impact of home gardens on production by targeted households. A commonly used indicator to measure the impact on production is the number of households who have adopted garden cultivation as a result of the intervention. For examle, in Nepal and Bangladesh the proportion of households producing vegetables and fruits increased as a result of the home gardening and farming education interventions (CARE/ Nepal 1995; Greiner and Mitra 1995). Few studies measured actual increases in the quantity of fruits or vegetables produced, although a number of studies showed an

TABLE 1. Summary of Intervention and Evaluation Designs of Recent Studies Reviewed (1995-1999).

Country	Reference/Year	Intervention			Target Groups	Evaluation		Findings			
		Target Nutrients	Production	Nutrition Education (NED)		Design	Methods	Production	Income	KAP + Dietary Intake	Nutritional Status
Nepal	CARE/Nepal, 1995	Vitamin A	• Home gardening • Irrigation • Agriculture extension • Seed distribution		1) HH 2) Children 3) 6-60 mo	• Before (1992) • After (1995)	HH Survey	Increase in % HH producing vegetables	—	Diet shows insufficient vitamin A intake by mothers and kids	Deterioration of nutritional status of kids (no control)
Bangladesh	Greiner and Mitra, 1995	Vitamin A	• Home gardening • Seeds • Farming education	NED	1) Women 2) Children	• Treatment/control • Before/after	• HH survey • Clinical assessment • 24-h recall	Increase in % HH growing vegetables and fruits in both treatment/control	—	Increased knowledge about the function of vitamin A	Slight decrease in night blindness
Vietnam	• English et al., 1997 • English and Badcock, 1998	• Vitamin A • Vitamin C • Iron • Iodine • Proteins, calories • Fat	• Home gardens • Fish ponds • Animals	NED	1) Mothers 2) Children < 6 yr	• Treatment/control • After	• HH survey • Morbidity recall • KAP • Anthropometry • Food intake	Increased production of vegetables, fruits, fish, and eggs	—	• Increased KAP • Greater intake of vegetables, fruits, energy, proteins, and vitamin A, C, and iron in kids, compared to control.	• Reduced severity and incidence of ARI • Improved growth of children
Bangladesh	IFPRI et al., 1998	• Vitamin A • Iron	• Vegetable production • Fish ponds • Credit and agricultural training	—	1) Women 2) Their household and kids	• 3 groups: Fish ponds Vegetables Control • Before/after	• HH survey • Anthropometry • Biochemical analysis	Increased production of vegetables and fish	Slight increase in income from adoption of fish or vegetables technol.	• No increase in consumption of fish among fish pond group • increase in vegetable intake among vegetable group	No effect on hemoglobin from fish ponds or vegetable production

Kenya	Hagenimana et al., 1999	• Vitamin A	• Introduction of new variety of sweet potatoes • Training in food processing techniques	NED to increase intake and use processing techniques	1) Women's groups 2) Kids 0-5 yr	• Treatment/control • Before/after	• HH survey • HKI vitamin A food frequency questionnaire • KAP	—	—	• Greater HKI score for frequency intake of vitamin A-rich foods in children (control group had decreased intake)
Thailand	Smitasiri and Dhanamitta, 1999 Smitasin et al., 1999	• Vitamin A • Vitamin C • Iron • Iodine	• Seeds distribution • Training of women farmers • Promotion of gardens, fish ponds, chicken	• Education • Social marketing	1) Pregnant, lactating women 2) 2-5 yr old 3) School girls	• Treatment/control • Before/After	• HH survey • 24-h recall • Biochemical assessment (in school girls)	—	—	• Increased KAP about vitamin A and iron • Increased vitamin A intake in all target groups • No increase in fat intake • Increase in iron intake in 2-5 yr old, 10-13 yr old, and lactating women • Increased intake of vitamin C in lactating women • Blood samples in school girls: • increased serum retinol • reduction in vitamin A deficiency • increased mean hb (not significant) • reduced anemia prevalence (not significant) • reduction in low serum ferritin

TABLE 1 (continued)

Country	Reference/ Year	Target Nutrients	Intervention Production	Intervention Nutrition Education (NED)	Target Groups	Evaluation Design	Evaluation Methods	Findings Production	Findings Income	Findings KAP + Dietary Intake	Findings Nutritional Status
Bangladesh	Marsh, 1998	Vitamin A	• Vegetable home garden • Ag. training • Seeds	NED	1) Women 2) Children	• Treatment/ control • Before/after	• HH survey • Vegetable production • Size of cultivated plot • Income • Intake of vegetables	• Increase in vegetable production • Increase in size of plot cultivated • Increase in year-round availability of vegetables	• Increase in income • Increase in women's control of income	• Increase in vegetable consumption per capita • Increase in vegetable consumption of children	—
Ethiopia	Ayalew et al., 1999	Vitamin A	• Ag. training • Food preparation • Seeds	Health education NED	1) Women 2) Children	• Treatment/ control • After	• HH survey • Qualitative research • HKI vitamin A food frequency questionnaire	—	—	• Increase in KAP about vitamin A, night blindness • More diversified diet • Higher HKI vitamin A food frequency scores	Reduced prevalence of night blindness and Bitot's spots

Abbreviations: ARI = acute respiratory infections; HH = household; HKI = Helen Keller International; KAP = Knowledge, Attitudes and Practices; NED = nutrition education.

increase in the availability of vegetables or fruits among producer households (English et al. 1997; English and Badcock 1998; IFPRI et al. 1998; Marsh 1998).

Only a few studies looked at the impact on income, farmer profits of home gardens or household market sales. The study by IFPRI and collaborators (1998) in Bangladesh looked at the profitability of vegetable or fish production compared to rice, and linked this profitability to changes in household income. They showed modest increases in income as a result of adoption. Also in Bangladesh, Marsh (1998) documented an increase in household income and women's control over income as a result of the home gardening promotion efforts. An earlier evaluation of a home garden project by Brun, Reynaud, and Chevassus-Agnes (1989) in Senegal also documented a positive impact on women's income.

In sum, although relatively few projects have quantified the impact of home gardening projects on household production, income, and women's control over income, those that have seem to indicate a trend for positive effects on these outcomes.

Impact on Knowledge, Attitude and Practices (KAP),
and on Intake of Vitamin A-Rich Foods

The absence of an integrated behavior change intervention with the home gardening strategy was notable in many of the earlier studies. Interventions tended to focus mainly on increasing adoption and promoting food production, but the role of nutrition education and communication was largely neglected (Ensing and Sangers 1986; Brun, Reynaud, and Chevassus-Agnes 1989). Not surprisingly, among these studies, most of those that looked at the impact on food intake or nutritional status, failed to demonstrate any significant change in these outcomes (Brun et al. 1989; CARE/Nepal 1995). By 1994, things had started to change and Gillespie and Mason (1994) in their review noted that more communication projects had been implemented in recent years, either as the main intervention or in combination with production activities.

Of the home gardening interventions we reviewed, several of them documented an increase in consumption that was attributed to the project. Among these was the HKI/AVRDC project in Bangladesh that demonstrated an increase in average weekly vegetable consumption per capita among the targeted households (Marsh 1998). Intra-household consumption data also showed a higher consumption of dark green leafy vegetables by infants and very young children. In Vietnam, a community nutrition project combining household garden production of carotene-rich fruits and vegetables, fish ponds, and animal husbandry with nutrition education (English et al. 1997; English and Badcock 1998) showed that participating mothers had a better understanding of the functions of vitamin A compared to mothers from the control commune. In addition, children from participating households consumed significantly more vegetables and fruits, and had greater intakes of energy, protein, vitamin A, and iron.

In Kenya, new varieties of β-carotene rich sweet potatoes were introduced to women's groups (Hagenimana et al. 1999). The control group participated in on-farm trials and received minimal agricultural support for the production of the new varieties of sweet potatoes, whereas the intervention group received nutrition education, lessons on food processing, and technical assistance. The intervention group experienced a statistically significant increase in the frequency of consumption of vitamin A-rich foods compared to a decrease among the control group.

In Ethiopia, a home gardening and health and nutrition education intervention was built on to a previous dairy goat project. The participants increased their knowledge, attitude, and practices related to vitamin A, child feeding practices, and prevention of night blindness (Ayalew et al. 1999). These changes were accompanied by increases in frequency of intake of vitamin A-rich foods.

Thus, the studies reviewed consistently show the success of well designed home gardening activities that integrate production and education activities. Compared to the traditional home gardening interventions carried out in the 1980s, which often did not include an education component, the new generation of integrated production and education interventions have been much more successful in improving knowledge, awareness, attitude, and practices related to vitamin A.

Impact on Nutritional Status

The question of whether home gardens have a positive impact on vitamin A status has been examined in prior reviews and in some of the more recent studies, but evidence is still scant. In the set of earlier studies, home gardens were positively associated with a decreased risk of vitamin A deficiency (Cohen et al. 1985) and reduced clinical eye signs of vitamin A deficiency (Solon et al. 1979). Gillespie and Mason (1994) also concluded from their review that there was evidence that food-based approaches could be effective in the control of vitamin A deficiency. In the review of recent work, undertaken for this chapter only a few of the home garden and nutrition education studies actually measured their impact on vitamin A status indicators. In Bangladesh, Greiner and Mitra (1995) documented a slight reduction in night blindness associated with an increase in intake of dark green leafy vegetables in young children. In Vietnam, preschool children's growth was increased and the severity and incidence of acute respiratory infections were reduced. These improvements were associated with a program that combined the promotion of home production of vegetables, fish, and animal husbandry with nutrition education (English et al. 1997; English and Badcock 1998). In Ethiopia, the prevalence of night blindness and Bitot's spots was lower among participants in the home gardening and nutrition education intervention compared to the control group.

Conclusions on Strategies to Increase Production and Intake of Vitamin A-Rich Foods

Consistent with the findings from earlier reviews, this synthesis of more recent literature points to the potential of home gardening and promotional and education interventions to improve vitamin A nutrition. The new studies have focussed on community participation aspects and the careful selection of appropriate set of interventions for specific contexts. They also use considerably improved design and implementation strategies compared to previous studies. The evaluation protocols and the statistical analysis of findings, however, remain weak and lacking scientific rigor even in the more recent work. Failure to correct this crucial aspect will continue to slow down progress in understanding the real potential of production and education interventions in controlling vitamin A deficiency.

Iron

Compared to vitamin A, production and education interventions to increase the supply and intake of iron from plant foods have not been popular. This unpopularity is not surprising since researchers have long raised questions about the potential for plant sources to make a major contribution to control iron deficiency in developing countries (Yip 1994; de Pee et al. 1996). Although many non-animal foods contain relatively large amounts of iron, the non-heme form of iron present in these foods has poor bioavailability. In addition, plant foods often contain a variety of powerful inhibitors of non-heme iron such as tannins, phytates and polyphenols. Thus, to increase the household supply of bioavailable iron, promotional efforts may have to support the production of animal products such as small animal husbandry or fishponds, which would increase the supply of more bioavailable heme-iron. A few recent experiences in this direction are included in Table 1. In fact, of the 8 new studies reviewed, all of those that targeted increasing iron intake or iron status promoted the production and consumption of animal products. The study in Vietnam, for example, promoted fishponds and animal husbandry (English et al. 1997); adoption of fishponds was promoted in Bangladesh (IFPRI et al. 1998); and the home gardening intervention supported fishponds and chicken production as well as vegetable production in Thailand (Smitasiri and Dhanamitta 1999).

Impact on Iron Intake and Iron Status

The Vietnam project documented an increase in the intake of iron among children of households in the intervention communities (home gardens, fish ponds and animal husbandry) compared with control communities (English et al. 1997; English and Badcock 1998). No mention was made of whether the increased iron was from vegetable or animal sources. Furthermore, iron status was not measured. In Bangladesh (IFPRI et al. 1998), preliminary results from the evaluation of the adoption of fishponds or commercial vegetable production suggest that there was no increase in the intake of fish or vegetables, respectively, among adopting households. There was also no evidence of improved iron status among members of adopting households. The evaluation is still on-going and longer-term impacts will be assessed. In Thailand, preschoolers, school children, and lactating women increased their iron intake. Lactating women also increased their intake of vitamin C, a promoter of non-heme iron absorption (Smitasiri and Dhanamitta 1999; Smitasiri et al. 1999). Biochemical indicators of iron status were measured, but only among schoolgirls, and significant improvements in serum ferritin were observed. Unfortunately, the effects of the food-based intervention could not be separated from the effects of the overall strategy targeted to school girls, which included the weekly distribution of iron tablets for 12 weeks and improved dietary quality of school lunches (Smitasiri and Dhanamitta 1999).

In Ethiopia, preliminary results of the effects of commercialization of crossbred cows found a 72% increase in household income among adopters, while their food expenditure increased by only 20% (Ahmed, Ehui, and Jabbar 2000). Both vitamin A and iron intake was higher among adopters compared to non-adopters, but the authors did not differentiate between animal and plant sources of micronutrients. Forthcoming analyses of the data will assess the impact on children's nutritional status.

Conclusions on Strategies to Increase Production and Intake of Iron-Rich Foods

Clearly, experience with food-based approaches to increase production and consumption of heme or non-heme iron-rich foods is very limited. In addition to the well-known problems of bioavailability with iron from plant sources, the experience with animal production suggests trade-offs between increased income from selling home-produced animal products and increasing own consumption of these products to improve dietary quality. Evidence from household studies in Bangladesh and Ethiopia showed that increases in income through the sale of animal products, did not successfully translate into significant improvements in dietary quality. The results of both studies are preliminary, but reinforce the observation that promoting animal production without a strong nutrition education component may not be sufficient to achieve improved dietary diversity. Households may chose to improve their income rather than their diet, and the increases in income may be invested in basic necessities other than food. Thus the question of what exactly can be achieved through well-designed integrated production and education interventions to promote increased intake of animal products and to improve iron status remains largely unanswered.

PLANT BREEDING STRATEGIES

The possibilities of improving micronutrient nutrition through plant breeding are numerous. They include: (1) increasing the concentration of minerals (iron or zinc), or vitamins (β-carotene); (2) reducing the amount of anti-nutrients such as phytic acid; and (3) raising the levels of sulfur-containing acids, which can promote the absorption of iron and zinc.

Traditionally plant breeding has been used primarily to improve farm productivity, usually by developing crops with higher yields. When crossing varieties with particular traits, scientists also attempt to monitor and maintain consumer characteristics such as taste, cooking qualities, and appearance. These characteristics are important because they have a bearing on market prices, and consequently on profitability, which motivates farmers to adopt the improved varieties. Until recently, breeding to enhance the nutrient content of crops for human nutrition purposes has rarely been an explicit objective, largely because of the presumption that nutrient-enhanced crops may be lower yielding, and thus, would jeopardize profitability and adoption by farmers. Recent research, however, indicates that at least in the case of trace minerals (iron and zinc, in particular), the objectives of breeding for higher yield and better human nutrition do largely coincide. That is, mineral-dense crops offer various agronomic advantages, such as greater resistance to infection, and thus lower dependence on fungicides, greater drought resistance, and greater seedling vigor, which in turn, is associated with higher plant yield (Graham and Welch 1996). With these new developments, one of the most serious barriers to combining human nutrition and plant breeding objectives has been lifted.

This section summarizes the potential nutritional benefits of the different plant breeding approaches that can contribute to the control of micronutrient malnutrition. More detailed information can be found in the literature (Graham and Welch 1996; Ruel and Bouis 1998; Bouis 1996).

Increasing the Mineral or Vitamin Concentration of Staple Crops

The main question about the potential benefits of using mineral- or vitamin-dense staple crops is whether the increased concentrations will in fact result in significant increases of bioavailable minerals (or vitamins) and conse-quently improve the nutritional status of deficient populations. For this im-provement to happen, vulnerable groups have to consume the improved varieties of staple crops in sufficient quantities, but even more importantly the net amount of bioavailable nutrients ingested must be increased relative to tra-ditional crops.

As indicated previously, the main sources of iron in impoverished popula-tions are staple cereals and starchy roots, tubers, and legumes. Thus, it is in the non-heme iron form and has low bioavailability (Gibson 1994). Estimates in-dicate that cereals contribute up to 50% of iron intake among households from lower socioeconomic groups (Bouis 1996). For zinc, the contribution from non-animal sources can be as high as 80%, as shown for preschoolers in Ma-lawi (Ferguson et al. 1989). Therefore, doubling the iron or zinc density of food staples could increase total intakes by at least 50%. The main problem, though, is that diets based on non-animal staples usually contain large amounts of phytic acid (Gibson 1994; Allen et al. 1992), which inhibits both non-heme iron and zinc absorption. Some argue that in circumstances where phytic acid is so prominent in the diet, raising the concentration of minerals in plants through plant breeding may not be sufficient to counteract the inhibitory effect of phytic acid on mineral absorption. The argument continues that even if, for instance, the non-heme iron concentration of the grain is increased two- to four-fold, there may still be enough phytic acid to bind the extra minerals, in which case, the net absorption of iron would not be increased.

Results based on animal (rat) models suggest that the percent of bioavail-ability remains constant when traditional crops are compared to mineral-en-hanced crops, and the final result is a net increase in bioavailable mineral. Rats, however, have substantially more intestinal phytase activity than humans (by a factor of about thirty), and therefore, are more able to absorb iron or zinc from high phytate foods than humans (Iqbal, Lewis, and Cooper 1994). Human bioavailability studies are urgently needed to address this critical question.

To date, most of the progress in developing mineral-dense staple crops has come from screening for genetic variability in the concentration of trace min-erals. The crops tested (wheat, maize, rice, and beans) have shown significant genotypic variation, up to twice that of common cultivars for minerals (Fig-ure 1) and even greater variation was found for β-carotene in cassava (Chavez et al. 2000). Positive correlations between mineral concentrations have been found, indicating that varieties with greater iron concentration are most likely to also contain greater concentrations of zinc.

Increasing seed ferritin is another plant breeding approach that has the po-tential to increase the content of bioavailable iron in plant foods (Theil, Burton, and Beard 1997). The approach is promising because ferritin, a common source of stored iron in seeds and developing plants, appears to be highly bioavailable (Theil, Burton, and Beard 1997). New genetic engineering exper-

FIGURE 1. Genetic variability in the concentration of trace elements (Panel A: Iron; Panel B: Zinc) for wheat, maize, rice, and beans (adapted from Welch and Graham, 2000).

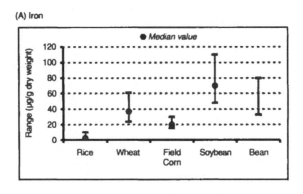

(A) Iron

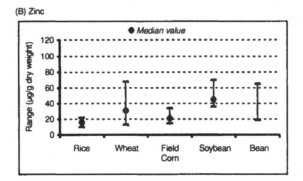

(B) Zinc

iments are also currently being conducted with rice to simultaneously increase their concentration of vitamin A and iron. The approaches include: (1) increasing the iron content of the rice with a ferritin transgene; (2) reducing the phytate content of cooked rice with a transgene for a heat-stable phytase (which allows enzymatic hydrolysis of phytates during cooking); (3) increasing the concentration of cystein in rice (a promotor of non-heme iron and zinc absorption) by increasing the resorption-enhancing effect from a transgenic sulfur-rich methallothionin-like protein; and (4) generating β-carotene production in rice grain by adding three genes (two from daffodil and one from the bacterium *Erwina uredovora*) (Potrykus et al. undated; Ye et al. 2000).

Although encouraging, this area of research is still at an early stage of development and much more extensive screening and genetic engineering must be undertaken before the potential impact on human nutrition can be assessed.

Reducing the Phytic Acid Concentration in the Plant

A complementary approach to increase the concentration of plant minerals is to act directly on their main inhibitor of absorption, phytic acid. Research in humans has shown that minimal amounts of phytic acid added to meals can produce a severe inhibition of non-heme iron absorption (Sandström, Lönnerdal, 1989). Although studies do not agree on the exact cut-off point at which non-heme iron absorption is significantly improved by the removal of phytic acid, some argue that almost complete removal (< 10 mg/meal) is necessary (Hurrell et al. 1992). Another study has shown as little as 50 mg of phytic acid in a meal can cause a 78 to 92% reduction in non-heme iron absorption (Reddy et al. 1996).

To provide an idea of the order of magnitude, daily intake of phytic acid among preschool children from populations whose staple diets are based on cereals, legumes, and starchy roots and tubers are estimated to range from 600 to 1900 mg, that is 200 to 600 mg per meal (Gibson 1994). Among Mexican adult men and women, whose diets are based on maize (tortillas), beans, and rice, intakes of phytic acid are in the order of 4,000-5,000 mg per day (Allen et al. 1992). Cereals such as whole wheat, corn, and millet contain approximately 800 mg of phytic acid per 100 gm of cereal.

A key issue, then, is whether plant breeding can achieve the magnitude of reduction in phytic acid that may be necessary to obtain significant improvements in absorption of both zinc and non-heme iron. If, as suggested by Raboy (1996), phytic acid in staple foods can be reduced by a factor of two-thirds, and if dietary phytic acid comes mainly from staple foods, it is likely that this strategy would impact bioavailability of zinc and iron simultaneously, and potentially calcium, manganese, magnesium, and possibly even other trace minerals.

A small pilot study was carried out recently to measure iron absorption from a low-phytate maize. The improved variety contained approximately 35% of the phytic acid content of regular maize, but its concentration of macronutrients and minerals was unchanged (Mendoza et al. 1998). Iron absorption was almost 50% greater from the low-phytic maize compared to the traditional maize. These results are encouraging for populations that consume maize-based diets and efforts to decrease the phytic acid content of staple cereals even further are underway.

Increasing the Concentration of Promoter Compounds (Sulfur-Containing Amino Acids)

Another potentially complementary approach to increase the bioavailability of minerals in staple crops is to increase the concentration of specific amino acids that may promote mineral absorption. These are sulfur-containing amino acids, namely methionine, lysine, and cysteine. At this time, there is little information about the agronomic advantages or disadvantages to increasing the concentration of sulfur-containing amino acids in staple foods. In terms of human nutrition, it appears that a small increase in amino acid concentration is needed to positively affect the bioavailability of iron or zinc, and therefore, it is unlikely to affect plant functions significantly (Welch 1996). Again, this is an area that is currently being researched.

Conclusions About Plant Breeding Approaches

Involving agricultural research in the fight against micronutrient malnutrition holds great promise. Because trace minerals are important not only for human nutrition, but for plant nutrition as well, plant breeding has the potential to make a significant, low-cost,[2] and sustainable contribution to reducing micronutrient malnutrition, and mineral deficiencies in humans. Furthermore, increasing farm productivity in developing countries is an important spin-off effect. There is increasing evidence that because iron, zinc, and provitamin A have such important synergies in absorption, transport, and function in the human body, enhancing all three nutrients simultaneously could achieve maximum impact (Graham and Rossner 1999; Garcia-Casal et al. 1998). The genetic resources needed to meet this challenge are available and research is ongoing to unveil the most promising and viable alternatives.

CONCLUSIONS AND RECOMMENDATIONS
FOR FUTURE RESEARCH

Food-based strategies are generally regarded as potentially sustainable because their overall goal is to empower individuals and households to take ultimate responsibility over the quality of their diet through own-production of nutrient rich foods and informed consumption choices (Howsen, Kennedy, and Horwitz 1998). A particularly attractive aspect of food-based strategies is that they can address multiple nutrients simultaneously, including calories, proteins, and various micronutrients, without the risk of antagonistic nutrient interactions or overload. This aspect is a major advantage of these approaches over the single nutrient types of interventions (such as supplementation programs), because it is well recognized that populations deficient in vitamin A or iron are more likely to also suffer from various other vitamin and mineral deficiencies.

Our review suggests that some food-based strategies, particularly home gardening and production interventions have been increasingly successful over the past few decades in addressing micronutrient deficiencies. The inclusion of a strong education and communication component seems to be key to the success and impact of food-based strategies involving behavioral changes.

Plant breeding strategies, on the other hand, are at a much earlier stage of development and information is not yet available on their contribution to the control of vitamin A and iron deficiencies. Studies on human bioavailability are urgently needed to understand the full potential of plant breeding. It is clear, nonetheless, that these strategies are promising because they have an enormous potential to improve the dietary quality of populations relying mainly on cereal staples. In addition, if new varieties are similar to traditional varieties in terms of organoleptic characteristics, these strategies will not require any behavior change from the part of the consumer, which relieves one of the main challenges of most food-based approaches.

Experience with gardening and other home production approaches for the control of vitamin A are also at a different stage of development compared to those aiming at alleviating iron deficiency. In spite of the current controversy over the bioavailability of provitamin A, there is increasing evidence that well-designed production interventions can play an important role in the control of vitamin A deficiency, especially when implemented in combination with effective education and communication strategies. The quality of the information to judge the effectiveness of these strategies, however, is still weak mainly because evaluation designs often lack scientific rigor. Evaluations should include a careful analysis of the role of different intervention components on all direct outcomes likely to be affected and gather information to document the mechanisms involved. They should also measure the multiple indirect effects that the interventions may have on aspects such as their contribution to the diet of other family members, or the benefits for other micronutrient deficiencies.

Similar to vitamin A, deficiency in iron faces information gaps on the potential efficacy of food-based approaches especially those relying on plant sources to improve iron status. Because of the low bioavailability of non-heme iron in plant products, other complementary interventions are needed to address iron deficiency. For instance, the efficacy of animal foods to control iron deficiency is well established, and there is no doubt that these products can improve absorption of non-heme iron and maintain iron status at least among certain population groups. The main concern about promoting animal products to improve iron status, however, is their prohibitive cost for most of the populations affected by the deficiency. Therefore, additional information on the minimum amounts of animal products that would be required to complement a plant-based diet to achieve a certain net amount of absorbed iron would be the first step towards assessing the feasibility of such approaches. The few studies that have looked at the effectiveness of promoting animal food production have encountered the predictable problem that increased income resulting from adoption may not result in improved dietary quality (IFPRI et al. 1998; Ahmed et al. 2000). Research should explore issues related to the supply and demand of animal products that affect both farmers' incomes and consumer prices. Additionally, research should look at the income and consumption trade-offs involved in animal production and how these affect the household's dietary quality. An additional consideration is the fact that promotion of animal products may be constrained by cultural and religious factors that prohibit their inclusion in the diet of at-risk populations.

This review did not cover the cost effectiveness of alternative food-based interventions, because such studies are noticeably absent from the literature. However, few exceptions exist that compared a single food-based strategy to supplementation and food fortification interventions (Popkin et al. 1980; Grosse and Tilden 1988; Phillips et al. 1996), using aggregate data. Cost-effectiveness analysis of alternative food-based interventions is needed in addition to studies that contrast food-based approaches with supplementation and fortification strategies. Analyses of food-based interventions should capture spill over effects and both short- and long-term costs that influence the sustainability of alternative interventions.

In conclusion, our review suggests that food-based interventions are an essential part of the long-term global strategy for the fight against micronutrient malnutrition, and that researchers, program planners, and policy implementers need to continue to explore their full potential.

NOTES

1. Approaches to increase intake of micronutrient-rich foods and strategies to increase the bioavailability of plant-based micronutrients through home processing techniques are reviewed elsewhere (Ruel and Levin 2000).

2. Estimates of the cost of plant breeding compared to other interventions to control iron deficiency are presented in Ruel and Bouis 1998.

REFERENCES

Ahmed, M.M., S. Ehui, and M. Jabbar. 2000. Household level economic and nutritional impacts of market-oriented dairy production in the Ethiopian highlands. *Food and Nutrition Bulletin* 21 (4), 460-465.

Allen, L.H., J.R. Backstrand, A. Chávez, and G.H. Pelto. 1992. *Functional Implications of Malnutrition.* Final Report, Mexico Project, Mexico, 290 p.

Allen, L.H. and N. Ahluwalia. 1997. *Improving Iron Status Through Diet. The Application of Knowledge Concerning Dietary Iron Bioavailability in Human Populations.* OMNI Opportunities for Micronutrients Interventions. John Snow, Inc./OMNI Project, Washington, DC, 83 p.

Ayalew, W.Z., Wolde Gebriel, and H. Kassa. 1999. *Reducing Vitamin A Deficiency in Ethiopia: Linkages with a Women-Focused Dairy Goat Farming Project,* OMNI Research Report Series No. 4, International Center for Research on Women, Washington, DC, 28 p.

Bouis, H. 1996. Enrichment of food staples through plant breeding: a new strategy for fighting micronutrient malnutrition, *Nutrition Reviews*, 54, 131-137.

Brun, T., J. Reynaud, and S. Chevassus-Agnes. 1989. Food and nutritional impact of one home garden project in Senegal, *Ecology of Food and Nutrition*, 23, 91-108.

CARE/Nepal. 1995. *A Study on Evaluation of home Gardening Program in Bajura and Mahottari Districts*, Katmandu, Nepal, September 1995.

Chavez, A.L., J.M. Bedoya, T. Sánchez, C. Iglesias, H. Ceballos, and W. Roca. 2000. Iron, carotene, and ascorbic acid in cassava roots and leaves, *Food and Nutrition Bulletin*, 21, 410-413.

Cohen, N., M.A. Jalil, H. Rahman, M.A. Matin, J. Sprague, J. Islam, J. Davidson, E. Leemhuis de Regt, and M. Mitra. 1985. Landholding, wealth and risk of blinding malnutrition in rural Bangladeshi households, *Social Science and Medicine*, 21(11), 1269-1272.

de Pee, S. and C.E. West. 1996. Dietary carotenoids and their role in combating vitamin A deficiency: a review of the literature, *European Journal of Clinical Nutrition*, 50 (suppl.), S38-S53.

de Pee, S., C.E. West, Muhilal, D. Karyadi, and G.A.J. Hautvast. 1996. Can increased vegetable consumption improve iron status? *Food and Nutrition Bulletin*, 17 (1), 34-36.

de Pee, S., C.E. West, Muhilal, D. Karyadi, and G.A.J. Hautvast. 1995. Lack of improvement of vitamin A status with increased consumption of dark-green leafy vegetables, *Lancet* 346, 75-81.

de Pee, S., M.W. Bloem, J. Gorstein, M. Sari, Yip R. Satoto, R. Shrimpton, Muhilal. 1998. Reappraisal of the role of vegetables in the vitamin A status of mothers in Central Java, *American Journal of Clinical Nutrition* 68, 1068-1074.

English, R. and J. Badcock. 1998. A community nutrition project in Viet Nam: effects on child morbidity, *Food, Nutrition and Agriculture*, 22, 15-21.

English, R., J. Badcock, Tu Giay, Tu Ngu, A.M. Waters, and S.A. Bennett. 1997. Effect of nutrition improvement project on morbidity from infectious diseases in preschool children in Vietnam: comparison with control commune, *British Medical Journal*, November 1, 315 (7116), 122-125.

Ensing, B. and S. Sangers. 1986. *Home Gardening in a Sri Lankan Wet Xone Village: Can It Contribute to Improved Nutrition*, Manuscript, The Netherlands, Wageningen, 41 p.

Ferguson E.L., R.S. Gibson, L.U. Thompson, and S. Ounpuu. 1989. Dietary calcium, phytate, and zinc intakes and the calcium, phytate, and zinc molar ratios of the diets of a selected group of East African children, *American Journal of Clinical Nutrition*, 50, 1450-1456.

Fairweather-Tait, S.J. 1995. Bioavailability of iron. *In*: P. Nestel ed., *Iron Interventions for Child Survival;* Proceedings of the 17-18 May 1995 conference, London. Opportunities for Micronutrient Interventions, Washington, DC, 13-30.

FAO/WHO (Food Agriculture Organization of the United Nations/Word Health Organization). 1988. Requirements of vitamin A, iron, folate and vitamin B12. *Food and Nutrition Series 23*. FAO, Rome, Italy.

Ferguson,\ E.L., R.S. Gibson, L.U. Thompson, and S. Ounpuu. 1989. Dietary calcium, phytate and zinc intakes and the calcium, phytate, and zinc molar ratios of the diets of a selected group of East African children, *American Journal of Clinical Nutrition*, 50, 1450-1456.

García-Casal, M.N., M. Layrisse, L. Solano, M.A. Barón, F. Arguello, D. Llovera, J. Ramírez, I. Leets, and E. Tropper. 1998. Vitamin A and β-carotene can improve nonheme iron absorption from rice, wheat and corn by humans, *Journal of Nutrition*, 128, 646-650.

Gibson, R. 1994. Zinc nutrition in developing countries, *Nutrition Research Reviews*, 7, 151-173.

Gillespie, S. and J. Mason. 1994. *Controlling vitamin A deficiency*. ACC/SCN State-of-the-art series. Nutrition Policy Discussion Paper No. 14. United Nations/Administrative Committee on Coordination–Subcommittee on Nutrition, Geneva, 81 p.

Gillespie, S. 1998. *Major Issues in the Control of Iron Deficiency*. The Micronutrient Initiative and UNICEF. The Micronutrient Initiative, Ottawa, ON, Canada, 104 p.

Graham, R.D. and R.M. Welch. 1996. *Breeding for Staple Food Crops with High Micronutrient Density*, Working Papers on Agricultural Strategies for Micronutrients No. 3, International Food Policy Research Institute, Washington, DC, April 1996, 79 p.

Graham, R.D. and J.M. Rossner. 2000. Carotenoids in staple foods: their potential to improve human nutrition, *Food and Nutrition Bulletin*, 21, 404-409.

Greiner, T. and S.N. Mitra. 1995. Evaluation of the impact of a food-based approach to solving vitamin A deficiency in Bangladesh, *Food and Nutrition Bulletin*, 16 (3), 193-205.

Grosse, R. and R. Tilden. 1988. Vitamin A Cost-Effectiveness Model, *International Journal of Health Planning and Management*, 3, 225-244.

Hagenimana, V., M. Anyango Oyunga, J. Low, S.M. Njoroge, S.T. Gichuki and J. Kabira. 1999. *Testing the Effects of Women Farmers' Adoption and Production of Orange-Fleshed Sweet Potatoes on Dietary Vitamin A Intake in Kenya*, OMNI Research Report Series No. 3, International Center for Research on Women, Washington, DC, 24 p.

Hallberg, L. 1981. Bioavailability of dietary iron in man. *Annual Review of Nutrition*, 1, 123-147.

HKI/AVRDC. 1993. *Home Gardening in Bangladesh: Evaluation Report*, Bangladesh, 9 p.

Howsen, C.P., E.T. Kennedy, and A. Horwitz, Eds. 1998. *Prevention of Micronutrient Deficiencies*. Tools for Policymakers and Public Health Workers, National Academy Press, Washington, DC, 207 p.

Hurrell, R.G., M.-A. Juillerat, M.B. Reddy, S.R. Lynch, S.A. Dassenko, and J.D. Cook. 1992. Soy protein, phytate, and iron absorption in humans, *American Journal of Clinical Nutrition*, 56, 573-578.

Immink, M., D. Sanjur, and M. Colon. 1981. Home gardens and the energy and nutrient intakes of women and preschoolers in rural Puerto Rico, *Ecology of Food and Nutrition*, 11, 191.

IFPRI (International Food Policy Research Institute), Bangladesh Institute of Development Studies, Institute of Nutrition and Food Science, Data Analysis and Technical Assistance and Research Department of Human Nutrition, Royal Veterinary and Agricultural University. 1998. *Commercial Vegetable and Polyculture Fish Pro-*

duction in Bangladesh: Their Impacts on Income, Household Resource Allocation, and Nutrition, Report, Volume 1, November 1998.

Iqbal, T.H., K.O. Lewis, and B.T. Cooper. 1994. Phytase activity in the human and rats small intestine, *Gut*, 35, 1233.

Jalal, F., M.C. Nesheim, Z. Agus, D. Sanjur, and J.P. Habicht. 1998. Serum retinal concentrations in children are affected by food sources of β-carotene, fat intake, and anthelmintic drug treatment, *American Journal of Clinical Nutrition*, 68, 623.

Marsh, R. 1998. Building on traditional gardening to improve household food security, *Food, Nutrition and Agriculture*, 22, 4.

McLaren, D.S. and M. Frigg. 1997. *Sight and Life Manual on Vitamin A Deficiency Disorders (VADD)*. Task Force SIGHT AND LIFE, Basel, Switzerland, 138 p.

Mendoza, C., F.E. Viteri, B. Lönnerdal, K.A. Young, V. Raboy, and K.H. Brown. 1998. Effect of genetically modified, low-phytic acid maize on absorption of iron from tortillas, *American Journal of Clinical Nutrition*, 68, 1123-1127.

Peduzzi, C. 1990. *Home and Community Gardens Assessment Program Implementation Experience: The Tip of the Iceberg*. Vitamin A Field Support Project (VITAL) Report No. TA-2, ISTI, Washington, DC, 16 p.

Phillips, M., T. Sanghvi, R. Suarez, J. McKigney, and J. Fiedler. 1996. The costs and effectiveness of three vitamin A interventions in Guatemala, *Social Science Medicine*, 42, 1661-1668.

Popkin, B.M., F.S. Solon, T. Fernandez, and M.C. Latham. 1980. Benefit-cost analysis in the nutrition area: a project in the Philippines, *Social Science and Medicine* 14, 207-216.

Potrykus, I., P. Lucca, X. Ye, S. Al-Babili, R.F. Hurrel, and P. Beyer. Research abstract: contributions to food security by genetic engineering with rice (Undated).

Raboy, V. 1996. Cereal low phytic mutants: a global approach to improving mineral nutritional quality, *Micronutrients and Agriculture*, 2, 15-16.

Reddy, M.B., R.F. Hurrell, M.A. Juillerat, and J.D. Cook. 1996. The influence of different protein sources on phytate inhibition of nonheme-iron absorption in humans, *American Journal of Clinical Nutrition*, 63, 203-207.

Ruel, M.T. and H.E. Bouis. 1998. Plant breeding: A long-term strategy for the control of zinc deficiency in vulnerable populations, *American Journal of Clinical Nutrition*, 68(Suppl.), 488S-494S.

Ruel, M. T. and C.E. Levin. 2000. *Assessing the Potential for Food-Based Strategies to Reduce Vitamin A and Iron Deficiencies: A Review of Recent Evidence*. Food Consumption and Nutrition Division Discussion Paper # 92, International Food Policy Institute, Washington, DC, 54 p.

Sandström, B. B. Lönnerdal. 1989. *Promoters and Antagonists of Zinc Absorption, in Zinc in Human Biology*. Human Nutrition Reviews, Mills C.F., Ed., Springer-Verlag, International Life Sciences Institute, United Kingdom, 57-78.

Smitasiri, S. and S. Dhanamitta. 1999. *Sustaining Behavior Change to Enhance Micronutrient Status: Community- and Women-Based Interventions in Thailand*, OMNI Research Report Series No. 2, International Center for Research on Women, Washington, DC, 28 p.

Smitasiri, S., K. Sa-ngobwarchar, P. Kongpunya, C. Subsuwan, O. Banjong, C. Chitchumroonechokchai, W. Rusami-Sopaporn, S. Veeravong, and S. Dhanamitta. 1999. Sustaining behavioural change to enhance micronutrient status through community- and women-based interventions in north-east Thailand: vitamin A, *Food and Nutrition Bulletin*, 20 (2), 243-251.

Soleri, D., D.A. Cleveland, and A. Wood. 1991. Vitamin A Nutrition and Gardens Bibliography, *Vitamin A Field Support Project (VITAL) Report No. IN-1*, ISTI, Washington, DC, 65 p.

Soleri, D., D.A. Cleveland, and T.R. Frankenberger. 1991. Gardens and Vitamin A: A Review of Recent Literature, *VITAL Report No. IN-2*, VITAL, Arlington, VA, 32 p.

Solon, F., T.L. Fernández, M.C. Latham, and B.M. Popkin. 1979. An evaluation of strategies to control vitamin A deficiency in the Philippines, *American Journal of Clinical Nutrition*, 32, 1445-1453.

Sommer, A. and K.P. West. 1996. *Vitamin A Deficiency. Health, Survival, and Vision.* Oxford University Press: New York and Oxford, 387 p.

Theil, E.C., J.W. Burton, and J.L. Beard. 1997. A sustainable solution for dietary iron deficiency through plant biotechnology and breeding to increase seed ferritin control, *European Journal of Clinical Nutrition*, 51, S28-S31.

UN ACC/SCN (United Nations Administrative Committee on Coordination/ Subcommittee on Nutrition). 1997. *Third Report on the World Nutrition Situation.* ACC/SCN, Geneva, 111 p.

WHO (World Health Organization). 1995. *Global Prevalence of Vitamin A Deficiency.* Micronutrient Deficiency Information System. *WHO MDIS Working Paper # 2.* WHO, Geneva, 116 p.

Welch, R.M. 1996. The optimal breeding strategy is to increase the density of promoter compounds and micronutrient minerals in seeds; caution should be used in reducing anti-nutrients in staple food crops, *Micronutrients and Agriculture*, 1, 20-22.

Welch, R.M. and R.D. Graham. A new paradigm for world agriculture: productive, sustainable, nutrition, healthful food systems. *Food and Nutrition Bulletin*, 21, 361-366.

Ye, X., S. Al-Babili, A. Kloti, J. Zhang, P. Lucca, P. Beyer, and I. Potrykus. 2000. Engineering the provitamin A (β-carotene) biosynthetic pathway into (carotenoid-free) rice endosperm, *Science* 287, 303-305.

Yip, R. 1994. Iron deficiency: contemporary scientific issues and international programmatic approaches, *Journal of Nutrition*, 125, 1479S-1490S.

Effects of Micronutrient Deficiencies on Human Health: Its Status in South Asia

T. Schaetzel

R. Sankar

SUMMARY. Vitamin A, iodine, and iron deficiencies affect large numbers of people worldwide. A deficiency of one or more of these micronutrients adversely affects the physical and mental abilities of humans. South Asia contains a high percentage of these individuals, not just because of its large population, but also the prevalence of deficiency is higher there than in many other parts of the world. The reasons for the high rates of deficiency in South Asia are many, but they include inadequate availability of micronutrient-rich foods, sub-optimal dietary habits, and high rates of infection. Across the region, national plans vary from (a) increasing availability of appropriate foods, (b) introducing new dietary behaviors, (c) improving health status, and (d) directly addressing deficiency through intervention programs. The extent to which each of the countries is making progress toward the goals of these plans can help in understanding the priorities for future efforts to address micronutrient malnutrition. This article discusses the adverse effects of micronutrient deficiencies in humans with special reference to South Asia. *[Article copies available for a fee from The Haworth Document Delivery Service: 1-800-HAWORTH. E-mail address: <getinfo@haworthpressinc.com> Website: <http://www. HaworthPress.com> © 2002 by The Haworth Press, Inc. All rights reserved.]*

T. Schaetzel is Senior Program Specialist, The Micronutrient Initiative, South Asia Regional Office, 208 Jor Bagh, New Delhi 110003, India (E-mail: tschaetzel@idrc.org.in).

Col. R. Sankar is Head, Thyroid Research Centre, Institute of Nuclear Medicine & Allied Sciences, Lucknow Road, Timarpur, Delhi 110054, India (E-mail: sankar@drinma.ren.nic.in).

[Haworth co-indexing entry note]: "Effects of Micronutrient Deficiencies on Human Health: Its Status in South Asia." Schaetzel, T., and R. Sankar. Co-published simultaneously in *Journal of Crop Production* (Food Products Press, an imprint of The Haworth Press, Inc.) Vol. 6, No. 1/2 (#11/12), 2002, pp. 55-98; and: *Food Systems for Improved Human Nutrition: Linking Agriculture, Nutrition, and Productivity* (ed: Palit K. Kataki, and Suresh Chandra Babu) Food Products Press, an imprint of The Haworth Press, Inc., 2002, pp. 55-98. Single or multiple copies of this article are available for a fee from The Haworth Document Delivery Service [1-800-HAWORTH, 9:00 a.m. - 5:00 p.m. (EST). E-mail address: getinfo@haworthpressinc.com].

KEYWORDS. Anemia, Bangladesh, deficiency, goiter, India, iodine, iodized salt, iron, malnutrition, micronutrient, Nepal, Pakistan, South Asia, vitamin A

INTRODUCTION:
MICRONUTRIENT DEFICIENCIES

At least one-quarter of children in developing countries suffer from sub-clinical vitamin A deficiency; about 74 million people suffer from iodine deficiency disorders (as judged by the prevalence of goiter); and an astonishing 2 billion people suffer from anemia (Mason et al., 2001). Certainly, micronutrient deficiency is not the only important nutritional problem the world faces today, as protein-energy malnutrition affects a greater number of people and remains the number one nutritional public health priority worldwide. Nonetheless, interventions to reduce protein-energy malnutrition historically have produced mixed results at high cost, and progress against protein-energy malnutrition, although steady, has been slow. In contrast, effective and relatively cheap interventions exist for addressing micronutrient deficiencies that can bring quick results. For this reason, the 1992 World Summit for Children focused attention on micronutrients, noting that (a) vast numbers of people either suffered from or were in danger of micronutrient deficiency, (b) deficiencies have devastating consequences for both individuals and societies, and (c) effective interventions exist to address the problem. The goals specific to "micronutrients" produced by the World Summit were as follows:

- Elimination of vitamin A deficiency and its consequences;
- Elimination of iodine deficiency disorders; and
- Reduction of iron deficiency anemia to 1/3 of 1990 levels.

While efforts to reduce protein-energy malnutrition continue apace, governments worldwide have undertaken special efforts to eliminate micronutrient deficiency.

VITAMIN A:
PHYSIOLOGICAL ROLE, DEFICIENCY SYMPTOMS,
AND CONSEQUENCES

Vitamin A is a fat-soluble vitamin stored in the liver. In different chemical forms, it has functions for proper vision, tissue differentiation, and immunity. Although its role in immunity is not well understood vitamin A is essential for maintaining the epithelium of any organ or organ system with rapid cell turnover, such as the eyes, skin, respiratory tract, and intestines. The physiological requirement for vitamin A is highest during life stages of rapid growth, such as during early childhood or pregnancy, and deficiency thus is most common during these life stages.

Vision

Vitamin A, in the form of retinal, is a structural component of the light-sensitive pigment rhodopsin, which is found in the rod cells of the eye. When excited by light, retinal dissociates from the molecule, initiating a series of steps that generate an electrical impulse to the optic nerve. Under low light conditions, rhodopsin accumulates to allow the rod cells to function for vision, but the formation of rhodopsin requires adequate retinal. Thus, a vitamin A deficient individual suffers from night-blindness because they lack sufficient retinal for this process to occur.

Cell Differentiation

Healthy epithelial tissues are in constant turnover. Vitamin A deficiency (VAD) leads to an inability to replace these cells normally, and they harden. This hardening is apparent in perhaps the best-known consequence of VAD, *xeropthalmia*, the progressive eye disease of vitamin A deficiency.

The Eye

The epithelial cells of the eye are constantly being replaced, and they must remain soft and moist to protect the eye from injury and to maintain transparency over the lens. When an individual is vitamin A deficient, cell turnover is limited, and the eye becomes dry resulting in xeropthalmia. The most common vitamin A deficiency disease of the eye.

The usual first indication of xeropthalmia is difficulty in seeing at night (see "Vision" above), when adequate rhodopsin is not available for rod cells to enable low-light vision. As the disease progresses, the conjunctiva and cornea become abnormally dry, taking on a dull luster. Further progression results in the development of foamy lesions on the conjunctiva called "Bitot's spots," followed by gradual opacity enveloping the cornea. At this last stage of the disease, the eye is very susceptible to damage–even from dust– and ulceration, which can result in *keratomalacia*, or scarring of the cornea. Eventually, this scarring can result in blindness. Because it results from vitamin A deficiency, blindness due to xerophthalmia thus is called *nutritional blindness*.

For clinical purposes, codes have been designated for each of the stages of xeropthalmia as follows:

- Night blindness: XN
- Corneal xerosis: X1
- Bitot's spots: X2
- Keratomalacia: X3

Immunity

Vitamin A's role in immunity is well documented, but not well understood. Children with vitamin A deficiency are more susceptible to infectious diseases, including diarrhea, respiratory disease, and measles (Blomhoff and Smeland, 1994). Several studies have shown the protective effects of vitamin A supplementation for children. For example, in the earliest randomized controlled trial, conducted in Sumatra, vitamin A supplementation reduced mortality among children 12-71 months by 34% (Sommer et al., 1986). Similarly, in India, supplementation was shown to reduce the risk of child mortality by one-half (Rahmathullah et al., 1990). A comprehensive meta-analysis of published vitamin A supplementation studies demonstrated that supplementation confers a 23% reduction in child morbidity (Beaton et al., 1993). Recent studies in Nepal (West et al., 1999) strongly suggest that vitamin A supplementation during pregnancy may also reduce maternal mortality, but further research is needed to confirm these findings.

VITAMIN A:
DIETARY REQUIREMENTS AND FOOD SOURCES

Vitamin A exists in two forms: preformed vitamin A (retinol) available only from animal sources, and provitamin A available from plant sources. Both require fat for their absorption, a nutrient most people in South Asia consume in inadequate amounts.

Provitamin A exists in the form of carotene compounds, pigments found in many plants, and among these provitamin A, β-carotene is the most important because it has the highest vitamin A activity. When absorbed, the body can convert carotenoids into vitamin A, but the efficiency of conversion varies due to the type and the mix of carotenoids. Green leafy vegetables, dark orange and red fruits, and vegetables are good food sources for carotenoids.

Preformed vitamin A is common in animal foods, especially liver and eggs. Milk is a relatively good source of vitamin A, and the vitamin A in breast milk provides the sole vitamin A source for exclusively breastfeeding infants and a major source for older children as long as their mother continues to breastfeed. The US Recommended Daily Intake of vitamin A is 1,000 retinol equivalents (RE; a microgram of retinol, either as preformed vitamin A or after *in vivo* conversion of provitamin A to retinol) for males and 800 retinol equivalents for females.[1] The vitamin A requirement for females is higher during pregnancy, and considerably higher during lactation.

Preformed vitamin A is toxic in high amounts, and it also has been linked with birth defects. Provitamin A is not toxic, since the body does not convert carotenoids to retinol when blood serum levels are adequate.

COMMON PROGRAMS TO ADDRESS VITAMIN A DEFICIENCY

Three major types of community-based programs are most common for addressing vitamin A deficiency: food-based approaches to increase the availability and consumption of vitamin A-rich (or β-carotene-rich) foods; supplementation and food fortification.

Dietary Diversification

The most common food-based approach to address vitamin A deficiency has been the introduction of vegetable consumption at the household level. While these programs have been successful in increasing household availability of β-carotene-rich foods and improving household incomes, they have had little success in controlling vitamin A deficiency.

Supplementation

Children

Vitamin A is safe for children even in massive doses, and, thanks to mass-dose vitamin A capsules donated by the Micronutrient Initiative (by means of a grant from the Canadian International Development Agency) to UNICEF for distribution; twice-annual supplementation of children under the age of six years has become a successful intervention worldwide. The most successful programs have linked vitamin A supplementation with immunization campaigns, often achieving coverage rates of over 80%. Although the age group of 6 months to 6 years is the urgent target for supplementation, many countries target a smaller age range to reduce program costs. Table 1 provides the WHO-recommended supplementation rates for children under the age of 6 years.

Women

Vitamin A has been linked with birth defects, so mass-dose supplementation is dangerous for pregnant women. At the same time, the requirement for vitamin A is high during fetal development, so pregnancy often induces vitamin A deficiency. The eight-week period following parturition, during which a girl/woman remains infertile, thus provides the only safe opportunity for mass-dose supplementation of girls and women of reproductive age. Table 2 details the WHO recommendations for post-partum vitamin A supplementation in areas where women's habitual vitamin A intakes do not exceed 2,400 RE (8,000 IU). The difficulty of implementing these recommendations in countries where a provider does not normally attend births is obvious.

Low-level daily supplementation during pregnancy is another option for addressing women's need for vitamin A during pregnancy. While the WHO has recommended up to 3,000 RE/day as a safe limit during pregnancy, many countries choose not to implement this recommendation out of (unfounded) fear of toxicity.

Fortification

As a means to provide nutrients to the general population, fortification offers the advantages of low cost, program-free (and program-cost-free) distribution, frequent dosing, and compatibility with established dietary habits. Because vitamin A is fat-soluble, oils and fats are the simplest vehicles for fortification, but other foods, such as sugar and flour, can provide an acceptable medium. Unfortunately, most of the poor who suffer from vitamin A deficiency consume limited amounts of centrally processed food, making fortification of the foods they consume more difficult and more expensive than fortification by means of central processing. Additionally, some outdated food purity laws in South Asia prevent the addition of any substance to a "pure food," thus preventing manufacturers from fortifying.

TABLE 1. WHO Recommendations for Supplementation of Children up to the Age of 6 Years (adapted from World Health Organization, 1998).

Age	Supplementation
< 6 months	None
6-11 months	30,000 RE*
12-59 months	60,000 RE** every six months

* 100,000 IU
** 200,000 IU

TABLE 2. WHO Recommendations for Safe Post-Partum Vitamin A Supplementation (adapted from World Health Organization 1998).

Breast-Feeding Status	Population Recommendation	Individual Recommendation
Breast-feeding	60,000 RE* within 8 weeks of delivery**	• If using reliable contraception, 60,000 RE any time • If practising post-partum abstinence, 60,000 RE any time • If amenorrhoeic, 60,000 RE within six months • If not amenorrhoeic, 60,000 RE at next menstruation or supplement child
Not breast-feeding	60,000 RE within 4 weeks of delivery	60,000 RE within 4 weeks of delivery

* 200,000 IU
** New recommendations under consideration suggest two 60,000 RE doses, one at delivery and one at four weeks after delivery.

IRON:
PHYSIOLOGICAL ROLE, DEFICIENCY SYMPTOMS AND CONSEQUENCES

Iron forms a key structural component of the oxygen-carrying molecules *hemoglobin*, found in red blood cells (RBCs), and *myoglobin*, found in muscle. Because hemoglobin can reversibly bind oxygen, it enables RBCs to carry oxygen to tissues, and iron thus plays an important role in cell metabolic processes. Iron also exists in association with proteins involved in its transport, and as storage iron in the liver. Iron also is a component of *cytochromes*, electron-transferring proteins involved in the liberation and use of energy from food.

Although anemia, or a low concentration of hemoglobin in the blood, usually is considered as a sign of iron deficiency, anemia actually may have many causes. For example, other nutrient deficiencies (e.g., folate, vitamin B_{12}), or blood loss due to parasitic infection can cause low hemoglobin even if an individual is consuming adequate iron in their diet. Anemia thus is not necessarily synonymous with iron deficiency.

Iron deficiency has three distinct stages: iron depletion, during which iron stores in the liver is depleted; iron-deficient erythropoiesis, which occurs when iron stores are completely depleted and insufficient iron reaches the erythropoietic cells in the bone marrow; and iron-deficiency anemia, which is characterized by a reduction in the concentration of hemoglobin in RBCs (Gibson, 1990). An individual may exhibit a combination of these stages because the body uses available iron to maintain hemoglobin concentration in the blood. For example, an individual may have inadequate iron stores due to poor iron consumption in the past, or iron loss (e.g., parasitic infection), but may not suffer anemia if their current diet contains sufficient iron to maintain an adequate hemoglobin level.

Significantly, only the most severe form of iron-deficiency anemia has clinical characteristics. Severe iron-deficiency anemia can be detected reliably by examination of the inner eyelids and fingernails for pallor, but no visible signs result from mild and moderate iron-deficiency anemia, iron-deficient erythropoiesis, or depletion of iron stores. Assessment of the level of serum ferritin, a protein that rises and falls in association with iron stores, is the best means to determine an individual's iron stores. Iron-deficient erythropoiesis can be assessed in two ways: the degree to which iron saturates the protein (i.e., transferrin) that binds it for transport is an indication of the circulating iron available for erythropoiesis; and secondly, the concentration of erythrocyte protoporphyrin, a precursor of heme, in RBCs indicates whether adequate iron is available for hemoglobin synthesis. The last stage iron deficiency anemia is assessed by the concentration of hemoglobin in whole blood.

Despite the universal use of hemoglobin to determine the public health importance of iron deficiency, hemoglobin concentration assessment does not provide information concerning the cause of iron deficiency anemia. Low hemoglobin status may have many causes other than inadequate iron consumption: low hemoglobin status in conjunction with inadequate iron stores most likely results from inadequate consumption and/or absorption of iron from the diet, and low hemoglobin status in conjunction with adequate iron stores indicates that a condition resulting in blood loss (e.g., parasitic infection) or destruction of blood cells (e.g., malaria) is the most likely cause of anemia. Since most anemia prevalence data rely on hemoglobin assessment alone, such data require careful interpretation.

Oxygen Transport

The hemoglobin molecule's unique ability to reversibly bind oxygen to itself makes possible the energy-requiring processes that sustain life. The weakness and lack of energy characteristic of anemia result from inadequate availability of oxygen required for these processes.

Immunity and Infection

The exact mechanism by which iron supports the immune function is not completely understood, but several studies have convincingly documented the increased susceptibility to infection that occurs when iron status is poor.

Too much iron, however, leads to an excess of free iron in the bloodstream, on which many bacteria can thrive. Inappropriate iron supplementation thus can spur infection, especially in cases where the individual has inadequate protein (transferrin) for binding the free iron in the blood. Case management of infants and toddlers suffering from severe protein-energy malnutrition, for example, requires a one-week delay in iron supplementation to replenish protein nutriture and ensure adequate transferrin for binding free iron.

Infant/Child Development

Anemic children experience delayed motor and mental development. Observational studies show that moderately anemic infants score 0.5 to 1.5 standard deviations lower than infants with sufficient iron stores (Ross and Horton, 1998). If the anemia is left untreated, the developmental delays may be irreversible. Additionally, anemic schoolchildren have reduced energy and depressed attention spans, limiting their active learning capacity. While reduced learning capacity is reversible, days of poor attention during school are irretrievable.

Pregnancy

During pregnancy, a girl/woman's blood volume increases substantially, diluting the hemoglobin in her bloodstream. This dilution is normal, but it significantly increases a woman's iron requirements. For this reason, even girls/ women with adequate iron intakes usually cannot consume enough iron to meet the iron demands of pregnancy and they develop iron deficiency anemia. Importantly, girls or women who suffer from anemia during pregnancy may deliver babies with inadequate iron stores who are predisposed to anemia.

Anemia during pregnancy also puts the mother at risk. Anemia leads to tiredness and reduced energy expenditure, which can reduce appetite and limit weight gain during pregnancy. Severe anemia, or very low body hemoglobin, is a dangerous condition at any time during pregnancy, and an emergency situation during the third trimester. An anemic, pregnant girl/woman, especially a severely anemic one, is particularly at risk of dying if she hemorrhages during or after delivery. Preferred treatment for severe anemia during the third trimester, or when hemorrhage occurs, is hospitalization and administration of parenteral iron. The percentage of maternal deaths due to anemia is difficult to estimate because it is partly a function of (a) the availability and quality of emergency obstetric services, and (b) the severity of anemia, which often is not quantified in hospital records. Nonetheless, a review of mainly hospital-based studies in Africa and Asia estimated that 23% of maternal deaths in Asia result from anemia (Ross and Thomas, 1996).

ECONOMIC CONSEQUENCES OF IRON DEFICIENCY

The functional consequences of iron deficiency have economic costs: motor and mental impairment of children, reduced work output of adults, poor pregnancy outcomes, detrimental effects on children's health, and taxing the resources of individuals and society.

Motor and Mental Impairment of Children

As mentioned above, numerous studies have demonstrated that infants and toddlers with moderate anemia do not score as well as non-anemic children on developmental tests. Although mental development scores are poorly correlated with intelligence later in life (Ross and Horton, 1998), scores on motor development test have been shown to predict cognitive ability later in childhood and at 18 years of age (Pollitt and Gorman, 1990). Children older than age two also may suffer an IQ deficit of one-half standard deviation due to iron deficiency (Seshadri and Gopaldas, 1989).

Reversal of anemia can reverse these developmental limitations, but few anemia programs exist worldwide for addressing children's anemia. Despite the many programs that exist to address anemia in pregnancy, adults who have high rates of childhood anemia, can suffer from intelligence and productivity deficits.

Reduced Productivity Among Adolescents and Adults

Iron deficiency anemia induces lethargy and fatigue, and therefore, reduces physical output (Davies, Chukweumeka, and van Haaren, 1973). For students, anemia also may limit school performance. Randomized studies have documented improvements in performance on tests of verbal learning and memory even among non-anaemic but iron-deficient adolescent girls (Bruner et al., 1996). Intervention studies also have demonstrated that (a) short-term iron supplementation of anemic individuals can produce rapid and substantial increases in work output even when hemoglobin levels are not affected (Ohira et al., 1981), (b) replenishment of iron stores in nonanemic individuals results in improved physical capacity (Zhu and Haas, 1998), and (c) increased hemoglobin among anemic individuals can increase productivity even among individuals involved in work that is not physically demanding (Li et al., 1994). Extrapolating from the results of studies such as these, estimates of productivity losses have been as high as 20% for all adult wage earners who suffer from anemia (Levin et al., 1994).

Maternal Mortality

As mentioned above, anemia during pregnancy significantly contributes to maternal mortality. Certainly the greatest tragedy of maternal mortality is human, not economic. This tragedy is further multiplied by the high mortality rates among living children of mothers who die during or around childbirth; mortality among these children is as high as 50% by five years of age (Rush, 2000).

In addition to these human costs, maternal mortality has economic costs such as the loss of women's productivity, and the costs of child care lost. Medical procedures employed in an attempt to save a girl or woman whose life is threatened during pregnancy (e.g., hospitalization, transfusion, transport to higher levels of health care) also have costs to households and society, whether or not the girl/woman survives.

COMMON PROGRAMS TO ADDRESS
IRON DEFICIENCY ANEMIA (IDA)

In comparison with the costs anemia exacts from individuals and society, programs for its control can be relatively inexpensive. The best long-term strategy to control IDA is improved diet, but this option requires time and is unaffordable in the short-term. Dietary improvement also cannot fully address the problem of iron deficiency during pregnancy, which requires supplementation even for individuals consuming iron replete diets.

Dietary Approaches

Iron from Food

Iron absorption varies greatly due to several factors, the most important of which is the form in which iron is consumed. The iron available to humans is of two forms: "heme" iron, which is found in animal food sources such as meat, fish, and poultry; and "non-heme" iron, which is available from plant sources as well as some animal sources. While all iron from plants is non-heme, iron in meat, fish, and poultry is only one-half to three-fifths non-heme (Monsen, 1988; Monsen and Balintfy, 1982). Humans can absorb both the heme and non-heme forms of iron, but heme iron is much more readily absorbed (15-35%) than is non-heme (2-20%).

Dietary iron absorption is further influenced by the presence of dietary factors that either enhance or inhibit absorption of non-heme iron. Heme iron from cellular animal proteins (beef, veal, pork, lamb, liver, and fish) and ascorbic acid (vitamin C) are the major enhancers of non-heme iron absorption. The effects of these enhancers are dependent on inclusion in the same meal with the non-heme iron source, and by the temperature and pH conditions of ascorbic acid (Monsen, 1988). Inhibitors of non-heme iron absorption include polyphenols (tannins) in tea and coffee, and phytates, which are found in fiber.

Additionally, an individual's iron status affects the absorption of iron. When iron nutriture is adequate, most individuals do not absorb dietary iron due to the "mucosal block" by which molecular sites for its uptake are unavailable. Genetic disorders, most notably thalassemia, interfere with some individuals' ability to stop absorbing iron, putting them at risk for over-absorption and the precipitation of iron in body tissues. When iron nutriture is inadequate, most individuals absorb a higher percentage of the iron in their diet; the body is able to increase absorption dramatically, even of non-heme iron (Cook, 1990).

Dietary approaches for reduction of iron deficiency anemia therefore must increase the amount of iron absorbed, not just the amount of iron consumed, through a combination of increased iron intake, increased consumption of animal foods and absorption-enhancing factors, and reduced consumption of absorption-inhibiting factors. The limitations of dietary approaches thus are: (a) increased iron intake from affordable plant sources is limited by their poor iron bioavailability; (b) increased consumption of animal food sources of iron is too expensive for most poor individuals who suffer from iron deficiency (and religious practices forbid the consumption of animal foods for many in South Asia); (c) increased consumption of absorption-enhancing factors, like vitamin C, requires availability of fruits, which are too expensive for most individuals to consume regularly, and usually are not available (affordably, at least) year-round; and (d) reduced consumption of iron absorption inhibiting factors is difficult because cereal grains constitute most of the diet of poor people and because wholesale dietary change is necessary.

Iron from Breast Milk

Milk is not an iron-rich food. Nonetheless, the iron in human breast milk is highly bioavailable, and for the first six months of life, while the infant's iron stores are still adequate, an exclusively breast-fed infant normally receives sufficient iron from her/his mother's milk to maintain adequate iron status. At around six months of age, however, infants' iron stores are depleted and they outgrow the amount of iron available from breast milk, so they require solid food, which is more iron-dense than breast milk, to maintain proper iron nutriture.

Late introduction of complementary solid food is a major cause of anemia among infants. Nutrition education programs that inform mothers about the appropriate time to introduce solid food to the infant, and the appropriate foods to introduce are an important intervention against iron deficiency anemia.

Supplementation

Pregnant and Lactating Women

The requirement for iron during pregnancy and lactation is such that nearly all pregnant girls and women are unable to satisfy it through dietary means. For this reason, anemia is extremely common during pregnancy.

The WHO and UNICEF have determined that universal supplementation of pregnant and lactating women is called for when the prevalence of anemia in pregnancy is 30% or greater. In situations such as this, iron supplementation is indicated from the time the woman is aware that she is pregnant through one-year post-partum. Although daily iron supplementation has been shown many times to be efficacious for the reversal of anemia during pregnancy, community-based programs for universal supplementation have achieved mixed results. The reasons for program failure may be related to program delivery (supplement availability, girls'/women's access to supplements, appropriate counseling) or lack of compliance with the daily regimen. Although weekly iron supplementation also has been shown to be efficacious, poor compliance with a once-weekly dosage results in 14 days without a supplement rather than just one or two days, and weekly supplementation is not recommended for community-based programs targeting pregnant girls and women (Beaton and McCabe, 1999).

Adolescent Girls

Early motherhood is common in South Asia because many marriages occur at a young age; therefore, adolescence is especially a critical time when girls need to build iron stores. Most girls, once they marry and become pregnant, will have little chance to build iron stores during their reproductive life due to frequent pregnancies that are also common in South Asia. For this reason, iron supplementation of unmarried adolescent girls may offer the best intervention for anemia during pregnancy because it allows them to build iron stores before they must cope with the nutritional demands of (frequent) pregnancy. Since the girls are not pregnant, weekly iron supplementation is recommended as adequate for the purpose of building iron stores.

Fortification

Several countries worldwide currently fortify staple foods with iron. Most fortify wheat flour, but fortification of other foods is also possible. The cost of iron fortification on large-scale production facilities is minimal, making it the most cost-effective community-based means to provide iron for individuals with inadequate iron intake. Unfortunately, iron fortification has several limitations for South Asia. First, most of the rural poor, who disproportionately suffer from anemia, consume flour and other fortifiable food products ground at small, local mills, where fortification is more difficult and less cost-effective. Second, many countries in South Asia have food purity laws that forbid the addition of any substance to a "pure food" or severely restrict the items that can be added legally. The passing of new legislation, a sometimes-lengthy process in South Asia, could eliminate the restrictions imposed by outdated food purity laws, but low consumption by the poor of centrally processed foods nonetheless will limit the reach of fortification for many years to come. Some new initiatives for fortification through small-scale mills offer promise, but they must overcome quality control constraints and higher costs in comparison with centralized fortification.

IODINE:
PHYSIOLOGICAL ROLE, DEFICIENCY SYMPTOMS AND CONSEQUENCES

Iodine is a micro-mineral, an element humans require in amounts less than 1 mg per day. Its primary role in human physiology is the synthesis of the thyroid hormones thyroxin and triiodothyronine, which regulate cell activity and growth in all tissues. Iodine is necessary for normal mental function and, while iodine deficiency affects mental performance at any age, its deficiency is especially damaging during fetal development when it can lead to fetal loss, or neurological damage to the fetus resulting in *cretinism*. Deficiency for children and adults has a broad range of consequences collectively known as *iodine deficiency disorders* (IDD) that include intellectual impairment, stunted growth, apathy, and impaired movement, speech or hearing.

Severe Deficiency for the Developing Fetus: Cretinism

The severe retardation of cretinism results from impaired fetal neurological development due to iodine deficiency. Obviously, fetus obtains iodine only from its mother, so a baby born with cretinism has a mother who suffers from iodine deficiency. Cretinism occurs less frequently than other iodine deficiency disorders, even in endemic populations, but it has tragic consequences for an individual and her/his family, and it imposes significant costs on society.

Deficiency from Childhood to Adulthood

The effects of iodine deficiency can vary depending on the life stage of the affected individual, but with the exception of stunted growth, they primarily affect mental performance. Communities with endemic IDD have been shown to suffer up to a 13 point loss in IQ scores, and studies in India comparing learning scores in severely iodine deficient villages (high rates of goiter and cretinism) with those from mildly iodine deficient villages (moderate rates of goiter and cretinism) revealed longer times for maze solving, lower scores for ordered recall of word lists and pictorial recognition, and poorer motivation to achieve (Tiwari et al., 1996). Adults also suffer from diminished mental performance, which results in reductions in productivity.

Prolonged iodine deficiency can also result in a clinically detectable enlargement of the thyroid gland called a goiter. The thyroid gland produces iodine-containing hormones that regulate cell activity and growth, and the amount of the hormones in the bloodstream controls their production. Without adequate iodine, levels of thyroid hormones decline, and the thyroid responds by trying to produce more hormones, gradually enlarging as it attempts an impossible task. A goiter is classified into grades according to size: goiter that is palpable and not visible (but may be visible with the neck in extension) is classified as Grade I, and a goiter that is visible with the neck in normal position is classified as Grade II. Goiters can range from a slight swelling in the neck to large and pendulous appendages.

Many misconceptions surround goiters, the most unfortunate of which is the belief that iodine deficiency exists only when a goiter is present. To the contrary, many of the effects of IDD manifest when no goiter is present. Similarly, many believe that goiter indicates current iodine deficiency, but, since goiters do not simply "go away" once proper iodine nutriture is restored, a goiter may indicate past rather than current iodine deficiency.[2]

Detection and classification of a goiter is highly subjective, dependent on the training and experience of the examiner. Nonetheless, goiter prevalence is the most commonly used measure of the level of iodine deficiency. While goiter prevalence is an important marker for iodine deficiency, its use as the sole indicator of iodine deficiency is unfortunate because (a) it neglects sub-clinical deficiency, (b) it is a poor measure of current iodine status, and (c) its assessment by palpation has poor agreement from observer to observer and depends largely on the examiner's skill and experience. Goiter prevalence is much more useful in combination with assessment of urinary iodine excretion.

Measurement of iodine excreted in the urine can reveal sub-clinical deficiency because it shows present iodine intake, and it does not depend on the skill of the examiner. As much as 90% of iodine consumed is excreted in the urine, so the amount in the urine correlates with current iodine consumption. Excretion values for individuals tend to vary greatly, so the measure is best applied to communities: the median urinary iodine excretion value of a population can indicate the extent of iodine deficiency in it.

Dietary Requirements and Food Sources

Humans require very small amounts of iodine, which is available from most foods, whether animal or plant, that are produced in an iodine-replete environment. Since the oceans are the earth's repositories of iodine, seafood is a good source of iodine, and soils in coastal areas nearly always contain enough iodine to support human needs. The further from the sea a food source is grown, the more likely will be low in iodine, and mountainous areas or regions with high rainfall are most likely to have inadequate iodine in the soil.

Some plants, particularly cabbage, brussels sprouts and, legumes contain *goitrogens* that inhibit iodine utilization by the thyroid gland. A diet high in these foods can precipitate iodine deficiency. The effects of goitrogens can be overcome either by increasing iodine intake or by reducing the intake of goitrogenous foods.

Iodine is toxic to humans if chronically consumed in excessive amounts. The symptoms of toxicity are hyperthyroidism and, in some cases, goiter. In populations where iodine consumption has been very low in the past, mild toxic effects have been seen after the introduction of iodized salt.

Common Programs to Remedy Iodine Deficiency

For most of the world, salt iodization provides the most effective means of ensuring adequate iodine nutriture. One of the goals of the World Summit for Children was to achieve universal salt iodization in every country by 2000. The goal has been nearly achieved. There are a few notable exceptions, however, such as the states that comprised the former Soviet Union, where effectiveness of salt iodization programs has fallen off following independence.

Unfortunately, an established policy for iodizing salt does not, of itself, ensure that all salt is adequately iodized. This scenario is particularly true in South Asia, where technical difficulties constrain adequate iodization at production facilities, and inadequate political will interferes with monitoring and enforcement of iodization guidelines.

In some areas where iodized salt is not available, supplementation programs, using iodized oil, have been effective. Because of the higher cost involved in comparison with salt iodization, most countries have abandoned these programs in favor of salt iodization.

SOUTH ASIAN (BANGLADESH, INDIA, NEPAL, AND PAKISTAN) MICRONUTRIENT SITUATION

South Asia is home to approximately 1.3 billion people representing many diverse cultural and religious groups, and widely divergent food production and consumption practices. The area also is geographically vast and varied, containing the world's highest mountains and sea-level river deltas, with ecological extremes from glaciers to rain forests to deserts.

Policy Environment for Micronutrient Nutrition

Effective policies for addressing micronutrient malnutrition are essential for successful and sustainable intervention programs. The National Plan of Action for Nutrition that countries adopt is probably the most important policy document that influences the types of programs implemented to address micronutrient malnutrition.

The National Nutrition Plan and the National Plan of Action on Nutrition

In 1992, representatives of 159 nations and the European Economic Community signed a "World Declaration on Nutrition" at the International Conference on Nutrition in Rome, to which was attached an international "Plan of Action on Nutrition." The final paragraph of the Declaration stated:

> With a clear appreciation of the intrinsic value of human life and the dignity it commands, we adopt the attached Plan of Action for Nutrition and affirm our determination to revise or prepare, before the end of 1994, our national plans of action, including attainable goals and measurable targets, based on the principles and relevant strategies in the attached Plan of Action for Nutrition. We pledge to implement it.

Thus each of the signatory nations pledged to create, by 1994, their own National Plan of Action on Nutrition (NPAN), patterned on the one drafted at the Conference, "to eliminate hunger and reduce all forms of malnutrition." All of the South Asian countries save Pakistan have ratified such a plan.

Nutrition is a multi-sectoral concern, influenced by agriculture and food, health, women's rights and status, and industry. Thus the priorities of a long-term plan to alleviate malnutrition can reflect the priorities of the Ministry responsible for penning the plan. The Indian plan, drafted by the Department of Women and Child Development of the Ministry of Human Resource Development, has no provision for increased production of micronutrient-rich foods, although it mandates extension of preservation technologies for vegetables and fruits, and emphasizes the need to achieve household food security through cereal crop production. In contrast, the Bangladesh plan, which was developed by the Ministry of Agriculture, underscores the need for increased production of micronutrient-rich foods, at the household level through home gardens, and at the national level by means of increased land area dedicated to horticultural crops.

NPAN SPECIFICS AND IMPLICATIONS FOR THE FUTURE

Bangladesh

The Bangladesh NPAN gives specific emphasis to production needs of micronutrient-rich foods, and, reflects the heightened awareness of the nutritional consequences of diarrheal disease; therefore, it gives important emphasis to micronutrient concerns of the primary health care and public works sectors.

Specific Bangladesh NPAN goals for micronutrients are as follows:

- Nutritional anemia

    To reduce the prevalence of anemia in women of the reproductive age group to 50% by 2000 and 25% by 2010.
    To reduce the prevalence of anemia in children under five years of age to 50% by 2000 and 25% by 2010.

- Vitamin A Deficiency (VAD)

    To reduce the prevalence of night-blindness in children aged 6-71 months to < 1% by 2000 and to eliminate it by 2010.

- Iodine Deficiency Disorders

    To reduce the prevalence of goiter in the entire population to 25% by 2000 and < 10% by 2010.
    To iodize all edible salt by the year 1996.

The Bangladesh NPAN focuses on all types of anemia, as the percentages indicated imply prevalence of severe, mild, and moderate anemia combined. Unfortunately, the plan limits its objectives for VAD and IDD only to levels of deficiency evidenced by goiter (the text does not specify whether "goiter prevalence" refers to total goiter rate, or only Grade II visible goiter), minimizing the need to eliminate excess child morbidity and mortality resulting from sub-clinical vitamin A deficiency, and the reduced productivity and mental development and performance resulting from non-goiter IDD.

The Government of Bangladesh conducts intensive programs for the elimination of VAD and IDD, although both of these programs are heavily dependent on foreign assistance. The Bangladesh VAD reduction program has achieved high supplementation coverage rates, and Government support for it remains strong–a fortunate situation, since supplementation alone cannot eliminate the causes of VAD. However, without specific objectives for the elimination of sub-clinical deficiency, it is possible that support for the program could wane after the elimination of clinical deficiency symptoms (see discussion below concerning India NPAN).

In addition, the program is highly dependent on foreign assistance. All vitamin A capsules are provided by UNICEF, which in turn receives them from the Micronutrient Initiative through a grant from the Canadian International Development Agency (CIDA). Should donor support collapse, as it did for a brief time in 1996, the program would cease operations and VAD would return.

Similarly, the Government of Bangladesh strongly supports the elimination of IDD through its Control of Iodine Deficiency Disorders program for the universal iodization of salt. Even without a specific objective for the elimination of sub-clinical (non-goiter) IDD, control of both clinical (goiter) and sub-clinical IDD is secure as long as the program for universal iodization of salt is in place. The program operates through industry, but UNICEF provides potassium iodate for fortification, so external support continues to be necessary to ensure the program's continuation.

India

The Indian NPAN is comprehensive in its integrated approach for improved nutrition through guaranteed food security, micronutrient supplementation and fortification, nutrition education, and improvements in the status of women. Nonetheless, language concerning the scope of direct micronutrient interventions is imprecise, diffusing focus for the elimination of deficiency.

The goals of the India NPAN that specifically relate to micronutrient malnutrition are as follows:

- Elimination of blindness due to vitamin A deficiency.
- Reduction in iron deficiency anemia among pregnant women to 25%.
- Universal iodization of salt to reduce iodine deficiency disorders to 10%.
- Promoting appropriate diets and healthy lifestyles.

The goals for vitamin A deficiency and iodine deficiency disorders reflect concern only for *clinical* deficiency.[3] Language in the introductory assessment of the present nutrition situation reinforces this clinical emphasis by stating that "specific overt clinical signs" characterize micronutrient deficiencies.[4] This oversight would be less worrisome if it were due to the plans' development prior to the discovery of the consequences of sub-clinical VAD. This is not the case, however, as another section of the document points out that:

> Recent scientific evidence reveal that disturbances produced by lack of these essential nutrients are not confined to a single organ as was formerly believed, but affects multiple organ systems. In other words, vitamin A deficiency does not result in just eye damage, nor iron deficiency in just nutritional anemia, and iodine deficiency in just the goiter. Even

the milder deficiency states of these micronutrients lead to adverse consequences in growth, development, and immunity.

This confusion recently found voice during India's "National Vitamin A Consultation" (see "Recent Developments" below), and it clouds the priorities of the VAD control program–especially in a climate where other compelling priorities compete for the resources of the primary health care system.

Nepal

The Nepal National Plan of Action for Nutrition, adopted in 1998, creates comprehensive strategies for addressing protein energy and micronutrient malnutrition, with an important emphasis on nutrition education and institutional development. The Nepal plan also specifies action steps to be taken for the achievement of its goals. The micronutrient-related goals adopted in the plan are as follows:

- To promote exclusive breast feeding to all infants until the age of five months.
- To promote the combination of breast feeding and proper foods for children between the age of five months and two years.
- To reduce IDD to 9 percent by the year 1998 through the provision of iodized salt and iodized oil injections/capsules to 95 percent of children and women of childbearing age and ensuring knowledge of causes and effects of IDD in 50 percent of the population in the 40 targeted districts.
- To establish an effective monitoring system to assure the adequate level of iodine in salt.
- To reduce child mortality and to prevent xerophthalima through dietary supplementation of high dose vitamin A capsules to children between 6 months to 60 months of age and to achieve reduction in vitamin A deficiency to a level that no longer constitute a public health problem (less than 0.5 percent).
- To bring about a change in dietary behavior so as to increase vitamin A intake of the target group through nutrition education, increased home production, consumption and preservation of vitamin A rich foods, proper breast feeding and child feeding practices and maternal literacy programs.
- To reduce maternal anemia to 55% by the year 1998 by ensuring iron foliate distribution to 10 percent of all pregnant and breast feeding mothers through the health posts and 90 percent from a ward based program, as well as ensuring knowledge of iron deficiency anemia among 33 percent of pregnant and lactating mothers (NPAN-Nepal, 1996, p. 36).

The goals of the Nepal plan have much stronger emphasis than the plans of Bangladesh and India for the role of child feeding practices in the control of micronutrient deficiency: emphasis on exclusive breastfeeding and timely introduction of complementary foods can help to focus behavioral change efforts for improved infant/child vitamin A and iron status. Additionally, the language of the vitamin A supplementation goal specifically mentions the role of vitamin A in reducing child mortality, which might ensure continued program intervention until sub-clinical deficiency has been controlled, but the goal also mentions a target prevalence for night-blindness, suggesting that the program may not focus on sub-clinical deficiency. The goal for IDD also suggests that only clinical deficiency need be targeted, as the prevalence target (9%) most likely refers to goiter prevalence and not the more common deficiencies resulting from sub-clinical iodine deficiency.

While the Nepal NPAN goal for the reduction of vitamin A deficiency targets "increased home production, consumption and preservation of vitamin A rich foods," food security goals from the plan actually could hamper progress in this area. One goal for food security suggests to "[s]witch-over-from the traditional food crops-oriented production system to diversification and commercialization wherever possible or-feasible and potential to help raise the purchasing power of the farmers of small land holding" (NPAN-Nepal, 1996, p. 19). Increases in purchasing power, if coupled with nutrition education, could have amplified benefits for nutrition, and crop diversification might be beneficial for the availability of micronutrient-rich foods, but shifting from "food crops-orientation" to "commercialization" likely would have a negative effect on household availability of micronutrient-rich foods. Similarly, another objective suggests that "nutritional objectives" should inform "orienting efforts at horticulture development on the basis of . . . market reaches" (NPAN-Nepal, 1996, p. 19), but home consumption of micronutrient-rich vegetables would be more likely to contribute to nutritional objectives for isolated communities.

In contrast to these food security goals that might lead to worsened micronutrient status for rural households, one food security goal unique to the Nepal plan that could have important consequences for reducing childhood anemia and protein-energy malnutrition is "to improve child feeding through the promotion of home and village prepared weaning food based on local cereals and legumes multimixes" (NPAN-Nepal, 1996 p. 20). The addition of vegetables to these foods would be even more preferable, but, if these cereal-pulse-based complementary foods replace traditional foods made from cereals alone, they could have significant potential for improving childhood anemia.

Pakistan

Of the four countries considered in this paper, only Pakistan has failed to adopt a National Plan of Action for Nutrition. This is the case despite strong support for nutrition by the Government, which gives nutrition a privileged position as a separate cell in the Ministry of Planning. The future consequences of the lack of an NPAN are difficult to assess, but the Nutrition Cell, despite its planning authority, lacks the mandate of a plan adopted by the National Assembly.

RECENT DEVELOPMENTS

Recent developments in each of the four South Asian Countries are of particular importance for the future of micronutrient status in the region. Some are extremely promising; others are ominous.

Bangladesh

In keeping with the tenets of its NPAN, the Government of Bangladesh (GOB) in 1995 initiated the Bangladesh Integrated Nutrition Project (BINP) for the elimination of malnutrition as a significant health problem. This project, which covers 60 of the nation's *upazillas*, signifies the GOB's commitment to the elimination of all forms of malnutrition, including micronutrient malnutrition. The project focuses on intensive counseling of mothers and families concerning child feeding practices, and on exclusive breastfeeding until the age of 6 months, followed by the introduction of appropriate complementary foods. This plan should have important effects on children's vitamin A and iron status. The BINP also seeks to improve maternal nutrition, and regular monthly contacts with pregnant and lactating women have enabled it to achieve remarkable coverage rates for iron/folate and post-partum vitamin A supplementation. Additionally, the project introduces household food security projects for home gardening and egg/poultry production that in addition to improving incomes, can improve the local availability of micronutrient-rich foods.

In 2000, the GOB decided to expand, the BINP model. The National Nutrition Project (NNP), a follow-up of the BINP, eventually will provide community-based nutritional services to all of the country. In addition to those mentioned above in the context of BINP, several aspects of the NNP, are significant for micronutrients. First, the project has budgeted for the purchase of all vitamin A and iron/folate supplements for its own interventions and those of the primary health care system. While the Government of Canada has agreed to provide the iron/folate requirement as a grant, and the Micronutrient Initiative, through UNICEF, has pledged to continue providing vitamin A capsules, the placing of micronutrient supplement purchase under the GOB revenue budget significantly reduces dependency on foreign aid for programs that distribute them, and bodes well for future sustainability.

India

Despite India being a long time regional leader for policies and programs addressing micronutrient malnutrition, some recent developments related to micronutrient malnutrition programs in India have not been positive. Most notably, the Central Government repealed in December 2000 the national ban on the sale of non-iodized salt. Additionally, a recent "National Vitamin A Consultation," under the authority of the Ministry of Health and Family Welfare produced a consensus document that weakens the position of the vitamin A supplementation program.

Repeal of the Ban on the Sale of Non-Iodized Salt

India under Prime Minister Indira Gandhi was the first country in the region to mandate universal iodization of salt. This legislation banned the sale of non-iodized salt for human or animal consumption. Over the last few years, however, community and nongovernmental groups protested against the compulsion to purchase iodized salt that is inherent in the legislation. Additionally, they constructed politically powerful parallels between large-scale production required for iodization and the prohibition on home-based salt production imposed by the British tax on salt which Mohandas Gandhi mounted a famous campaign of civil disobedience. Importantly, their arguments focused on the higher price of the iodized product and suggested that the ban discriminated against small-scale producers.

Currently, all but two Indian states (Kerala and Andhra Pradesh) have their own bans against the sale of non-iodized salt, so most of the Indian population continues to have access to iodized salt. Similar campaigns against individual state bans are possible, however, and could have important consequences for the availability of iodized salt.

Vitamin A and Child Morbidity/Mortality

The Ministry of Health and Family Welfare organized a "National Vitamin A Consultation" in September 2000 to establish consensus on the scope of vitamin A deficiency and to assess the need for a vitamin A supplementation program. Representatives from the Government, nutrition community, medical (pediatric) community, and implementing agencies (e.g., UNICEF, WHO, MI, NGOs) reviewed available data and research findings and concluded that, despite trends showing a reduction in clinical signs of vitamin A deficiency among children, vitamin A deficiency remains a serious threat to the well-being of children and pregnant women. In addition, participants in the Consultation refused to accept an association between sub-clinical vitamin A deficiency and child morbidity and mortality, stating: "available data are not robust enough to persuade us to recommend a policy of vitamin A supplementation for the purpose of mortality reduction in children" (Kapil and Sachdev, 2001).

As the reduction of clinical vitamin A deficiency is a worldwide trend, clinical VAD likely will continue to decline in India whether or not the Government of India continues to implement a program to control VAD. With this rejection of the findings that sub-clinical VAD causes infant mortality, findings that are universally accepted outside of India, the results of this consultation eventually may jeopardize the vitamin A supplementation program before it can address the serious problem of sub-clinical VAD.

Nepal

His Majesty's Government of Nepal (HMG/N) released, in December 2000, the country's first comprehensive national micronutrient status survey. As expected, this survey revealed substantial micronutrient malnutrition problems, and the Ministry of Health of HMG/N has already begun discussions for programs to address the identified problems. Specific issues likely to be addressed under these new initiatives include iron/folate supplementation for pregnant and lactating women for addressing the high levels of anemia identified throughout the country, and further expansion of the vitamin A supplementation program for children to reach currently un- or under-served areas.

Nepal continues to have an effective program for the universal iodization of salt, since, for practical purposes, the nation imports all of the salt it consumes from India.[5] Thus the ban on the sale of non-iodized salt in India effectively guaranteed that all salt consumed in Nepal would be iodized, and the lifting of the Indian ban on the sale of non-iodized salt could have important consequences for Nepal.

Pakistan

Few new developments are taking place for micronutrient malnutrition in Pakistan, yet changes in the universal salt iodization program may have important consequences for improved service delivery. Previously, the Government of Pakistan (GOP) contracted all Universal Salt Iodization (USI) activities to a Non-Governmental Organization (NGO), a scheme that met with limited success. For example, the salt production industry still has no formal organization, making coordination of activities difficult. Additionally, an unfortunate association between iodized salt and family planning occurred in the minds of many, resulting in refusal to purchase the iodized product.

Under a new scheme, the GOP has undertaken to organize the salt industry and to control USI activities itself in cooperation with Provincial governments. By working with an association of salt producers, the GOP should be able to better coordinate compliance with USI production goals, and the involvement of Provincial governments should enhance government authority to mandate iodization.

MICRONUTRIENT DEFICIENCY PREVALENCE BY COUNTRY

Bangladesh

While the Government of Bangladesh conducts nation-wide nutrition surveys approximately every ten years, these surveys do not assess micronutrient status. Information on iodine deficiency prevalence is available from surveys conducted by the International Consultative Committee on Iodine Deficiency Disorders (ICCIDD) and UNICEF for IDD, and information on vitamin A and iron deficiency is available from National Vitamin A Deficiency surveys conducted by Helen Keller International in collaboration with the Bangladesh Institute of Public Health Nutrition.

Iron Deficiency Anemia

Anemia prevalence is just over 50% among children in Bangladesh, and slightly lower among unmarried adolescent girls. Similarly, roughly 50% of pregnant and lactating women suffer from anemia, with prevalence approximately 10% lower outside of pregnancy. The survey reported in Table 3 that 43% of unmarried adolescent girls are anemic, while another study (Sahabuddin et al., 2000) reported a much higher prevalence at 95%. Judging by the results of Table 3, Bangladesh has nearly reached its year 2000 NPAN goal of 50% anemia among children and girls/women of reproductive age.

Anemia among children in Bangladesh may result from many factors, especially from poor feeding practices, parasitic infection, and low iron intake. The results showing higher prevalence among 6-11-month-old infants than among 12-23-month-olds strongly suggests that feeding practices have an important influence on infants' iron status. Delayed introduction of complementary foods past six months will precipitate anemia as the infant would have exhausted its iron stores from birth and breast milk is not sufficient in fulfilling its iron requirement. The Bangladesh 1997 Demographic and Health Survey reported that 30.5% of mothers are feeding only breast milk or infant formula at 6-7 months, 30.4% at 8-9 months, and 25.0% at 10-11 months. Neither breast milk nor infant formula is sufficiently iron-dense to provide for an infant's needs after six months. Poverty is an unlikely cause for this failure to introduce solid complementary foods, since older children (who consume more food) are receiving solid foods and have a lower prevalence of anemia. Additionally, infant formula is more expensive than locally available and appropriate solid foods, yet a large percentage of mothers (21.2% at 6-7 months, 22.9%

TABLE 3. Anemia Prevalence Among Preschool Children, School-Aged Children, Unmarried Adolescent Girls and Women in Bangladesh, 1997-98 (adapted from HKI, 1992).

Mild, Moderate and Severe Anemia	Prevalence (%)
Children 6-59 months*	52.7
6-11 months	78.0
12-23 months	64.0
Children 6-11 years**	55.5
Unmarried adolescent girls 11-16 years**	43.0
Women (ever-married, 15-49 years)	
Pregnant*	49.2
Lactating (non-pregnant)**	48.7
Non-pregnant non-lactating**	38.9

* Hb < 11.0 g/dl; ** Hb < 12.0 g/dl

at 8-9 months, and 20.5% at 10-11 months) choose to purchase it or continue to breastfeed rather than to produce solid foods. Nutrition education for improved feeding practices would likely provide the best solution for addressing the high prevalence of infant anemia and the anemia later in childhood to which it predisposes Bangladeshi children.

The high prevalence of anemia among adolescent girls emphasizes the potential to address anemia in pregnancy by providing supplementation to girls prior to marriage: supplementation to increase iron stores prior to pregnancy could build iron stores in preparation for reproductive life. The National Nutrition Project plans to introduce an intervention for weekly iron supplementation of unmarried adolescent girls.

Iodine Deficiency Disorders

The findings shown in Table 4 require one important caveat: this survey, conducted in 1993, reports the situation just as the universal salt iodization program in Bangladesh took hold. During 1995, UNICEF with support from CIDA, provided salt iodization plants along with potassium iodate for fortification to all salt producers. The situation today is likely much different than in 1993. According to these 1993 results, however, Bangladesh had a huge task ahead to reach its Year 2010 NPAN goal of goiter prevalence below 10%.[6]

The prevalence of goiters is highest in the flood prone areas of Bangladesh, where heavy monsoon rains leach the iodine from the soil. Nonetheless, prevalence is high in all areas and it tends to be higher among females, especially

TABLE 4. Prevalence of Goiter, Median Urinary Iodine, and Prevalence of Low Urinary Iodine for Children and Adults in Bangladesh (adapted from Yusuf et al., 1993).

Indicator	Geographic Zone			
	National	Hilly	Flood Prone	Plains
*Goiter**				
Adolescents and Adults (15-44 years)				
Male	33.6	27.2	36.7	34.2
Female	55.6	56.1	59.8	51.3
Total	45.4	43.0	48.8	45.6
Children (5-11 years)				
Male	47.0	43.4	50.5	46.0
Female	53.0	50.4	55.8	52.0
Total	49.9	46.8	53.1	48.9
Urinary Iodine				
Adolescents and Adults (15-44 years)				
Median (µg/l)				
Male		45.0	64.7	80.5
Female		27.5	49.7	57.1
Total		34.0	54.7	69.8
Prevalence < 100 µg/l (%)	67.4	84.4	63.7	60.8
Children (5-11 years)				
Median (µg/l)				
Male		37.3	49.2	90.5
Female		27.5	43.4	60.9
Total		33.3	46.8	77.5
Prevalence < 100 µg/l (%)	70.7	84.5	71.7	59.8

* Total goiter rate (visible and palpable)

adults. This prevalence may be due to the low overall food consumption among adult women, which corresponds to lower iodine intake.

Median urinary iodine shows a serious problem with iodine deficiency in all population groups in all regions (> 100 µg/l indicates normal iodine status), with the lowest median values in the plains region. Similar to the prevalence of goiter, median urinary iodine excretion is considerably lower among females in both age groups.

The data in Table 5 support the assumption that the situation for iodine deficiency disorders is considerably different today than it was in 1993 (Table 4).

TABLE 5. Distribution of Household Salt Samples by Iodine Content in Bangladesh.

Iodine Concentration (ppm)*	Percent of Samples
No Iodine	0.9
Iodine present at < 20 ppm	41.6
20-49.9 ppm	22.6
50-99.9 ppm	14.9
100-999.9 ppm	17.0
1000 + ppm	3.1

* Iodine content of 20+ ppm at the household level is mandated by law.

Ninety-nine percent of salt sampled at households contained iodine, a remarkable achievement and a resounding success in meeting NPAN goals for iodizing all edible salt. Unfortunately, quality control problems persist in the USI program, because nearly 43% of samples showed inadequate iodine levels, and just over 3% contained worrisomely high iodine levels.

Vitamin A Deficiency

Because the prevalence of night-blindness among school-aged children falls below the WHO cutoff of 1%, clinical VAD no longer is a public health problem in Bangladesh and the country has achieved its Year 2000 NPAN goal to reduce the prevalence of night blindness to below 1% (Table 6). This result strongly suggests that success has resulted from the biannual mass-dose supplementation programs, as prevalence was 3.5% in 1982-1983 when the program was not operating successful. A serious clinical VAD problem remains, however, among women–even non-pregnant non-lactating women. The difficulties of vitamin A supplementation during pregnancy, and the low percentage of births that occur in the presence of a trained attendant who could administer mass-dose vitamin A post-partum, and the low percentage of new mothers who receive post-natal care within one month of delivery all complicate the possibilities for addressing the problem among women.

Despite the elimination of clinical VAD as a public health problem, Table 6 clearly shows that sub-clinical VAD poses a serious threat to pre-school and school-aged children in Bangladesh, resulting in excess morbidity and mortality. The level of sub-clinical deficiency among children is similar to that of pregnant women, for whom clinical deficiency is much higher. Biannual mass-dose vitamin A supplements have proven effective in Bangladesh for reducing the threat of clinical deficiency (Bloem et al., 1995), and coverage rates

TABLE 6. Prevalance of Night-Blindness and Low Serum Retinol Status Among Preschool and School-Aged Children, Unmarried Adolescent Girls, and Women in Bangladesh (adapted from WHO, 1998).

Indicator	Prevalence (%)
Night-blindness (%)	
Children 12-59 months	0.62
Women	2.2
Pregnant	2.7
Lactating	2.4
Non-pregnant, non-lactating	1.7
Serum retinol (% < 0.70 µmol/l*)	
Children 6-59 months	21.8
Children 6-11 years	21.6
Adolescent girls (12-16 years)	11.6
Women	
Pregnant	23.7
Lactating	14.3
Non-pregnant, non-lactating	4.8

*0.70 µmol/l corresponds to 20 µg/dl

now are reaching exceptional levels through campaign approaches (HKI, 1992).

Improvements in health status and dietary changes will be required to further improve the vitamin A status for children in Bangladesh. Night blindness is more common among children who have infrequent consumption of animal foods (fish, meat, milk, and eggs), dark green leafy vegetables, and yellow fruits. Improved diets, however, require widespread changes in cultivation patterns, which will be especially difficult since the trend in cropping patterns over the last 10 years shows that rice production is expanding faster, and at the expense of crops that are more rich with micronutrients.

Although Bangladesh has met its NPAN goal of increasing land devoted to horticultural crops (Table 7), the large increase in land area given to rice coupled with the decrease in area given to pulses indicates that agricultural policy does not favor micronutrient-rich crop production. While irrigation has made land use possible during dry seasons and converts land previously not suited for cultivation, the gain of land to rice cultivation has been very high and land in pulse production has decreased.

The remarkably high rates of both clinical and sub-clinical vitamin A deficiency among Bangladeshi women pose a great challenge for the Government. Dietary changes to address the problem require significant improvements in incomes and in the status of women, who normally are the last in a household to take food, leaving them undernourished in food insecure households.

TABLE 7. Production of Selected Crops in Bangladesh, 1991-2000 (adapted from FAO, 2000).

Year	Paddy Rice (Ha)	Fresh Vegetables (Ha)	Pulses (Ha)
1991	10,244,503	95,910	725,368
1992	10,178,417	95,911	718,854
1993	9,905,600	98,744	713,115
1994	9,919,300	99,149	709,760
1995	9,951,700	100,360	741,360
1996	10,200,000	104,000	698,450
1997	10,263,000	106,000	669,321
1998	10,113,130	108,457	664,344
1999	11,700,000	108,457	667,569
2000	12,000,000	108,457	667,569
1991-2000 change (%)	17.1	13.1	−8.0
1991-2000 change (Ha)	1,755,497	12,547	−57,799

Low-level vitamin A supplementation during pregnancy and food fortification may offer cost-effective options.

India

Iron Deficiency Anemia

The 1998-99 National Family Health Survey (NFHS-2) provides the first-ever nation-wide assessment of anemia status for women and children. Previous surveys exist that provide prevalence data, but no survey prior to the NFHS-2 took representative samples from all Indian states.

Anemia is extremely common among children under 3 years of age in India, as only approximately 25% of children have normal iron status (Table 8). Similar prevalence would be expected among older children as well. These high prevalence figures suggest that a high percentage of Indian children suffer from mental and motor developmental delay, their immune systems are compromised, and active learning capacity is diminished.

Anemia also is common among Indian women, still far higher than the NPAN goal of reduction to 25%. Approximately 50% of non-pregnant women of reproductive age have some type of anemia (mild, moderate or severe), with prevalence slightly higher among pregnant women. Prevalence during preg-

TABLE 8. Anemia and Severe Anemia Among Preschool Children and Women in India.

Indicator	Prevalence (%)
Anemia (% Mild, Moderate and Severe)	
Children 6-35 months*	74.3
Women (ever-married, 15-49 years)	
Pregnant**	49.7
Lactating (non-pregnant)†	56.4
Non-pregnant, non-lactating†	50.4
All‡	51.8
Severe anemia (Hb % < 7 g/dl)	
Children 6-35 months**	5.4
Women (ever-married, 15-49 years)	
Pregnant**	2.5
Lactating (non-pregnant)†	1.6
Non-pregnant, non-lactating†	1.9
All‡	1.9

* Hb < 11.0 g/dl; ** Hb < 11.0 g/dl
† Hb < 12.0 g/dl;
‡ Hb < 11.0 or 12.0 g/dl depending on pregnancy status.
Source: International Institute for Population Sciences (IIPS) and ORC Macro (2000).

nancy at 50%, remains far higher than the NPAN goal of 25%. Severe anemia rates are not remarkably high, although the prevalence of severe anemia is considerably higher among pregnant women than lactating or non-pregnant, non-lactating women.

Iodine Deficiency

As shown in Table 9, the south region of India has the lowest goiter prevalence, yet some of the worst percentages of households consuming non-iodized salt and adequately iodized salt. Each of the states in the south region has seashore; perhaps iodine in the soil is adequate to prevent iodine deficiency. Unfortunately, no urinary iodine values are available for further investigation of this apparent contradiction.

Overall, the goiter prevalence in India remains quite high, far above the 10% goal of the NPAN and the percentage of households consuming non-iodized salt remains unacceptably high (28.4%), again falling short of the NPAN goal of universal salt iodization. The recent withdrawal of the national ban on the sale of non-iodized salt could have a ruinous effect if individual States now repeal their bans, and the percentage of households not taking iodized salt would rise even higher.

TABLE 9. Goiter Rates and Coverage of Iodized Salt by State in India.

Region/State	Total Goiter Rate[a] (%)	Households with Salt Containing No Iodine[b] (%)	Households with Adequately Iodized Salt[b] (%)
North	**22.7**		
Delhi	14.6	6.1	89.2
Haryana	17.9	19.5	71.0
Himachal Pradesh	13.0	3.2	90.5
Jammu & Kashmir	37.6	24.8	52.9
Punjab	30.3	16.7	75.3
Rajasthan	21.7	37.1	46.3
Central	**24.5**		
Madhya Pradesh	31.2	25.0	56.7
Uttar Pradesh	21.3	22.7	48.8
East	**21.7**		
Bihar	13.2	22.9	47.0
Orissa	18.7	29.6	35.0
West Bengal	34.5	11.3	61.8
Northeast	**19.9**		
Arunachal Pradesh	11.8	0.8	84.1
Assam	17.4	1.8	79.6
Manipur	25.9	2.3	87.9
Meghalaya	5.4	6.7	63.0
Mizoram	68.6	0.7	91.2
Nagaland	30.0	10.9	67.2
Sikkim	36.8	3.1	79.1
Tripura	28.7	--	--
West	**18.4**		
Goa	16.6	37.3	41.9
Gujarat	10.9	29.5	56.1
Maharashtra	22.4	32.0	60.1
South	**16.7**		
Andhra Pradesh	17.7	36.8	27.4
Karnataka	10.2	24.1	43.4
Kerala	17.8	47.6	39.3
Tamil Nadu	20.7	62.7	21.2
INDIA	**20.9**	**28.4**	**49.4**

[a] Source: Pandav, C.S.; Moorthy, D.; Sankar, R.; Anand, K.; and M.G. Karmarkar (2001).
[b] Source: International Institute for Population Sciences (IIPS) and ORC Macro (2000).

Vitamin A Deficiency

No national surveys of vitamin A deficiency exist for India, so an assessment of the progress toward meeting the NPAN goal of elimination of nightblindness due to vitamin A deficiency cannot be made. In the absence of vitamin A status data, dietary assessment data becomes the best proxy of vitamin A status. Fortunately, the National Nutrition Monitoring Bureau (NNMB) has been collecting dietary intake data for 25 years, and Table 10 presents the findings from the 1995 NNMB survey.

The Indian RDA for vitamin A is 600 RE/day,[7] and the 1995 NNMB results show that mean intake falls far below that amount (Table 10). Although at first glance these data suggest that vitamin A intakes are seriously low, their interpretation unfortunately is problematic.

First, the RDA is a consumption recommendation based on the distribution of nutrient needs. The RDA value represents the average daily nutrient requirement of the 99th percentile of the population: 1% of the population must consume more than the RDA to meet their nutrient needs, and 99% of the population requires the RDA amount or less. The distribution of individuals' nutrient requirements is a normal distribution, so the mean requirement for the nutrient thus is lower than the RDA value. If the mean *requirement* is lower than the RDA, then a mean *intake* lower than the RDA is not necessarily alarming.

Secondly, the NNMB report does not provide any information on the variability among individual intakes in the population. If the distribution is narrow, then few individuals in the population will be consuming the RDA

TABLE 10. Mean Vitamin A Intake for 10 States Assessed by the National Nutrition Monitoring Bureau in 1995.

State	Mean Vitamin A Intake (RE)
Andhra Pradesh	352
Gujarat	263
Karnataka	286
Kerala	214
Madhya Pradesh	343
Maharashtra	222
Orissa	436
Tamil Nadu	184
Uttar Pradesh	233
West Bengal	368
All States Combined	288

Source: National Institute of Nutrition, Indian Council of Medical Research, 1997.

amount. If the distribution is wide, then a significant proportion of individuals' daily intakes may exceed the RDA, and an even larger proportion of individuals might be consuming amounts of vitamin A adequate to meet their individual requirement, despite the *mean* intake being lower than the RDA.

Although reporting of prevalence of intakes below the RDA might be a more useful presentation for the NNMB data, these interpretation problems highlight the need for valid vitamin A status data in India. India urgently needs a nationally representative survey to determine the actual prevalence of VAD, both clinical and sub-clinical.

Without nationally representative data, prevalence information from smaller studies must suffice. Several small studies have found high prevalence of deficiency, as high as 8.7% among children in urban slums (Khandait, Vasudeo, and Zodpey, 1998; Khandait and Vasudeo, 1999) and 20.6% in rural areas of Tamil Nadu. Sub-clinical deficiency has been reported as high as 35.7% among slum children (Khandait et al., 1999).

Despite the low intake of vitamin A/β-carotene-rich foods, and reports of high prevalence of clinical and sub-clinical deficiency among children and women, many in India question the need for vitamin A supplementation programs. Importantly, a recent National Consultation on vitamin A issued consensus statements rejecting the internationally recognized association between vitamin A deficiency and mortality among children and the WHO recommendation to provide post-partum supplementation for mothers (Kapil and Sachdev, 2001). These statements suggest that vitamin A supplementation programs, although shown to be a cost-effective means to reduce its deficiency and address mortality in numerous other countries, can run the risk of closure due to competition from other primary health care priorities. In fact, a decision in 1992, presumably responding to cost concerns, to limit vitamin A supplementation to children under 3 years rather than the ages of 6 months to 6 years as recommended by WHO, leaving a highly-vulnerable group of children with high vitamin A deficiency prevalence unserved by a life-saving program (Khandait et al., 1999).

Nepal

In December 2000, His Majesty's Government of Nepal released the results of the 1998 *National Micronutrient Status Survey* conducted by the Ministry of Health, the Planning Commission, UNICEF, the Micronutrient Initiative and New Era Ltd., a research company.

Iron Deficiency Anemia

Iron deficiency anemia is extremely high among preschool children in all areas of Nepal, and its prevalence is most likely comparable among school-aged children (Table 11). Clearly, Nepalese children are experiencing mental and motor developmental delay, and active learning capacity suffers similarly. Additionally, the high rates of anemia indicate that the children's immune status is compromised.

Many factors may contribute to anemia among children in Nepal, such as parasitic infection, poor iron intake or poor iron availability in the diet, and inadequate feeding practices. As shown in Table 12, anemia among preschool children is highest in the 6-12-month-old age group, most likely indicating that mothers are not providing enough solid food. Results from the 1996 Demographic and Health Survey show that 28.3% of mothers are still only feeding breast milk at 6-7 months, 13.2% at 8-9 months, and 13.2% at 10-11 months (Pradhan, Aryal, and Regmi, 1996). Table 12 also shows that anemia gradually declines from 6 months to 59 months, indicating that poverty does not compel mothers to avoid feeding solid food (older children consume more solid food, at greater cost, than younger children). Clearly, nutrition education efforts are required to address this problem if Nepal is to meet its NPAN goal of exclusive breastfeeding for all infants up to the age of five months.

Anemia prevalence is also quite high among Nepali women, pregnant and non-pregnant alike, with prevalence slightly higher among pregnant women.

TABLE 11. Anemia and Severe Anemia Among Preschool Children and Women by Geographic Area in Nepal.

Indicator	Geographic Area			
	National*	Terai	Hills	Mountains
Anemia (% Mild, Moderate and Severe)				
Children 6-59 months**	78.0	79.7	76.2	78.9
Women (mothers)				
Pregnant[†]	74.6	80.3	68.4	77.1
Non-pregnant[‡]	66.7	72.6	61.1	65.0
All[§]	67.7	73.5	61.9	66.9
Severe anemia (Hb % < 7 g/dl)				
Children 6-59 months**	3.1	3.7	2.2	4.6
Women (mothers)				
Pregnant	5.7	3.6	7.9	5.7
Non-pregnant	1.7	1.4	2.1	1.5
All	2.2	1.6	2.8	2.0

* Sample sizes weighted to account for sample design–based on analysis at ecological zone level.
** Hb < 11.0 g/dl
† Hb < 11.0 g/dl
‡ Hb < 12.0 g/dl
§ Hb < 11.0 or 12.0 g/dl depending on pregnancy status
Source: Adapted from Ministry of Health, Child Health Division, HMG/N, New ERA, Micronutrient Initiative, UNICEF Nepal, and WHO, 2000.

TABLE 12. Anemia Prevalence by Age for Preschool Nepali Children.

Age Group	Prevalence		
	Total	Moderate*	Severe**
6-11 months	90.0	85.6	4.4
12-23 months	87.2	82.6	4.6
24-35 months	74.9	72.7	2.2
36-47 months	70.2	68.3	1.9
48-59 months	59.3	58.1	1.2

* Hb < 11.0 g/dl; ** Hb < 7.0 g/dl

The prevalence among pregnant women remains 20% higher than the NPAN goal of 55%. Anemia during pregnancy most likely contributes to the problem of anemia among preschool children, since children born to anemic mothers are more likely to have poor iron stores. Severe anemia is substantially higher among pregnant than among non-pregnant women, increasing the danger of maternal mortality. Although severe anemia is a serious condition for women in any part of Nepal, the danger is perhaps highest for those in the mountains, where access to emergency obstetric care is the lowest.

Iodine Deficiency

Because of the high inter-observer variability inherent in goiter assessment by palpation, goiter prevalence is not as reliable an indicator of community iodine status as is median urinary iodine concentration. Goiter rates are useful, however, for comparison with previous and other national surveys. As might be expected, the prevalence of goiter among women of reproductive age and schoolchildren is highest in the mountains of Nepal, where the iodine content of the soil is lowest (Table 13). The Terai area, which is a low-lying floodplain, and the Hills area have roughly the same goiter prevalence for women, while the rate among schoolchildren was slightly higher in the Terai than in the Hills. Using goiter prevalence as an indicator for iodine deficiency disorders (although iodine deficiency is possible even if a goiter is not present), Nepal has not achieved its NPAN goal to reduce IDD to 9% by the year 1998.

The WHO has established a minimum cutoff value for median urinary iodine of 100 µg/l indicating adequate iodine status (> 100 µg/l indicates normal iodine status) in a community. According to these urinary iodine excretion results, HMG/N's policy to control iodine deficiency disorders has eliminated IDD as a public health problem for Nepal as a whole. This elimination is an important achievement for such a mountainous, land-locked country. Nonethe-

TABLE 13. Prevalence of Goiter, Median Urinary Iodine, and Prevalence of Low Urinary Iodine for Children and Women (mothers) in Nepal.

Indicator	Geographic Zone			
	National*	Terai	Hills	Mountains
Goiter				
Women (mothers)				
Total goiter rate (% Grade I + II)	50.0	49.2	48.9	60.6
Visible goiter rate (% Grade II)	1.3	2.0	0.6	1.3
Children 6-11 years				
Total goiter rate (% Grade I + II)	40.0	38.5	40.7	44.6
Visible goiter rate (% Grade II)	0.0	0.1	0.0	0.0
Urinary Iodine				
Women (mothers)				
Median (µg/l)	114.1	85.0	142.7	168.6
Percent individuals < 100 µg/l	43.6	57.8	32.0	29.6
Children 6-11 years				
Median (µg/l)	143.8	108.9	183.0	196.6
Percent < 100 µg/l	35.1	46.7	40.7	44.6
Percent households with adequately iodized salt (> 15 ppm)	55.2	50.2	59.1	61.3
Percent households with salt containing no iodine	17.2	21.5	13.2	14.5

* Sample sizes weighted to account for sample design–based on analysis at ecological zone level.
Source: Adapted from Ministry of Health, Child Health Division, HMG/N, New ERA, Micronutrient Initiative, UNICEF Nepal, and WHO, 2000.

less, the median urinary iodine value for women living in the Terai area remains below the WHO cut-off.

The apparent contradiction between the goiter prevalence results, which show higher total goiter prevalence in the mountains and the urinary iodine results (Table 14), which show higher median urinary iodine concentration in the mountains, most likely is not a contradiction, but rather a testament to recent progress in HMG/N's IDD control efforts. Higher goiter rates in the mountains most likely reflect previous IDD and the urinary iodine values reflect current iodine status resulting from consumption of iodized salt.

The Terai region has the highest percentage of households consuming salt with no iodine and the lowest percentage consuming salt with adequate iodine. As mentioned above, Nepal imports essentially all the salt it consumes from India. Salt enters the country at a number of "entry sites" maintained by the Salt Trading Corporation (STC), a quasi-governmental body responsible for purchasing, distributing, and ensuring the quality of salt. The STC tests all salt

TABLE 14. Goiter Prevalence, Median Urinary Iodine Concentration, and Prevalence of Low Urinary Iodine by Pregnancy Status for Women (mothers) in Nepal.

Indicator	All Women*	Pregnant*	Non-Pregnant*
Goiter			
Total Goiter Rate (% Grade I + II)	50.0	55.5	49.3
Visible (% Grade II)	1.3	1.1	1.3
Urinary iodine			
Median (µg/l)	114.1	134.0	112.0
Percent < 100 µg/l	43.6	44.4	41.9

* Sample sizes weighted to account for sample design–based on analysis at ecological zone level.
Source: Adapted from Ministry of Health, Child Health Division, HMG/N, New ERA, Micronutrient Initiative, UNICEF Nepal, and WHO, 2000.

entering Nepal at these border sites to ensure the iodine content. The Terai region, which has, for all intents and purposes, an open border with India, and non-iodized salt may be entering Nepal across this porous border–and most likely available at a lower price than iodized salt.

The neurological development of a developing fetus suffers the most devastating consequences of iodine deficiency, so the iodine status of pregnant women is an especially important consideration. Although the total goiter rate is slightly higher among pregnant women than among non-pregnant, the median urinary iodine value is higher among pregnant women. The reason for this discrepancy is unknown, but the value of the urinary iodine median indicates that, as a group, pregnant women in Nepal have adequate iodine status.

Vitamin A Deficiency

The WHO has established a night-blindness prevalence cutoff of 1% or higher to indicate a public health problem. Results from the 1998 Nepal Micronutrient Status Survey indicate that VAD has ceased to be a public health problem for Nepal among children under the age of 6 years (Table 15), most likely due to bi-annual mass-dose vitamin A supplementation of this age group. This supplementation program represents a success according to NPAN goals, which targeted a reduction in prevalence of night-blindness in children 6-60 months of age to less than 0.5% by 1998. Among school-aged children and women, however, clinical signs of vitamin A deficiency remain extremely high.

In addition to the effects on them as individuals, vitamin A deficiency results in pregnant women giving birth to babies with low vitamin A stores, who

TABLE 15. Prevalance of Night-Blindness, Bitot's Spots, and Low Serum Retinol Status Among Preschool and School-Aged Children and Women (mothers) in Nepal.

Indicator	Geographic Area			
	National*	Terai	Hills	Mountains
Night-blindness (%)				
Children 24-59 months	0.27	0.45	0.10	0.17
Children 6-11 years	1.2	1.5	0.9	0.8
Women (mothers) current	4.7	5.5	3.9	4.5
Women (mothers) last pregnancy	16.7	19.3	13.3	20.4
Bitot's spots (%)				
Children 6-59 months	0.33	0.58	0.11	0.07
Children 6-11 years	1.9	2.7	1.2	1.7
Serum retinol (% < 0.70 µmol/l)**				
Children 6-59 months	32.3	40.0	23.4	35.5
Women (mothers)	16.6	20.8	10.5	22.9

* Sample sizes weighted to account for sample design–based on analysis at ecological zone level.
** 0.70 µmol/l corresponds to 20 µg/dl.
Source: Adapted from Ministry of Health, Child Health Division, HMG/N, New ERA, Micronutrient Initiative, UNICEF Nepal, and WHO, 2000.

are then predisposed to VAD early in life. VAD is remarkably prevalent among pregnant Nepali women (Table 16), a situation compounded by the difficulties of providing vitamin A during pregnancy and the low percentage of births that occur in the presence of a trained attendant who could administer vitamin A post-partum.

Pakistan

Less information related to micronutrient status is available from Pakistan than from any other country in the region. The Government conducted its last National Nutrition Survey in 1985-87, which did not assess IDD or VAD.

Iron Deficiency Anemia

As in the other countries of the region, anemia prevalence is quite high among preschool children (Table 17). Although these data represent the situation in 1985-87, no compelling reasons exist for assuming that the situation is different today. Unfortunately, the survey sample does not separate pregnant and lactating women, for whom differing cutoffs exist for determination of anemia, but anemia in this group is no higher than it is for other countries in the region.

TABLE 16. Prevalance of Night-Blindness and Low Serum Retinol Status by Pregnancy Status for Women (mothers) in Nepal.

Indicator	All Women*	Pregnant*	Non-Pregnant*
Night-blindness (%)			
Current	4.7	6.1	4.5
Previous pregnancy	16.7	16.7	16.6
Serum retinol (% < 0.70 µmol/l**)	16.6	31.5	15.0

* Sample sizes weighted to account for sample design-based on analysis at ecological zone level.
Source: Adapted from Ministry of Health, Child Health Division, HMG/N, New ERA, Micronutrient Initiative, UNICEF Nepal, and WHO, 2000.

TABLE 17. Anemia and Severe Anemia Among Preschool Children and Women in Pakistan (adapted from GOP, 1987).

Indicator	Prevalence
Anemia (% Mild, Moderate and Severe)	
Children 7-60 months*	65.2
Pregnant and lactating women*	45.2
Severe anemia (Hb % < 7 g/dl)	
Children 7-60 months	5.2
Pregnant and lactating women	0.9

* Hb < 11.0 g/dl

Severe anemia was a significant problem among children in 1985-87 and likely remains so today. According to these report results, however, severe anemia is essentially unknown among pregnant and lactating women, a situation hard to imagine. If poorer and perhaps more conservative households were more difficult to sample for hemoglobin status, then this sample may have overlooked those households where the severest forms of anemia are more likely to be found. At any rate, a new National Nutrition Survey is planned for within the next year and the results from the new survey may clarify the situation for severe anemia among women.

CONCLUSIONS

Micronutrient deficiency remains a serious public health problem in South Asia, but some of the countries of the region are making significant progress toward its elimination. In particular, Bangladesh and Nepal have eliminated vitamin A deficiency as a public health problem and have met their NPAN prevalence goals. This success, however, depends on continued external support for biannual vitamin A supplementation for children and longer-term food-based approaches will be necessary to achieve sustainable elimination of the problem. Because national prevalence data does not exist for India and Pakistan, it is not possible to determine whether either country is making progress toward the elimination of vitamin A deficiency among children.

Nepal has also eliminated iodine deficiency (as determined by median urinary iodine excretion) as a public health problem by WHO criteria, despite having not met its NPAN goals. Bangladesh may also be making progress, since 99% of salt samples from a 1999 survey showed at least some iodine present, but an IDD prevalence survey will be necessary to determine whether NPAN goals have been met or are likely to be met soon. India has not met its NPAN goals for reduction of IDD, but prevalence of goiters remains lower in that country than in nearby Nepal. The effect that the recent withdrawal of the national ban on the production and sale of non-iodized salt will have on IDD prevalence remains to be seen. Because data on IDD prevalence does not exist for Pakistan, assessment of progress in that country is not possible.

Anemia remains the most widespread micronutrient deficiency in all the countries of South Asia. None of the countries has achieved NPAN goals for its reduction and few if any signs of progress exist. Improved programs for iron supplementation during pregnancy and new programs for iron fortification of staple foods will require immediate priority throughout the region.

NOTES

1. A previous classification of vitamin A provided amounts in "international units" (IU). One retinol equivalent is equal to 3.33 IU.

2. The size of a goiter can gradually be reduced once proper iodine nutriture is restored, especially for children, but the process is slow and adult goiters rarely disappear.

3. The low 10% prevalence mentioned in the NPAN text for "iodine deficiency disorders" suggests clinical manifestations of iodine deficiency (goiter) rather than the more common disorders resulting from sub-clinical deficiency.

4. This statement also could be interpreted to indicate that only severe anemia is of public health concern for iron deficiency anemia. Mild and moderate anemia are invisible but have been linked with decreased productivity, delayed child mental and motor development, and reduced school performance.

5. Small amounts of salt consumed in Nepal enter the country from Tibet, but the number of individuals consuming this salt is small.

6. Assuming the "goiter prevalence" as mentioned in the Bangladesh NPAN refers to the total goiter rate, not just Grade II goiter.

7. The USA vitamin A RDIs for females and males older than 10 years are 800 IU/day and 1,000 IU/day, respectively.

REFERENCES

Beaton, G.H., and G. McCabe. 1999. *Efficacy of intermittent iron supplementation in the control of iron deficiency anemia in developing countries: an analysis of experience.* Final report to the micronutrient initiative, Ottawa, ON, Canada.

Beaton, G.H., R.T. Martorell, K.J. Aronson, B. Edmonston, G. McCabe, A.C. Ross, and B. Harvey. 1993. *Effectiveness of vitamin A supplementation in the control of young children morbidity and mortality in developing countries.* World Health Organization, Geneva, Switzerland. ACC/SCN nutrition policy discussion paper 13. 120 pp.

Bloem, M.W., A. Hye, M. Wijnoks, A. Raite, K.P. West, and A. Sommer. 1995. The role of universal distribution of vitamin A capsules in combatting vitamin A deficiency in Bangladesh. *American Journal of Epidemiology,* 142(8), 843-855.

Blomhoff, H., and E. Smeland. 1994. Role of retinoids in normal hematopoiesis and the immune system. In Blomhoff, R., (ed.), *Vitamin A in health and disease.* Marcel Dekker, New York, pp. 451-484.

Bruner, A., A. Joffe, A. Duggan, J. Casella, J. Brandt. 1996. Randomized study of cognitive effects of iron supplementation in non-anaemic, iron deficient adolescent girls. *The Lancet,* 348, 992-996.

Cook, J.D. 1990. Adaptation in iron metabolism. *American Journal of Clinical Nutrition,* 51,301-308.

Davies, C.T.M., A.C. Chukweumeka, and J.P.M. vanHaaren. 1973. Iron deficiency anaemia: its effect on maximum aerobic power and responses to exercise in African males aged 17-40 years. *Clinical Science,* 44, 555-562.

FAO. 2000. Food and Agricultural Organization (FAO) Statistical Databases, Rome, Italy: FAO. *<http://apps.org/cgi-bin/nph-db.pl>*.

Gibson, R.S. 1990. Assessment of iron status. In R.S. Gibson, ed., *Principals of nutritional assessment.* Oxford University Press, New York, NY, USA, 708 pp.

GOP (Government of Pakistan). 1987. *National nutrition survey report 1985-87.* Nutrition Division, National Institute of Health, Government of Pakistan.

HKI (Hellen Keller international). 1992. *Nutritional surveillance for disaster preparedness and prevention of nutritional blindness.* Handbook, Dhaka, Bangladesh:HKI.

International Institute for Population Sciences (IIPS) and ORC Macro. 2000. *National Family Health Survey (NFHS-2), 1998-99: India.*

Kapil, U., and H.P.S. Sachdev. 2001. National consultation on benefits and safety of administration of vitamin A to pre-school children and pregnant and lactating women. *Indian Pediatrics,* 38(1), 37-42.

Khandait, D.W., and N.D. Vasudeo. 1999. Vitamin A intake and xerophtalmia among Indian children. *Public Health,* March, 113(2), 69-72.

Khandait, D.W., N.D. Vasudeo, and S.P. Zodpey. 1998. Subclinical vitamin A deficiency in under-six children in Nagpur, India. *South East Journal of Tropic Medicine and Public Health.* June, 29(2), 289-292.

Khandait, D.W., N.D. Vasudeo, S.P. Zodpey, D.T. Kumbhalkar, and M.R. Koram. 1999. National Vitamin A Prophylaxis Programme: need for change in current age strategy. *Indian Journal of Pediatrics,* 66, 825-829.

Levin, H.M., E. Pollitt, R. Galloway, and J. McGuire. 1994. Micronutrient deficiency disorders (Chapter 19). In Jamison, D.T. and W.H. Mosely eds., *Disease control priorities in developing countries*. Oxford University Press, New York, NY. Pp. 421-451.

Li, R., X. Chen, H. Yan, P. Deurenberg, L. Garby, and J.G. Hautvast. 1994. Functional consequences of iron supplementation in iron-deficient female cotton mill workers in Beijing, China. *American Journal of Clinical Nutrition*, 59(4), 908-813.

Mason, J.B., M. Lofti, N. Dalmiya, K. Sethuraman, and M. Deitchler. 2001. *The Micronutrient Report: Current progress and trends in the control of vitamin A, iodine, and iron deficiencies*. The Micronutrient Initiative, Ottawa, ON, Canada.

Ministry of Health, Child Health Division, HMG/N, New ERA, Micronutrient Initiative, UNICEF Nepal, and WHO. 2000. *Nepal Micronutrient Status Survey 1998*. Kathmandu, Nepal, 131 pp.

Monsen, E. 1988. Iron nutrition and absorption: Dietary factors which impact iron bioavailability. *Journal of the American Dietetic Association* 7, 786-790.

Monsen, E., and J. Balintfy. 1982. Calculating dietary iron bioavailability: Refinement and computerization. *Journal of the American Dietetic Association*, 80, 307-311.

National Institute of Nutrition. 1997. *25 Years of National Nutrition Monitoring Bureau*. Indian Council of Medical Research, Hyderabad.

NPAN-Nepal. 1996. *National Plan of Action on Nutrition in Nepal*. National Nutrition Coordination Committee, Kathmandu, Nepal: National Planning Commission, 11th October, 1996.

Ohira, Y., V.R. Edgerton, G.W. Gardner, K.A. Gunawardena, B. Senewiratne, and S. Ikawa. 1981. Work capacity after iron treatment as a function of hemoglobin and iron deficiency. *Journal of Nutritional Science and Vitaminology*, 27(2), 87-96.

Pandav, C.S., D. Moorthy, R. Sankar, K. Anand, and M.G. Karmarkar. 2001. *Prevalence of IDD in India*. ICCIDD Technical Publication.

Pollitt, E., and K. Gorman. 1990. Long term developmental implications of motor maturation and physical activity in infancy in a nutritionally at risk population. In Schürch, B. and N.S. Scrimshaw, eds., *Activity, energy expenditure and energy requirements of infants and children*. International Dietary Energy Consultative Group, Lausanne, Switzerland, pp. 279-296.

Pradhan, A., R.H. Aryal, and G. Regmi. 1996. *Nepal Family Health Survey:1996*, Kathmandu, Nepal: Calverton, Maryland and Ministry of Health, Nepal; New ERZ and Macro International.

Rahmathullah, L., B.A. Underwood, R.D. Thulasiraj, and R.C. Milton. 1990. Reduced mortality among children in Southern India receiving small weekly doses of vitamin A. *New England Journal of Medicine*, 323, 929-935.

Ross, J., and S. Horton, ed. 1998. *Economic consequences of iron deficiency*. The Micronutrient Initiative, 44 pp.

Ross, J.S. and E.L. Thomas. 1996. *Iron deficiency anemia and maternal mortality*. Academy for Educational Development, Washington, DC, PROFILES Working Notes Series, No. 3.

Rush, D. 2000. Nutrition and maternal mortality in the developing world. *American Journal of Clinical Nutrition*, 72(suppl), 212S-240S.

Sahabuddin, A.K., K. Talukder, M.Q.K. Talukder, M.Q. Hassan, A. Seal, Q. Rahman, A. Mannan, A. Tomkinds, and A. Costello. 2000. Adolescent nutrition in a rural community in Bangladesh. *Indian Journal of Pediatrics*, 67(2), 93-98.

Seahadri, S., and T. Gopaldas. 1989. Impact of Iron supplementation on cognitive function in pre school-aged children–The Indian experience. *American Journal of Clinical Nutrition (Suppl.)* 50(3), 675-684.

Sommer, A., I. Tarwotjow, E. Djunaedi, K.P. West Jr., A.A. Loeden, and L. Mele. 1986. Impact of vitamin A supplementation on childhood mortality: A randomized controlled community trial. *The Lancet*, 1986(1), 1169-1173.

Tiwari, B.D., M.M. Godbole. N. Chattopadhyay, A. Mandal, and A. Mithal. 1996. Learning disabilities and poor motivation to achieve due to prolonged iodine deficiency. *American Journal of Clinical Nutrition*, 63, 782-786.

West, K.P. Jr., J. Katz, S.K. Khatry, S.C. LeClerq, E.K. Pradhan, S.R. Shrestha, P.B. Connor, S.M. Dali, P. Christian, R.P. Pokarel, and A. Sommer. 1999. Double blind, cluster randomized trial of low dose supplementation with vitamin A or beta carotene on mortality related to pregnancy in Nepal. The NNIPS-2 study group. *British Medical Journal*, 318 (7183), 570-575.

WHO (World Health Organization). 1998. *Safe vitamin A dosage during pregnancy and the first six months postpartum.*

Yusuf, H.K.M., Q. Salamatullah, M.N. Islam, T. Hoque, M. Baquer, and C.S. Pandav. 1993. *Report of the national iodine deficiency disorders survey in Bangladesh-1993.* Dhanaka University, United Nations Children's Fund, and International Council for the Control of Iodine Deficiency Disorders, Dhaka, Bangladesh.

Zhu, Y.I., and J.D. Haas. 1998. Altered metabolic response in iron-depleted non-anemic women during a 15km time trial. *Journal of Applied Physiology*, 84, 1768-1775.

Rapid Economic Change, the Nutrition Transition and Its Effects on the Structure of Consumption: The Nutrition Transition in China

B. M. Popkin
L. Bing
X. Guo

SUMMARY. Economic, demographic, and technological changes have led to a marked shift in the diet structure and the distribution of body composition in many regions of the world. Such changes include rapid reduction in fertility and aging of the population, urbanization, epidemiological transition, and the uneven distribution of the effect of economic reform. Research presented for China shows that it is undergoing a marked shift in its diet, activity, and nutritional status patterns. This paper presents data on the shifts in the structure of food decision-making and the associated body composition shifts. *[Article copies available for a fee from The Haworth Document Delivery Service: 1-800-HAWORTH. E-mail address: <getinfo@haworthpressinc.com> Website: <http://www.HaworthPress. com> © 2002 by The Haworth Press, Inc. All rights reserved.]*

B. M. Popkin is Professor of Nutrition, L. Bing is Research Assistant, Department of Nutrition, University of North Carolina at Chapel Hill, Carolina Population Center, 123 West Franklin Street, Chapel Hill, NC 27516.

X. Guo is Senior Research Epidemiologist, Statistics & Public Health Research Division, Analytical Sciences, Inc. (ASI), 2605 Meridian Parkway, Durham, NC 27713.

[Haworth co-indexing entry note]: "Rapid Economic Change, the Nutrition Transition and Its Effects on the Structure of Consumption: The Nutrition Transition in China." Popkin, B. M., L. Bing, and X. Guo. Co-published simultaneously in *Journal of Crop Production* (Food Products Press, an imprint of The Haworth Press, Inc.) Vol. 6, No. 1/2 (#11/12), 2002, pp. 99-118; and: *Food Systems for Improved Human Nutrition: Linking Agriculture, Nutrition, and Productivity* (ed: Palit K. Kataki, and Suresh Chandra Babu) Food Products Press, an imprint of The Haworth Press, Inc., 2002, pp. 99-118. Single or multiple copies of this article are available for a fee from The Haworth Document Delivery Service [1-800-HAWORTH, 9:00 a.m. - 5:00 p.m. (EST). E-mail address: getinfo@haworthpressinc.com].

KEYWORDS. China, food demand, nutrition transition

INTRODUCTION

Human history is characterized by a series of changes in the diet and nutritional status. This pace of change has quickened considerably over the last three centuries (Popkin, 1993, 1994). Before that, major changes in diet and nutritional status occurred infrequently and the shifts in diets occurred slowly over the first several million years of existence of the human race. In this article, we focus mainly on current stages in the nutrition transition. The concept of transitions or movement from one state or condition to another, is used to capture the dynamic nature of diet, particularly large shifts in its overall structure. Many of the same factors that explain the shifts in diet also explain those in physical activity and body composition. This work is based on the premise that the transitions that have occurred in nutrition are avoidable and that an understanding of the patterns and sources of change will serve as a basis for future interventions at the population level to lead to more healthful transitions.

A similar concept of transitions is embodied in the theory of the demographic transition–the shift from a pattern of high fertility and mortality (typical of less developed countries decades ago and of 18th century Europe) to one of low fertility and mortality (typical of modern, industrialization nations today). Even more directly relevant is the concept of the epidemiologic transition, which focuses on changes in patterns of disease and causes of mortality. As first conceptualized by Omran (1971), the epidemiologic transition moves from a pattern of a high prevalence of infectious diseases and malnutrition to one in which chronic and degenerative diseases predominate. Accompanying this progression from an earlier stage of pestilence, famine, and poor environmental sanitation to the later stage of chronic and degenerative diseases strongly associated with life-style, is a major shift in age-specific mortality patterns and life expectancy. Both of these concepts of transitions share a focus on how populations move from one stage or condition to the next.

There have been large changes over time in diet and physical activity, especially their structure and overall composition. These changes are reflected in nutritional outcomes such as stature and body composition. Further, these changes are paralleled by changes in life-style and health status, as well as by major demographic and socio-economic changes. For example, during the early stages of human evolution (from about 3 million to about 10 thousand years ago), human's subsistence was based primarily on a pattern of gathering, scavenging, and hunting. The diet these early humans consumed was varied, low in fat, and high in fiber. Physical activity levels were high. In consequence, early Homo sapiens hunter-gatherers tended to be taller and more robust, and suffered fewer nutritional deficiencies than humans who lived in settled communities during the period of early agriculture. These early agriculturalists' diet were much simpler and subject to tremendous fluctuations. After 10-12 thousand years of this second stage, the industrial revolution, a second agricultural revolution led to a considerable reduction in problems of famine, large shifts in diet, and increased stature. This period was followed by a marked shift to the high-fat, refined carbohydrate, low-fiber diet that marks most high-income societies today. There has been an increase in obesity and all the degenerative diseases of Omran's final stage has occurred during this stage. There is some indication that a new stage of behavioral change related to the reaction to man-made diseases is occurring in selected populations. We term these five periods: the age of collecting food, the age of famine, the age of receding famine, the age of degenerative diseases, and the age of behavioral change. For this article, we focus mainly on the periods that relate to the circumstances that most of the lower- and middle-income countries face–that is a period where famine has receded and degenerative diseases are rapidly emerging.

The theory of the nutrition transition posits that these changes or stages relate to the complex interplay of changes in patterns of agricultural, health, and socio-economic factors among others (for further detail see Popkin, 1993, 1994, 1998; Drewnowski and Popkin, 1997; Monteiro et al., 1995). This chapter focuses on the interplay of demographic and economic changes with affect China's food demand and nutritional status.

China is a critical case. While the nature of the economic and demographic changes affecting China differ from those of other Asian countries, the shifts in its dietary and physical activity patterns and nutritional status and health seem to be examples of quite similar changes that have occurred in SE Asia and are beginning to occur in South Asia. Furthermore, the emergence of obesity as an epidemic in China in the last decade is an issue unknown to many but one that is changing the face of Chinese health and well-being. It will have profound effects not only for the way it reflects major shifts in the structure of consumption but also on the health system of China and the welfare of its population.

DATA AND METHODS

This article pulls together a number of studies on trends in the Chinese diet, body composition patterns, and determinants of these changes. The data either comes from nationwide or large-scale surveys conducted among Chinese households and individuals.

National Household Level Food Consumption Data

The only source of national trends in food consumption over several decades for China is the income and expenditure survey system of the State Statistical Bureau. These data include estimates of household food consumption for a large national sample of households, based on consumption of a large number of commodities. The Bureau has collected food expenditures and in-kind food consumption in a reliable manner since 1970. The conversion of these data to macronutrients is based on many simplifications about the preparation of food for consumption. A food composition table developed by the Institute of Food Hygiene and Nutrition is used for this work. The results overestimate considerably the actual food available for intake. Food preparation and wastage, cooking losses, and other losses are not measured so a 15-30% overestimation of food consumption in possible.

China Health and Nutrition Survey

The China Health and Nutrition Survey (CHNS) is a longitudinal survey of health and nutrition in China, conducted jointly by the China Academy of Preventive Medicine and the University of North Carolina at Chapel Hill. The initial survey was in 1989 and included 8 provinces (Shangdong, Jiangsu, Hunan, Hutei, Henan, Guizhou, Guangxi, and Liaoning). Follow-up surveys were conducted in 1991, 1993, and 1997 (a fall 2000 survey is currently unavailable for analysis). The Liaoning province did not participate in the 1997 survey, but and was replaced by Helongjiang province. The survey is not nationally representative although the provinces vary considerably in geography, stage of economic development and health status. This variation was achieved using a multistage, random-cluster sampling process. Four counties were selected within each of the above provinces. Within each county/urban area, neighborhoods were randomly selected from suburbs, townships, and villages. Twenty randomly selected households were targeted within each neighborhood.

Dietary intake data were collected by nutritionists using 24-hour recalls and condiments and added oils were measured and weighed over the same three consecutive days. Daily energy intake was calculated using 1991 Chinese Food Composition Tables. The dietary data came from two sources–household survey instrument and individual dietary surveys. Detailed weighed inventory change of household food data was combined with three consecutive days of repeated 24-hour recalls. Detailed descriptions of the dietary survey are presented elsewhere (Zhai et al., 1996; CHNS website).

The income variable used in this study represents per capita household income. It included all cash and noncash income components. The data have been deflated to the 1988 value. Doing this for urban and rural China involved a complex process. Working with the national expenditure survey from 1989, we developed a 57-item consumer basket and have priced this out over time to create our deflator (Ren et al., 1989). The full documentation for this variable creation is presented on the CHNS website.

The CHNS collected food prices from each sample community. We examined three sources for food prices: state store prices, free market prices, and authority price records published by SSB, which provide the provincial average. Free market prices were found to be the most meaningful prices, in terms of affecting consumption decisions. We use these prices in this analysis.

Health workers visited each survey household with questionnaires on socio-demographics, health and nutrition that were directed at both the household and individual level. Anthropometric data were also collected, using standard measurement techniques. Height was measured without shoes to the nearest 0.2 cm using a portable stadiometer. Weight was measured without shoes and in light clothing to the nearest 0.1 kg on a calibrated beam scale. Body mass index was calculated as weight (in kilograms) divided by height (in metres) squared.

TRENDS IN DIET IN CHINA

Background

China represents one of the world's most rapidly developing economies. With its 1.2 billion people, China has achieved major advances in her socio-economic development within the space of less than a generation. Chinese per capita income grew at a remarkable 8.2 percent annual rate between 1978 and 1996 (World Bank, 1997). During this period there has been a significant reduction in the number of absolute poor in China, in conjunction with a rapid increase in income inequality. Accompanying these economic changes has been a rapid improvement of food supply and consumption. China has attained a high measure of food security and has seen marked changes in dietary structure (Ge, Zhai, and Yian, 1996; Popkin et al., 1993).

Change has not always been steady in China, and evidence of increased poverty among some subpopulation groups exists. For example, among the rural poor in some areas there has been an increase in chronic energy deficiency while, particular among higher income groups, the incidences of high-fat diets and obesity have increased rapidly (Popkin et al., 1995; Guo, Popkin, and Zhai, 1999b).

Long-Term Consumption Shifts

Household food consumption data from the national income and expenditure series can be used to understand the longer-term shift in food consumption patterns. The picture that emerges is of a shift upwards in cereal intake in urban areas during the early 1980s followed by a decline in cereal intake from 1985 to 1999. Vegetable intake also declined from 1980-99. In contrast there is a marked increase in meat, poultry, egg, and fish consumption in rural areas (Figure 1 Panels A and B).

FIGURE 1. Long-term trends in food consumption in Chinese diet: 1952-99.

A.

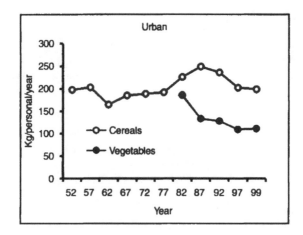

B.

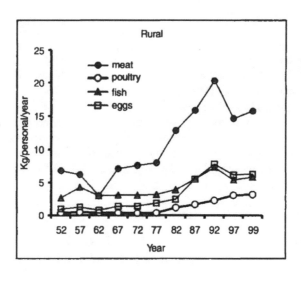

Related is an important shift in the proportion of energy from carbohydrate, protein, and fat sources in both urban and rural areas. By 1997 over 30% of energy came from fat in urban areas and over 23% in rural areas (Bing et al., in press).

Short-Term Dietary Intake Shifts

Income inequality has increased in China, which is reflected in quite different dietary patterns for each income class. Several studies have shown that fat intake is much higher among higher income groups (Popkin 1998; Bing et al., in press). In Table 1, data on food consumption patterns for low-, middle- and high-income tertiles in China is presented. CHNS data from 1989 and 1997, highlights the faster shift in the structure of food intake for the rich than the poor. Similar shifts, however, occur at varying magnitudes in the other two income tertiles. These include:

- A shift from coarse to refined grains and a reduction in total grain intake,
- A reduction in vegetable consumption, and
- A large increase in consumption of all animal products, in particular egg and egg products and poultry.

TABLE 1. Shift in Consumption in the Chinese Diet, CHNS 1989-1997 for Adults Aged 20-45 (Mean Intake Grams/Capita/Day).

Food	Low Income Tertile		Mid Income Tertile		High Income Tertile	
	1989	1997	1989	1997	1989	1997
Total Grains	811	615	642	556	595	510
• Coarse	226	68	98	43	78	30
• Refined	585	546	544	513	517	479
Fresh Vegetables	436	356	360	357	335	325
Fresh Fruit	5.5	8.0	13.2	18.1	26.1	37.5
Meat & Meat Products	36.3	40.2	57.5	63.9	66.5	96.2
Poultry & Game	4.1	7.0	6.6	10.2	7.7	20.3
Egg & Egg Products	6.0	13.9	10.6	21.7	15.8	31.5
Fish/Seafood	11.8	16.4	28.7	26.0	33.4	40.1
Milk & Milk Products	0.8	0.1	0.2	1.4	3.5	3.6
Plant Oil	12.9	32.1	15.8	37.1	16.4	41.5

Adapted from Bing et al., in press.

Related Shifts in Activity Patterns and Obesity

With the sectoral distribution of the labor force toward industry and service accelerating around the world, the changes in Chinas overall activity profile is remarkable. Occupational data obtained from the World Bank are used to study the structure of the occupations. A priori, one would expect that there would be few agricultural jobs in urban areas relative to rural areas. There is an expectation that there would be a much more rapid increase in the proportion of service jobs in urban areas. A time series analysis using OLS weighted by the total workforce in each low income country for the years 1972-1995 produced significant year, proportion urban, and urban interacted with year coefficients ($p > .001$ for all three sets of regressions for service, manufacturing, and agricultural occupations). The analysis simulated the occupation time trends for two scenarios–25% and 75% of the population is urban.

The results, as expected, show a much higher and more rapid shift towards service and away from agriculture in urbanized countries (see Popkin, 1999). In contrast, less urbanized countries have a larger agricultural sector, and there has been a much slower shift toward service and manufacturing employment. One of the most inexorable shifts with modernization and industrialization is the reduced use of human energy to produce goods and services. The result is obviously a marked shift in activity patterns at work, a trend particularly associated with the shift into increasingly capital-intensive production, sedentary service, and commercial work in more urbanized populations.

Unfortunately, there are only a few studies of this shift in activity and energy expenditures. One quite simple measure of overall activity has been collected in each survey of the CHNS. In Table 2, we grouped physical activity measures into categories of low, middle, and high with low being the least stressful and active patterns (Popkin, 1998). Activity patterns for Chinese adults shifted remarkably between 1989 and 1997, in particular, urban residents were more likely to have adopted a more sedentary activity pattern in 1997. In contrast, rural residents, particularly low-income residents showed a significant change from low and moderate activity patterns to a high physical activity pattern.

STRUCTURAL CHANGES IN FOOD DEMAND

To show the effects of income on food consumption patterns fairly complex two stage longitudinal estimation methods was employed. Individual level and random effect estimators were also used to obtain more accurate estimators. This approach considerably enhances the reliability of the estimated parameters. Bootstrap procedures were used to obtain standard errors. These methods controlled for within-household unobservables influencing food and nutrient

TABLE 2. Shifts in Energy Expenditure Levels at Work Among Chinese Adults Ages 20-45. (The Proportion of Adults Whose Occupations Place Them in the Light and Heavy Activity Categories.)

		Light Activity Patterns		Heavy Activity Patterns	
		1989	1997	1989	1997
Urban	Male	32.7	38.2	27.1	22.4
	Female	36.3	54.1	24.8	20.8
Rural	Male	19.0	18.7	52.5	59.9
	Female	19.3	25.5	47.4	60.0

Adapted from Bing et al., in press.

demands through time. The full discussion of these methods can be found in Guo et al. (1999a, 2000).

Multivariate Longitudinal Analysis

The most important and interesting estimates relate to the differences in income elasticities for foods and nutrients across income levels and across time. Since nonlinear income effects were estimated, it is most convenient to characterize the variations in elasticities through graphs. These graphs present estimates of income elasticities for 1989, 1991, and 1993 along with 95% confidence bands for the income elasticities of selected foods and macronutrients. The analysis also examined the changes in income elasticities and confidence bands about these temporal changes in elasticities from 1989 to 1993. Figures 3-7 present some of the more important results about the variations in income effects uncovered in this analysis.

The income elasticities for wheat flour and wheat flour products are quite informative. The first three panels in Figure 2 display the income elasticities for the probability of consuming any wheat flour products in 1989, 1991, and 1993 as a function of the income level. The lower right hand panel displays the change in elasticity between 1989 and 1993 as a function of income. The dashed lines indicate pointwise 95% confidence bands about the graphed regression lines.

Figure 2 shows that the probability of consuming any wheat flour is weakly but positively related to income in 1989. The estimated elasticity is statistically significant only about the mean income level. By 1991, wheat flour had become a statistically significant inferior good for individuals in the lower half of the income range, and by 1993 wheat flour had become an inferior good over nearly the entire range of incomes. The lower right panel in Figure 2 indicates

FIGURE 2. Income elasticities for the probability of consuming wheat flour, among adults aged 20-45 in China, 1989-93.

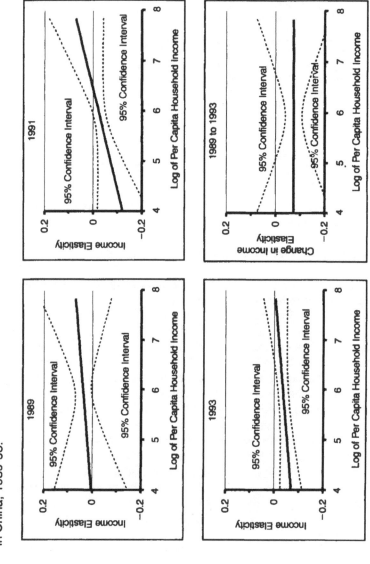

that the elasticity of the probability of consuming any wheat flour fell at all income levels and that this fall was statistically significant over the central portion of the income distribution. During these four years, higher income individuals became increasingly less likely to consume any wheat flour products.

Figure 3 presents nearly identical information about the amount of wheat flour products consumed given positive consumption. By 1993, the income elasticity is significant and negative for all incomes below the 90th percentile. The fall in the income elasticity across time is significant for most income levels. This illustrates that wheat flour products have clearly become inferior goods over just a four-year time span.

The demand functions for other grain products have also shifted in somewhat similar ways. Rice, the other major staple food, had stable income elasticity for the likelihood of consuming any rice. But there was a significant reduction from 1989 to 1993 in the income elasticity for the amount of rice consumed by those who consume it, and this reduction was much greater among the lower income groups. The income elasticity for rice fell at the 10th percentile of income from 0.20 to 0.04, while at the mean income level the elasticity shifted from 0.05 to 0.00. These downward shifts in income elasticities for rice were significant over most of the income range. Coarse grains were an inferior good both in terms of the likelihood of consuming them and the quantity consumed among those who ate them in 1989 and 1993, with only a slight downward shift in the income elasticity for the quantity of coarse grains consumed by consumers of coarse grains between 1989-93.

To simplify the presentation for pork and edible oil, only the summary changes in income elasticities are presented in Figures 4 and 5. There was positive income elasticity for the probability of consuming any pork in 1989. This income elasticity increased significantly from 1989-1993 with the increase being somewhat larger among lower income groups (Figure 4, upper panel). The income elasticity for the quantity of pork consumed (conditional on positive consumption) became more positive among all income groups, but higher income groups experienced the greatest increases in elasticities (Figure 4, lower panel). These shifts are statistically significant for all per capita incomes above the first quartile. For edible oil, the income elasticity for the probability of consuming this product is quite small, and there has not been a significant change over time (Figure 5, upper panel). The income elasticity for the amount of oil consumed (given positive consumption), surprisingly, was negative in 1989, but it was insignificantly different from zero over almost the entire income range. The income elasticity for edible oils rose significantly by 1993, and it was positive at all income values and significantly different from zero for all, but the top few percent of the income distribution.

The income elasticities for total energy intake (kcals) and total protein consumption also increased over these four years. Income elasticities for both nu-

FIGURE 3. Income elasticities for the amount of wheat products consumed, among adults aged 20-45 who consume any wheat products in China, 1989-93.

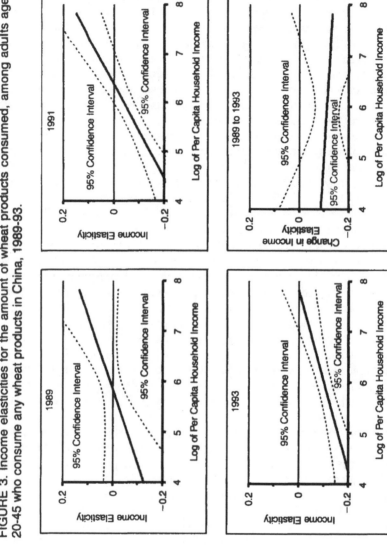

FIGURE 4. Changes in income elasticities pork consumption among adults aged 20-45 in China from 1989 to 1993.

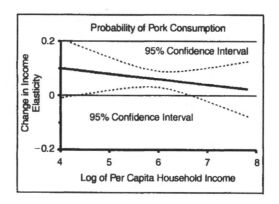

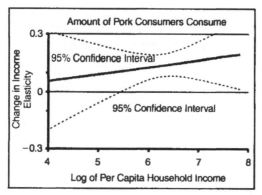

trients were small and negative in 1989. They increased slightly by 1993 and became positive at higher income levels. The magnitudes of these 1993 income elasticities, however, were less than 0.02 in absolute value at all income levels.

As a convenient and relevant summary measure, consider the income elasticities for the total amount of fat consumed in the diet as depicted in Figure 6. The estimated income elasticity for fat intake was not significantly different from zero in 1989. However, this elasticity increased and became significantly positive over almost the entire range of income by 1993. The increase in the income elasticity for fat was about 0.08 at all income levels, and it was significant about the center of the income distribution (Figure 6, lower right panel).

FIGURE 5. Changes in income elasticities for edible oils consumption among adults aged 20-45 in China from 1989 to 1993.

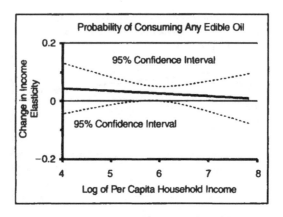

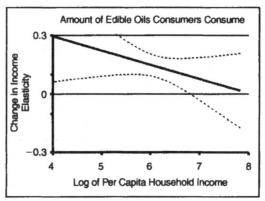

In summary, there were remarkable shifts in how Chinese diets varied with income over just these four years. The income effects for low fat, high fiber foods, such as wheat flour products, rice, and coarse grains, fell from 1989 to 1993. These foods became much less important in Chinese diets, especially at higher income levels. During the same time span higher fat foods became much more responsive to income levels. Pork, edible oils, and eggs had significant increases in their income elasticities. The quantity of fat in the diets increased significantly and now appears to increase much more rapidly with increases in incomes. Overall, these changes portend an important deterioration in the healthiness of the Chinese diets that could burgeon as the Chinese economy continues its expansion.

FIGURE 6. Income elasticities for dietary fat intake among adults aged 20-45 in China, 1989-93.

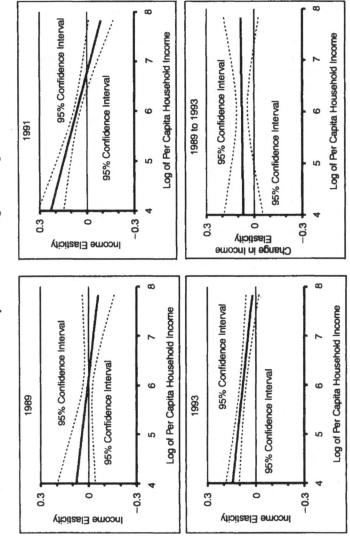

HEALTH IMPLICATIONS

These shifts in the diet in China, combined with equally rapid changes in physical activity during work and leisure have been linked with rapid changes in the obesity patterns in China. Among Chinese adults, the proportion of overweight men tripled and women doubled during the eight-year period of 1989-97. Today about 20% of Chinese adults are overweight or obese.

The shape of the BMI distribution curve also changed over the 8-year period (Figure 7) (see Bell, Ge, and Popkin, 2001). Mean BMI increased from 21.5 kg/m^2 to 22.4 kg/m^2 between the two time periods and the curve shifted to the right. However, it also flattened out and expanded at higher levels of BMI implying that the increase in overweight was greater than the decrease in underweight. This observation was borne out in a comparison of weight status categories between the two years of 1989 and 1997. From 1989 to 1997, the proportion of underweight men and women dropped by 2.3% and 4.4%, respectively. On the flip side, by 1997 14.1% of men and 20.7% of women were overweight or obese compared to 5.0% and 10.5%, respectively, in 1989.

Equally insightful for understanding the dynamic shifts in diet and activity and obesity are the changes within each Chinese household. One study used CHNS 1993 data to show that 23% of Chinese households with an underweight member also had an overweight member (Doak et al., 2000).

FIGURE 7. Eight-year change in Body Mass Index distribution curves for two cross-sections of Chinese adults aged 20-45 years.

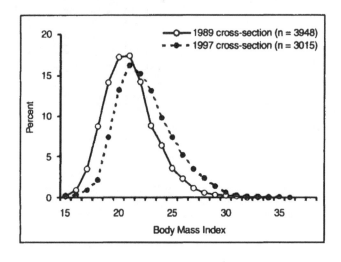

The health effects of these shifts in diet, activity patterns and obesity are large. Popkin et al. (2001) have studied the shift in the burden of diseases from problems of dietary deficit to excess in China as well as the shift in economic costs linked with this transition. The study estimated that by 1995 the costs of undernutrition and diet-related noncommunicable diseases were of similar magnitude in China, and the latter will predominate in 2025 (Popkin et al., 2001). Several broader reviews of these topics exist (WHO,1990; World Cancer Research Fund, 1997).

DISCUSSION

China is undergoing a marked transition in its diet, activity, and nutritional status patterns. The descriptive data provide a strong sense of the shifts that are occurring food consumption. Similarly, this research on the changing relationship between income and the structure of diet and total nutrient intake points out a number of important issues. First, the long-term trends show that the proportion of diet coming from what were previously viewed as superior grain and grain products–rice and wheat–is being reduced. Second, more pork and oil are being consumed. The largest increases in pork consumption are taking place among higher income adults and the larger increases in edible oils are happening among lower income adults. Concomitantly, there was a pronounced increase in the income elasticity for calories from fat from 1989 to 1993. This upward shift takes place over most of the income range, resulting in positive income elasticity for fat at all income levels in 1993. The increased income elasticities for total energy and for energy from fat suggest a worsening of the composition of diet, in ways that are linked to obesity and obesity related diseases, as incomes continue to rise. This represents one of the negative dimensions of the transitions taking place in China.

This study highlights two important issues. First, lower income people can afford more fat (from edible oils). This upward shift in fat consumption is important for explaining part of the nutrition transition in China, but the structural shift in the decision making related to edible oils and other fatty foods cannot be easily explained.

Second, it is clear that the nutrition transition in China is not decelerating, but actually accelerating. What is not clear is why. The shifts in the nature of work and leisure are straightforward, but the changes in diet and the reasons for the structural shifts in diet are what cannot be explained. Is it the rapid spread of mass media? In Asia between 1984 and 1989, the ownership of television sets increased from 62 million to 211 million. In the CHNS sample, TV ownership nearly doubled from 43% to 82%, for households in the lowest income tertile between 1989 and 1993. TV ownership went from 56% to 94% among the middle-income tertile during this same period of time. While television programming inside China is highly controlled, most individuals are now exposed to Western advertising and Western TV shows, and Hong Kong cable with its international perspective now reaches a large share of households. Perhaps this marked shift in television viewing is part of the explanation for the dietary change. While speculative, this may be an important link to explore to help understand the rapid changes in diets.

There are great concerns about this dietary change inside China. A national consensus meeting on obesity was held in May 2000. Earlier, the National Commission for Food Reform and Development was formed. The State Council issued the first document that addressed future food production and marketing in terms of its significance for nutritional well-being. In effect, they revised the Chinese dietary guidelines to create the current (1997) version. Updated guidelines focus both on the need to eliminate undernutrition and on what they term "diseases of affluence" or dietary excess and obesity. Education campaigns have been initiated; however, major shifts in other factors such as food prices are needed to affect the adverse components of dietary change more systematically.

The size and strength of relationships such as income and dietary fat, are of particular importance for these governmental efforts particularly as they relate to income and price increases over time. The changes in income elasticities that are documented in China forebode rapid increases in diet-related noncommunicable diseases. If incomes continue to grow and the elasticities continue to shift toward an increasing prominence of high fat diets, then it might be necessary to consider counteracting these changes with macroeconomic instruments such as price, credit, and tax policies. At the same time, it is important to realize that these changes in income elasticities could represent a major threat to the Chinese and world food supply if they foretell a major shift towards increased demand for grain-intensive livestock and poultry for China.

REFERENCES

Bell, C., K. Ge, and B.M. Popkin. 2001. Weight gain and its predictors in Chinese adults. *International Journal of Obesity* 25: 1-8.

Bing, L., S. Du, F. Zhai, and B.M. Popkin. (In press). The Nutrition Transition in China: a New Stage of the Chinese Diet. *Public Health Nutrition*.

CHNS Website: <http://www.cpc.unc.edu/projects/china/china_home.html>.

Doak, C., L.S Adair, C. Monteiro, and B.M. Popkin. 2000. Overweight and underweight co-exists in Brazil, China, and Russia. *Journal of Nutrition* 130: 2965-2980.

Drewnowski, A. and B.M. Popkin. 1997. The nutrition transition: New trends in the global diet. *Nutrition Reviews*, 55:31-43.

Ge, K., F. Zhai, and H. Yian. 1996. *The Dietary and Nutritional Status of the Chinese Population: 1992 National Nutrition Survey.* Beijing, China: People's Medical Publication House.

Guo, X., B.M. Popkin, T.A. Mroz, and F. Zhai 1999a. Food price policy can favorably alter macronutrient intake in China. *Journal of Nutrition* 129: 994-1001.

Guo, X., B.M. Popkin, and F. Zhai 1999b. Patterns of change in food consumption and dietary fat intake in Chinese adults, 1989-1993. *Food and Nutrition Bulletin* 20(3): 344-353.

Guo, X., T.A. Mroz, B.M. Popkin, and F. Zhai. 2000. Structural changes in the impact of income on food consumption in China, 1989-93. *Economic Development & Cultural Change* 48: 737-760.

INFH-CAPM (Institute of Nutrition and Food Hygiene, Chinese Academy of Preventive Medicine). 1991. *The Food Composition Tables.* Beijing, China: People's Medical Publication House.

Monteiro, C.A., L. Mondini, A.L.M. de Souza, and B.M. Popkin. 1995. The nutrition transition in Brazil. *European Journal of Clinical Nutrition* 49: 105-113.

Omran, A.R. 1971. The epidemiologic transition: A theory of the epidemiology of population change. *Milbank Memorial Fund Quarterly.* 49(4, pt. 1): 509-538.

Popkin, B.M. 1993. Nutritional patterns and transitions. *Population and Development Review* 19(1): 138-157.

Popkin, B.M. 1994. The nutrition transition in low-income countries: An emerging crises. *Nutrition Reviews* 52(9): 285-298.

Popkin, B.M. 1998. The nutrition transition and its health implications in lower income countries. *Public Health Nutrition* 1: 5-21.

Popkin, B.M. 1999. Urbanization, lifestyle changes and the nutrition transition. *World Development* 27: 1905-1916.

Popkin, B.M., K. Ge, F. Zhai, X. Guo, H. Ma, and N. Zohoori. 1993. The nutrition transition in China: A cross-sectional analysis. *European Journal of Clinical Nutrition* 47: 333-346.

Popkin, B.M., S. Paeratakul, F. Zhai, and K. Ge. 1995. Body weight patterns among the Chinese: Results from the 1989 and 1991 China health and nutrition surveys. *American Journal of Public Health* 85(5): 690-694.

Popkin, B.M., S. Horton, S. Kim, A. Mahal, and J. Shuigao. 2001. Diet-related noncommunicable diseases in China and India: The economic costs of the nutrition transition. (Unpublished manuscript, University of North Carolina, Chapel Hill.)

Ren, C.F., C.F. Liao, L.H. Huang, X.J. Chen, X. Ren, and Y.J. Wang. 1989. *The Income and Expense Survey in Chinese Urban Households,* Beijing: Chinese Statistical Press.

World Bank. 1997. *Sharing Rising Incomes: Disparities in China.* Washington, DC: World Bank China 2020, Series: 1-79.

WHO–World Health Organization. 1990. *Diet, Nutrition, and the Prevention of Chronic Diseases–Report of a WHO Study Group.* Geneva: WHO, Technical Report Series no. 797, pp. 108-181.

World Cancer Research Fund in association with American Institute for Cancer Research. 1997. *Food, Nutrition and the Prevention of Cancer: A Global Perspective.* Washington, DC: American Institute for Cancer Research.

Zhai, F., X. Guo, B.M. Popkin, L. Ma, Q. Wang, W. Yu, S. Jin, and K. Ge. 1996. The evaluation of the 24-hour individual recall method in China. *Food and Nutrition Bulletin* 17: 154-161.

Shifts in Cropping System
and Its Effect on Human Nutrition:
Case Study from India

P. K. Kataki

SUMMARY. More than twenty cropping systems are practiced in India. Rice-wheat and rice-rice are the major cropping systems practiced in an estimated 120 districts and 50 districts of the country, respectively. The rice-wheat cropping system (RWCS) of the Indo-Gangetic Plains (IGP) region of South Asia (Bangladesh, India, Nepal, and Pakistan) is the creation of the agricultural green revolution. Higher production of rice and wheat was necessary to meet the calorie needs of an increasing population in this region; as a result, the percent of malnutrition amongst children and adults decreased during the green revolution era. However, in recent years, there has been a reduction in both the rate of malnutrition decline and of the partial and total factor productivity of the RWCS in India. One of the many reasons for the decreased rate of malnutrition decline is micronutrient deficiency. Malnutrition amongst children and adults is a silent emergency in South Asia, including India. This review compares the food consumption habits, nutritional status, and cropping system practiced for different states of India to provide reasons for shifting the rice-wheat cropping system through crop diversification. Diversification of the RWCS will increase the supply of legumes and vegetables,

P. K. Kataki is currently at the Department of Plant Agiculture, Crop Science Building, University of Guelph, Guelph, Ontario, Canada N1G 2W1 (E-mail: pkataki@uoguelph.ca).

The author would like to acknowledge the assistance of Drs. John Duxbury and Julie Lauren of Cornell University, and R. Pokharel, K. R. Dahal, and S. M. Shrestha of IAAS, Rampur, Tribhuvan University, Nepal.

[Haworth co-indexing entry note]: "Shifts in Cropping System and Its Effect on Human Nutrition: Case Study from India." Kataki, P. K. Co-published simultaneously in *Journal of Crop Production* (Food Products Press, an imprint of The Haworth Press, Inc.) Vol. 6, No. 1/2 (#11/12), 2002, pp. 119-144; and: *Food Systems for Improved Human Nutrition: Linking Agriculture, Nutrition, and Productivity* (ed: Palit K. Kataki, and Suresh Chandra Babu) Food Products Press, an imprint of The Haworth Press, Inc., 2002, pp. 119-144. Single or multiple copies of this article are available for a fee from The Haworth Document Delivery Service [1-800-HAWORTH, 9:00 a.m. - 5:00 p.m. (EST). E-mail address: getinfo@haworthpressinc.com].

help to diversify the diets consumed, and increase micronutrient intake. This approach is important for a largely vegetarian population of India, and is therefore, considered to be one of several important Food Systems strategy to address the silent emergency of malnutrition in the region. *[Article copies available for a fee from The Haworth Document Delivery Service: 1-800-HAWORTH. E-mail address: <getinfo@haworthpressinc.com> Website: <http://www.HaworthPress.com> © 2002 by The Haworth Press, Inc. All rights reserved.]*

KEYWORDS. Cropping system, diversification, India, Indo-Gangetic Plains, malnutrition, nutrition, rice, South Asia, wheat

INTRODUCTION

There are five broad-based strategies available in a "Food Systems" approach to meet the nutritional requirements of various population groups: food production, food fortification, communication, planning, and monitoring (surveillance and evaluation). Crop diversification is envisaged to be an integral component of a Food Systems–Food Production strategy (FAO, 1997), though diversification *per se* is as old as agriculture. This need to diversify has become urgent to correct the changes brought about by an earlier need for increased staple cereal grain production, e.g., rice and wheat, in India, during the 1960s and 1970s. This emphasis on increasing cereal production has created new cereal-based cropping systems that displaced cultivation of other crops, especially the high-risk but beneficial legumes from the system. The rice-wheat cropping system (RWCS) of South Asia is the creation of the agricultural green revolution that started in the 1970s.

Across the Indo-Gangetic Plains (IGP) of South Asia (Bangladesh, India, Nepal, and Pakistan), wheat is grown immediately following rice in the same field. This rice-wheat (cereal-cereal) cropping system is currently being practiced in an estimated 12 million hectares, meeting the calorie needs of over a billion people in the region (Kataki, Hobbs, and Adhikary, 2001). The trends, productivity, constraints, and the strategies for efficient production management of the RWCS have been analyzed and discussed in several recent publications (Kataki, 2001a and b; Paroda, Woodhead, and Singh, 1994; Hobbs and Morris, 1996).

During the adoption and spread of RWCS, the percent of malnutrition in India decreased (Figure 1A), though the numbers of malnourished people in India are still high compared to other countries due to its higher population base. Increased production of rice and wheat (during the green revolution era) has been acknowledged for its role in reducing severe incidences malnutrition

FIGURE 1. Percent change in underweight and stunting for children below 5 years of age (Panel A) and percent shift in the nutritional status (Panel B) in India (Source: Measham and Chatterjee, 1999; and WHO, 2000).

(A)

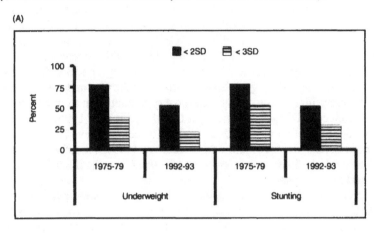

(B)

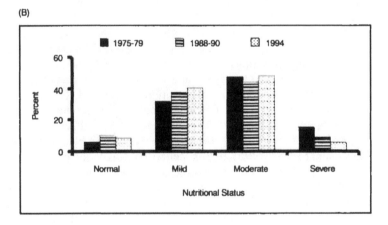

in India between 1970 and 1990, however, the percentage of mild to moderate incidences of malnourishment has increased (Figure 1B), creating a silent emergency. This increase has partly been due to a decrease in the diversity of diets thereby reducing micronutrient intake.

Malnutrition of any category reduces human productivity, and therefore, warrants corrective measures. The overall decrease in malnutrition within the last three decades in India can be attributed to two major factors: higher food grain production leading to improved food security and adequate cereal consumption and aggressive government programs for the reduction of malnutrition and improving human nutrition. However, the question remains, has the increased food grain prodution and government health program been enough?

Agricultural practices for cereal production in India has been guided by policies for higher production, productivity, and economics as were the needs for the period following the 1960s. During this same period, effort to reduce malnutrition in India has been primarily in the form of major programs including the Public Distribution System (PDS), Integrated Child Development Program (ICDP), National Mid-Day Meals Program (NMMP), and food for work programs. In spite of the progress made in food production and the reduction of overall malnutrition in the country, the cost of malnutrition to India's gross domestic product (GDP) was estimated at US$ 10 billion for 1996. Moreover, the nutritional goals set for the year 2000 may not be achieved even by the year 2010 (for more details see Measham and Chatterjee, 1999). Therefore, the crisis of malnutrition in India is far from over, and for its rapid reduction strategic thrusts in several areas are needed.

Since the RWCS contributed to the decrease in malnutrition during the 1970s and 1980s in India, this cropping system will be the focus of discussion in this chapter. The RWCS in India is largely practiced in the states of Punjab, Haryana, Uttar Pradesh, Bihar, and West Bengal from the northwestern to the eastern end of the IGP. Other states of India contribute to a lesser extent with respect to the RWCS acreage in the IGP. However, provinces in Bangladesh, Nepal, and Pakistan extend the RWCS region of the IGP. The nutritional status of these neighboring countries is very similar to that of India's.

The initial momentum of the 1970s and 1980s, both in terms of food grain production and rate of reduction in malnutrition, has slowed. Though the total food grain production still shows an annual increasing trend, the total and partial factor productivity of the RWCS has decreased during this period, after an initial high of the 1970s (Kataki 2001a and b; Kataki, Hobbs, and Adhikary 2001; Hobbs and Morris, 1996). In this scenario of stagnation or decrease productivity of the RWCS and the fall in the rate of declining malnutrition, the concept of Food Systems or Food-Based strategies can play a vital role in linking agriculture and human nutrition. This chapter discusses the importance of crop diversification as an important component of a Food Systems strategy for a long-term sustainable approach towards reducing malnutrition in the IGP.

A NOTE ON DATA SOURCES FOR ANALYSIS

An ideal data set should allow for a comparative yearly trend analysis on the nutritional status of population groups versus rice and wheat production and food consumption in the rice-wheat producing states of the IGP. However, such data sets are not available. Moreover, data on nutritional status for different states of India have been collected at different times and from different population groups in these states, and hence, analysis and interpretation of data should be done with care, though the overall trends and conclusions made in subsequent sections will hold. Quality and standardization of data is always a concern for making appropriate conclusion. For the subsequent discussions, data has been sourced from FAO (1998), and WHO global database for child growth and malnutrition (2000b). Data on per capita supply of cereal, pulses, vegetables and fruits in India was obtained from FAOSTAT (2000) from field surveys from Chitwan district in Nepal were used to highlight management problems of growing pulses in the IGP (Kataki et al., unpublished data). Information for drawing the schematic maps on cropping systems adopted and the soil and climatic environments within the IGP has been sourced from several sources (see maps for sources).

CONTRIBUTION OF THE RICE-WHEAT CROPPING SYSTEM TO NUTRITION

The Cycle of Malnutrition in the Indian IGP

The percent of underweight children for 21 states of India significantly correlates with the percent of malnourished adults (Figure 2). The percent of malnourished adults in this analysis is the sum of all the Body Mass Index (BMI) categories below and above the normal-range category (18.5 to 25) for adults, but not the normal category itself. This graph (Figure 2) highlights several truths for different states of India:

- First, states with higher percentages of malnourished children have higher percentages of malnourished adults. The probability of malnourished children getting caught in the malnourishment cycle is, therefore, high.
- Second, the malnutrition status between the states are highly variable.
- Third, within the Indian IGP, the higher rice-wheat producing states of Punjab and Haryana have a fairly high rate of malnourished children and adults, though it is comparatively lower than the other states of India.

Variability in Consumption Pattern and Nutritional Status Between States and Cropping Systems Practiced

A recent analysis (Kumar and Joshi, 2000) based on data collected by the National Sample Survey Organization between July 1993 and June 1994 studied calorie intake as a function of four major cereal based cropping systems of India: coarse cereal, rice, wheat, and rice-wheat based cropping system. In this study, the percent of undernourished for households in the rice-wheat (20%)

FIGURE 2. Correlation between percent children underweight (aged below 5 years) and adult malnutrition. The percent of adults malnourished is the sum of all Body Mass Index categories, except for the normal-range category of adults (Source: FAO, 1998; and WHO, 2000).

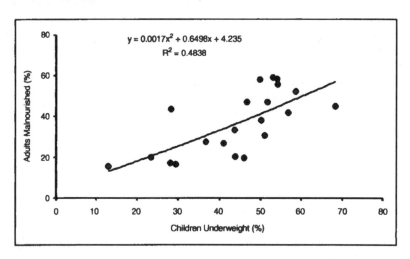

and wheat-based (21%) cropping system of the Indian-IGP was lower than the rice (35%) and coarse cereal (41%) based cropping system of eastern and southern India. The calorie intake in this study showed a decreasing trend of 3061, 2779, 2742, 2693, and 2495 kcal for the northern, western, eastern, southern, and north-eastern states of India, respectively. This trend in calorie intake followed the trends in the cropping system practiced in these regions; i.e., rice-wheat, wheat-based, rice-based, and coarse-cereal based, respectively. This study concluded that higher production of rice and wheat improved calorie intake, increased income, and increased the diversity in food consumption (milk, milk products, and vegetables) in the rice-wheat and wheat producing areas compared to the rice-based or coarse cereal-based cropping system areas. However, this conclusion should be looked at in a wider perspective, as discussed below.

There are several determinants of nutritional status of population groups (see Kataki 2002, this volume). Within the context of India, available data shows (Figure 3) that a few rice-based states (Meghalaya and Mizoram) that are economically poorer than the richer states of Punjab and Haryana in the rice-wheat growing areas have a much lower percentage of child (Figure 3A and B) and adult malnutrition (Figure 3C). In this review, for comparative purposes based on the cropping system practiced, data from four regions are being presented: (1) the RWCS-High; (2) RWCS-Low; (3) RB-East; and,

FIGURE 3. Comparison between the Indian states of Punjab, Haryana, Bihar, Meghalaya, Mizoram, and Kerala (Panels A to F) for percent children underweight; and stunted; adults malnourished; and consumption unit per day of cereals, energy, and pulses (adapted from FAO, 1998).

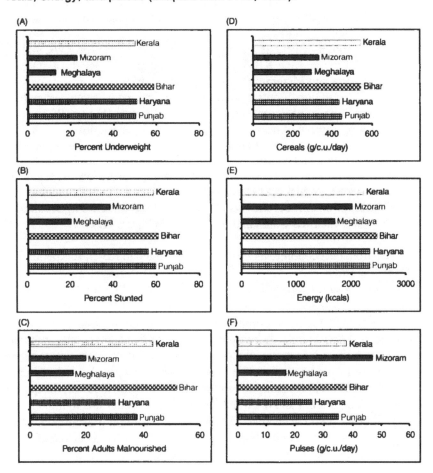

(4) RB-South. The RWCS-High refers to the higher rice and wheat producing states of Punjab and Haryana compared to the lower (RWCS-Low) producing state of Bihar. States from outside (RB-East and RB-South) the RWCS region (RWCS-High and RWCS-Low) of the IGP have been included for making comparisons and discuss important aspects of nutritional status of population groups in these regions. Details of this classification are described in Table 1.

There are several existing differences between these regions with respect to child and adult malnutrition and food consumption patterns:

- Food consumption pattern for ethnic children and adults in the state of Meghalaya and Mizoram are much more diverse than any other state of India (Figures 3 and 4).
- Consumption of cereals and hence, energy, is higher for RWCS-High, RWCS-Low and the RB-South region compared to RB-East states of Meghalaya and Mizoram (Figures 3 D and 3 E).
- The consumption of pulses, an important component of vegetarian diets, is lowest (except Mizoram) for the RB-East region (Figure 3F).
- The consumption of meat, fish, eggs, vegetables, and fruits consumed in the RB-East state of Meghalaya and Mizoram is many folds higher than the other regions (Figures 4 A and 4 B).
- Milk and milk product production and consumption are low in Meghalaya compared to Punjab and Haryana (Figure 4C).
- Consumption of roots and tubers in RB-East and RWCS-High is similar, but lower than RB-South and RWCS-Low (Figure 4D).

In addition, the economic independence of women in RB-East is better than other Indian states.

The northwestern states of Punjab and Haryana with a higher production (rice-wheat) and consumption of cereals, milk, and milk products have undoubtedly contributed to improving human nutrition in the region. However, the rice-based states of Meghalaya and Mizoram with a higher consumption of diverse food (though economically poorer than the northwestern states) have a significantly lower level of malnourished people compared to other Indian states. Though cereal consumption in the RB-East region is lower, the quality of the diet (i.e., protein and micronutrient supply) is better due to higher consumption of meat and vegetables in this region. Information from population groups from these highly nutritionally variable states of India can therefore be utilized to understand and formulate strategies to overcome malnutrition in India.

Correlation Between the Variety of Foods Consumed and Nutritional Status

Greater the variety of foods consumed, better will be the nutritional status of population groups and hence, lower will be the incidence of malnutrition in these groups, especially micronutrient-deficiency related malnutrition. For this analysis, Pearson's correlation was used to analyze food consumption and

TABLE 1. Characteristics of Categories of Cropping Systems for Analysis of Differences in Food Consumption and Nutritional Status of Population Groups.

Category	Cropping System Region	States	Characteristics
RWCS-High	Rice-Wheat Cropping System (RWCS)	• Punjab • Haryana	Higher levels of • Production • Productivity • Yield • Input use within the rice-wheat cropping system areas of the IGP region
RWCS-Low	Rice-Wheat Cropping System (RWCS)	• Bihar	Lower levels of • Production • Productivity • Yield • Input use of rice and wheat.
RB-East	Rice-based Cropping System (RB)	• Meghalaya • Mizoram	• Primarily a rice-based cropping system region in the northeastern part of India. Rice is the primary staple food.
RB-South	Rice-based Cropping System (RB)	• Kerala	• A rice-based cropping system region but in the southern part of India. Diet consists primarily of rice as the staple food.

nutritional status of population groups from 21 Indian states (Table 2). The population groups in these 21 states are nutritionally highly variable, which highlights some interesting results:

- Adult malnutrition was negative (Table 2) but significantly correlated with the consumption of fruits and vegetables ($p < 0.025$), and meat and fish ($p < 0.0418$). Therefore, apart from the production and consumption of cereals, variety in the foods consumed is important to meet the macro and micronutrient needs of humans.
- Adult malnutrition was positively and significantly correlated (Figure 2; Table 2) with the percent of children underweight ($p < 0.001$). A malnourished child is therefore likely to get caught in the malnutrition cycle.
- Consumption of cereal (staple grains) provide significant amounts of energy ($p < 0.0006$; Table 2). Increased food-grain production through the rice-wheat and rice-based cropping systems of the green revolution, therefore, contributed significantly to the nutritional well being of population groups in India.
- Interestingly, consumption of cereals also correlated positively and significantly with percent of stunting ($p < 0.008$) and underweight ($p < 0.0013$) amongst children of these 21 states (Table 2). This result indicates that cereal consumption alone is not sufficient to meet all the nutri-

tional needs of humans, specially children, and a lack of a balanced diet (i.e., a highly cereal-based diet) will increase the numbers of stunted and underweight children, though the incidences of severe malnourishment (hunger related) due to deficiency of energy would have decreased.

- The percent of fat consumed depended positively on the amount of milk and milk products ($p < 0.0036$), and oil and fat ($p < 0.001$) consumed, and it had a desirable negative impact on stunting ($p < 0.0089$) and underweight ($p < 0.0089$) of children (Table 2).
- In states where meat consumption was culturally acceptable, the consumption of fruits and vegetables was significantly high and both correlated significantly ($p < 0.0001$; Table 2) and were therefore a good source of quality proteins (percent, $p < 0.0003$; and on consumption unit/day, $p < 0.0013$).
- The consumption of oil and fat correlated significantly ($p < 0.0252$) with pulses, which is an indication of the preference of population groups of the 21 Indian states for vegetarian diets and a higher preference for oil (vegetable) and fat (milk and milk products) simultaneously (Table 2).

Though the results of the above analysis is in a broad sense as expected, it provides quantitative information for drawing firm conclusions, that can be used for nutritional strategies within the context of Food Systems in India. Foods that can be produced and stored for a long time (e.g., cereals and pulses to a lesser extent), versus those that are perishables (e.g., fruits, vegetables, etc.) can influence consumption behavior, keeping in view the cultural and social acceptabilities.

PRODUCTION FOR CONSUMPTION

Diversity in dietary consumption can largely be met by diversity in crop production, especially for a large population group preferring vegetarian diets for religious and cultural reasons, as is the case in South Asia. Crop diversification essentially needs to consider two factors: produce different foods and produce enough of each food to reduce its price and increase its supply, availability, and consumption. After all, the calorie demands of the past were met by strategies (scientific and policy changes) to increase staple food grain production in South Asia leading to shifts towards the adoption and spread of the rice-wheat cropping system. The drive to meet the calorie needs through cereal production in India resulted in less attention being given to other crops. This neglect has been corrected to some extent but falls short of meeting the silent emergency of malnutrition, especially micronutrient malnutrition in the country. This scenario is also true for other countries in South Asia (Bangladesh, Nepal, and Pakistan).

FIGURE 4. Comparison between the Indian states of Punjab, Haryana, Bihar, Meghalaya, Mizoram, and Kerala (Panels A to D) of consumption unit per day of meat, fish and egg; fruits and vegetables; milk and milk products; and roots and tubers (adapted from FAO, 1998).

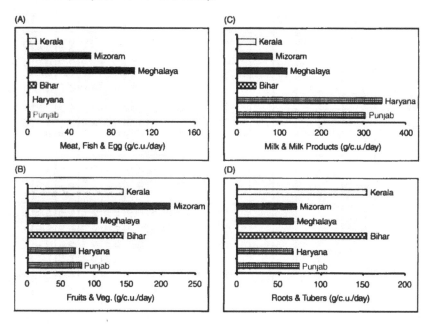

Diversity in Cropping System

In India, 30 major cropping systems have been identified (Yadav, Prasad, and Singh, 1998), of which, 20 cropping systems ranked first in four or more districts, and therefore, considered important (Figure 5). Cereal-cereal cropping system contributed 35% of the 20 most important cropping systems, followed by 30%, 20%, and 15% by the cereal-pulse/legume; cereal-oilseed; and other (i.e., cotton-wheat, sugarcane-wheat, cotton-safflower) cropping systems, respectively.

The cereal-cereal cropping system consisted mainly of rice-wheat; rice-rice; maize-wheat; sorghum-sorghum; pearlmillet-sorghum; and rice-sorghum system. The cereal-pulse/legume cropping system included rice-gram; soybean-wheat; pigeonpea-sorghum; maize-gram; pearl millet-gram; and soybean-gram systems. The cereal-oilseed rotation either included mustard in rotation with rice or pearl millet, and rice with groundnut. Thus, a range of cropping systems exists; however, green revolution technologies favored rice and wheat production. Politically, India is divided into states, and states into districts of different

TABLE 2. Correlation Between the Variety of Foods Consumed and Nutritional Status. Data for This Analysis Has Been Sourced from FAO, 1998.

	ADULT MAL-NUTRITION	CEREALS	ENERGY	FAT (G)	FAT (%)	FRUITS & VEG.	MEAT & FISH	MILK & MILK PRODUCT	OIL & FAT	PROTEIN (G)	PROTEIN (%)	PULSES	ROOT & TUBER	STUNTING (%)
CEREALS	0.2205													
P-VALUE	0.2894													
ENERGY	0.1014	**0.6405**												
P-VALUE	0.6296	**0.0006**												
FAT (G)	0.1105	−0.1006	0.1501											
P-VALUE	0.5988	0.6325	0.4740											
FAT (%)	−0.1044	**−0.6177**	0.1190	0.3203										
P-VALUE	0.6195	**0.0010**	0.5709	0.1186										
FRUITS & VEGETABLES	**0.4472**	−0.1045	0.0113	−0.1333	−0.1078									
P-VALUE	**0.0250**	0.6192	0.9574	0.5252	0.6082									
MEAT & FISH	**0.4100**	−0.2276	−0.2422	−0.2877	−0.0372	**0.6894**								
P-VALUE	**0.0418**	0.2739	0.2435	0.1632	0.8598	**0.0001**								
MILK & MILK PRODUCT	−0.0721	−0.2083	0.3092	0.2576	**0.5598**	−0.2735	**0.4206**							
P-VALUE	0.7321	0.3176	0.1326	0.2139	**0.0036**	0.1859	**0.0362**							
OIL & FAT	−0.1226	−0.3628	0.2883	0.1450	**0.7676**	0.0867	−0.0963	0.3763						
P-VALUE	0.5593	0.0747	0.1623	0.4892	**0.0000**	0.6804	0.6470	0.0638						
PROTEIN (G)	−0.2381	0.1203	**0.4265**	0.0656	0.0527	**0.6063**	**0.4736**	0.2127	0.0874					
P-VALUE	0.2518	0.5668	**0.0335**	0.7553	0.8024	**0.0013**	**0.0167**	0.3074	0.6778					
PROTEIN (%)	−0.3040	−0.2875	−0.1958	0.0203	0.0256	**0.6590**	**0.7013**	0.0078	−0.1019	**0.7991**				
P-VALUE	0.1395	0.1635	0.3482	0.9231	0.9035	**0.0003**	**0.0001**	0.9704	0.6279	**0.0000**				
PULSES	0.1108	−0.2632	0.0690	0.2306	0.1805	0.0892	0.3099	0.1139	**0.4465**	0.0742	0.0104			
P-VALUE	0.5981	0.2037	0.7431	0.2675	0.3879	0.6714	0.1317	0.5878	**0.0252**	0.7245	0.9605			
ROOTS & TUBERS	−0.2406	−0.0355	0.1968	0.2217	0.0070	**0.4863**	0.0673	0.1783	0.0131	0.0822	0.3569	0.1792		
P-VALUE	0.2465	0.8661	0.3457	0.2868	0.9734	**0.0137**	0.7491	0.3937	0.9506	0.6959	0.0799	0.3915		
STUNTING (%)	0.2001	**0.5182**	0.3272	−0.2488	−0.3734	−0.1318	−0.1109	−0.1086	0.0254	0.0822	−0.1255	−0.0065	0.0375	
P-VALUE	0.3376	**0.0080**	0.1104	0.2304	0.0660	0.5300	0.5977	0.6055	0.9039	0.6959	0.5500	0.9755	0.8588	
UNDER WEIGHT (%)	**0.6170**	**0.6057**	0.3011	0.1811	**−0.5119**	−0.1544	−0.1961	−0.1648	−0.3260	0.0614	−0.1162	−0.0007	−0.0951	**0.6907**
P-VALUE	**0.0010**	**0.0013**	0.1436	0.3862	**0.0069**	0.4612	0.3474	0.4310	0.1118	0.7705	0.5801	0.9974	0.6511	**0.0001**

FIGURE 5. Schematic map showing approximate distribution (not to scale) of different cropping systems practiced. The rice-wheat cropping system is shown for Bangladesh, India, Nepal, and Pakistan while the rest of the cropping systems are shown for India only. The pearl millet based cropping system includes its rotation with gram, mustard, sorghum, and wheat. The cropping system category "others" refers to the rest of the cropping system practiced (see text for details) in India, the areas being small and scattered across the country and is, therefore, not shown in this map to improve the visual clarity of the major cropping systems (Source: Kataki, 2001a; Yadav, Prasad and Singh, 1998; Ali and Pande, 1999).

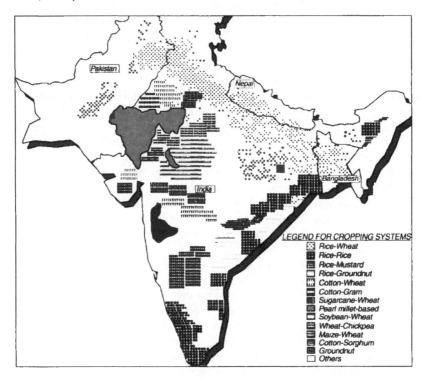

numbers per state. Approximately, 120 districts in the country practice the rice-wheat cropping system, followed by 50 districts with the rice-rice system. The rice-mustard and maize-wheat system are practiced between 20 to 30 districts each. The rest of the 20 important cropping systems are practiced in varying numbers of 4 to 20 districts each. Though crop production data is collected on an individual crop basis and not by the cropping systems practiced, the above description is a fair estimate of the cropping systems adopted in different states in India.

Per Capita Food Supply

The number of cropping systems described above, masks the neglect of several crops other than rice and wheat. The rice-wheat followed by the rice-rice cropping system is therefore the most important in acreage and production. Where summer rain or assured irrigation is available, rice and wheat cultivation in a sequence and on the same field has been favored, pushing other crops to be grown mostly under high-risk, low-input, and low-yielding, rainfed conditions. The number of high yielding varieties cultivated is more than double for rice and wheat compared to any other crop. The result of three decades of emphasis on cereal-production technologies is reflected in the supply of different crops. The per capita supply of cereals, including rice and wheat has increased steadily over the last three decades (Figure 6A), while that of pulses has decreased gradually (Figure 6B). Supply of oilseed crops (Figure 6B) has risen slightly in recent years, boosted by imports. Per capita supply of vegetables has risen faster than that of fruits (Figure 6B), but is far below the required levels of supply and consumption in India (for more details see the article by M. Ali, in this publication). In addition, poor storage and transit facilities result in 10 to 100% post-harvest losses of vegetables and fruits (Figure 6D). Therefore, the crop production and management system in India has tremendous scope for improvement. The existing knowledge of production technologies coupled with proper management and policy support, can significantly improve production and supply of other crops important to the diet. These intentional but strategic changes can bring about an increase in the supply and consumption of legumes (including pulses), vegetables and fruits to this largely vegetarian population.

As discussed earlier in this article (for details see Kataki, 2002, of this publication), there are five Food Systems strategies. Of these five, the food-production strategy can be classified into six categories (Table 1, Kataki, 2002 of this publication): crop diversification, breeding staple crops for higher micronutrient enriched grains, commercial vegetable and fruit production, community vegetable and fruit production, improved post-harvest storage, and production of small animals, poultry, and fish. The first two categories of the food-production strategy involve issues related to field crops. The following sections discuss the crop diversification category.

Major Constraints to Shifting the Rice-Wheat Cropping System (RWCS)

Shifting of the rice-wheat cropping system, i.e., crop diversification, can be brought about by breaking the cycle of growing rice in the summer or monsoon season, or of wheat in the winter season by introducing pulse (grain legumes), vegetable, oilseed or other cash (e.g., cotton, sugarcane, etc.) crops. There are very few options for replacing monsoon rice when water stagnation in fields is

FIGURE 6. Trends in the supply of cereals, wheat, rice, vegetables, fruits, pulses, and oil seeds; and the estimated range of storage losses of fruits and vegetables in India (Panels A to D) (Source: FAOSTAT, 2000; and Sehgal, 1999).

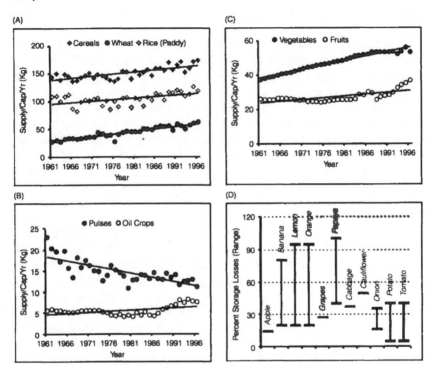

common. The focus of diversification in this section are pulses, i.e., the grain legume crops, since they are the key to the supply of micronutrients by adding variety to the diets for a large vegetarian population in India and also due to the decrease in per capita supply of pulses (Figure 6B) in India within the last three decades. (For analysis and discussion on diversification through vegetables, see article by M. Ali, in this publication.)

The two important constraints for enhancing pulse production are policy support and poor crop management. Compared to rice, wheat and oilseeds, pulse cultivation in India has been neglected in the past due to the lack of a good policy for remunerative price support mechanism. The government has provided minimum price support for 4 of the 12 pulses generally cultivated in India (Sehgal, 1999). Moreover, the open market price of pulses in recent years has always been higher than the support or procurement prices fixed by the government for these pulses; therefore, pulse cultivation has remained confined largely to marginal lands. Coupled with low yields, pulse production remains a high-risk venture. As a result, management of pulses by farmers is generally poor, adding to the constraints of enhancing its production. To highlight the management problems of pulses, data are presented from a survey of lentil crop from Chitwan district of Nepal, which is part of the rice-wheat growing IGP region of South Asia.

Lentil can replace wheat as a winter crop immediately following the monsoon rice. In the Chitwan district of Nepal, lentil cultivation has generally shifted from eastern Chitwan to western Chitwan over the years. During the 1999-2000 winter season, a survey of 53 lentil fields in the district (Figure 7) was conducted due to reports stating yearly yield decline of lentil in the district; generally low yields; poor crop stand; high plant mortality rate during the crop growing season; and poor second year lentil crop when grown in the same field as the first year lentil crop. Therefore, the objective of the survey was to quantify lentil crop stand in farmers field; assess root health and foliar diseases of lentil; estimate the extent of macro- and micro-nutrient deficiency problems; and to isolate, characterize, and assess the pathogenicity of the diseases identified during the survey.

The results of the survey were very striking. The recommended seed rate for sowing lentil in Chitwan is 40 kg/hectare. Though the mean seed rate used by the 53 surveyed farmers was 44 kg/hectare, however, the range varied (Figure 8A) from a mean of 25 (71% of farmers) to 150 kg/hectare (2% farmers). Seed quality and availability was a major concern for the farmers and the use of higher seed rate by some farmers was a form of insurance for better plant stand. However, lentil plant population varied from 100 to more than 1000-plants/4 sq. meters, with a mean of 372-plants/4 sq.m (Figure 8B). In addition, the correlation between the seed rate used and plant population was very poor (Figure 8C), due to variable soil moisture at sowing, variable planting dates (very late planting), poor or no tillage practice, little or no use of fertilizers, and disease (wilts) problems leading to an increase in plant mortality rates with progress of the growing season. Root and foliar samples collected from the surveyed fields showed regions within the district dominated either singly or by a combination of *Rhizoctonia solanaii*, *Sclerotium rolfsii*, and *Fusarium* sp. There were areas with no apparent disease incidences, but with soil micronutrient deficiency problems. Most of the surveyed farmers preferred to grow lentil on the same field for only a year due to a poor crop if grown for more than a year (Figure 8D). Though wilting was the main reason cited by farmers for lentil plants grown in the same field for more than a year, correction of soil B deficiency yielded a good crop of lentil. In a subsequent observational study in a farmers field, the second year chickpea (Plate 1) and lentil crop with soil applied B had a larger root volume, biomass, flower, pod, and seed set, and hence, higher yield, compared to the −B plots.

FIGURE 7. Map showing location of lentil fields surveyed in the Chitwan district of Nepal during 1999/2000-winter season. Chitwan district is a rice-wheat growing region of the Indo-Gangetic Plains region of South Asia (Bangladesh, India, Nepal, and Pakistan). The locations of the surveyed fields (latitude and longitude) were recorded using GPS, and plotted in the Geographic Information Systems Unit of SSD, NARC, Khumaltar, by Mr. Kamal Sah.

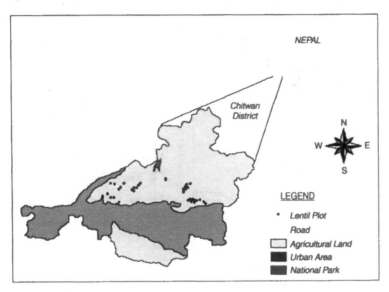

In conclusion, such wide variations in the use of inputs, crop establishment, and management methods is unacceptable in a post-Green Revolution era and at a time when increase in land area for agricultural purposes has peaked in South Asia. In addition, for the cultivation of rice and wheat, excessive and unbalanced input use has reduced its total and partial factor productivity (Kataki, 2001a and b; Hobbs and Morris, 1996). The survey results highlighted above for lentil are generally true for most pulses grown in the IGP region of Bangladesh, India, Nepal, and Pakistan. Management techniques to address most of the problems established through this survey are known, and access to good quality inputs and policy support can alleviate these production problems and enhance its supply.

Shifting Areas of Production

Shifting of the rice-wheat cropping system will shift the areas where crops are cultivated, probably following the principal of growing crops in lands where it is most suited. Within the IGP, annual precipitation varies between

FIGURE 8. Variations in the use of seed rate (for sowing lentil) and plant population (Panels A and B); correlation between seed rate used and plant population (Panel C); and preference for the number of years farmers grow lentil on the same field (Panel D). Such wide variations in crop establishment techniques are unacceptable for enhancing production of grain legumes in South Asia. This survey was conducted during the 1999/2000-winter season in farmers' fields in the Chitwan district of Nepal.

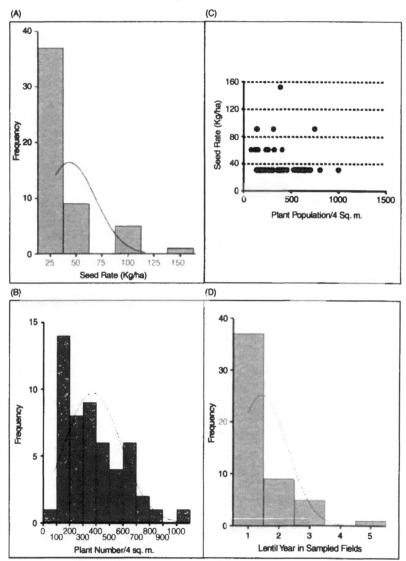

PLATE 1. Response of chickpea to soil B application in Chitwan district of Nepal. Poor crop establishment (therefore low grain yield) is a major constraint for growing legumes in this region of Nepal. Soil micronutrient deficiency limits crop growth and yield in Chitwan. Application of B significantly increased root and above ground vegetative growth (plant to the right) compared to B (plant to the left) chickpea plots.

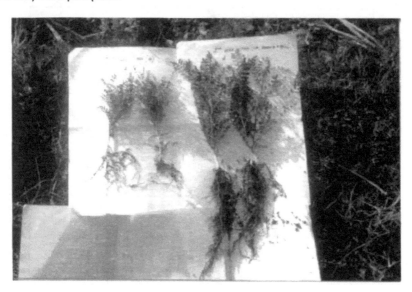

400 to 1600 mm (Figure 9) from the western to the eastern IGP (White and Rodriguez-Aguilar, 2001). Therefore, during the pre-Green Revolution period, rice was only grown in the monsoon season in the eastern IGP and wheat during the winter season in the western parts of the Indian IGP, primarily due to the lack of irrigation facilities. However, assured irrigation through canal and deep tube wells has allowed cultivation of rice in the western IGP. Free electricity has resulted in excesive pumping of ground water for irrigation to crops, thereby, lowering the water table at a rate faster than its recharge through rainwater, and increased soil salinity in some areas of the western IGP (Figure 10). If water and electricity for agricultural purposes is correctly priced in the northwestern IGP of India, fertilizer and pesticide subsidizes removed, and investments in farmer education made (Pingali and Shah, 2001), the economics of growing rice-wheat will not be attractive and will induce changes in the cropping system to more favorable systems. An example of economics inducing changes in a cropping system can be seen in Bangladesh.

After an initial increase, wheat production stagnated at a growth rate of only 0.4% in Bangladesh between 1983 and 1992 (Kataki, Hobbs, and Adhikary,

FIGURE 9. Schematic map showing the range of average annual precipitation (mm) distribution across the Indo-Gangetic Plains region of South Asia. Dotted area shows the spread of the rice-wheat cropping system in South Asia (Bangladesh, India, Nepal, and Pakistan). Information for this map was combined from Kataki, 2001a and P. Jones, CIAT, unpublished data.

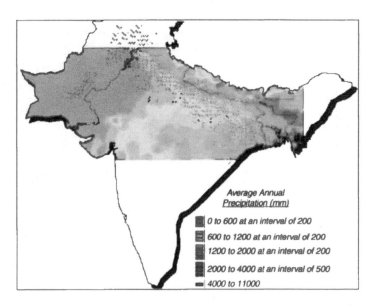

2001). This increase in wheat production was primarily due to the popularity and installation of shallow tube wells across the country, allowing farmers to irrigate their fields independently of others. This single factor change prompted an 87% and 51% acreage increase of winter and spring off-season rice cultivation, respectively. Winter rice competed with wheat for land, and therefore, wheat production became stagnant. However, post-1992, the cost of growing winter rice had increased substantially due to increased cost of irrigation, therefore, fields with coarser textured soils were then planted with wheat. Wheat production in Bangladesh then increased post-1992 at a rate of 11.1% per year (Kataki, Hobbs, and Adhikary, 2001). It is, therefore, possible to shift established cropping systems like rice-wheat.

In the context of the Indian IGP, shifting cropping systems by crop diversification will have to be strategic for the eastern, middle, and western IGP based on the agroclimatic zones that exist. Within the Indian IGP, changes that can be brought about without decline in the total cereal production would include:

FIGURE 10. Schematic map showing the range of soil pH distribution across the Indo-Gangetic Plains region of South Asia. Dotted area shows the spread of the rice-wheat cropping system in South Asia (Bangladesh, India, Nepal, and Pakistan). Information for this map was combined from Kataki, 2001a and FAO 1995.

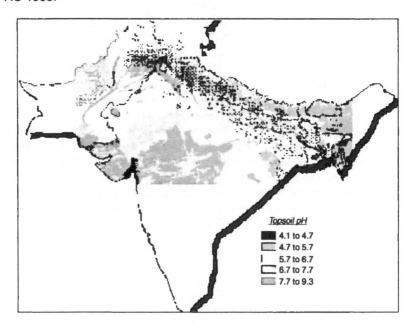

- Use of beds (either permanent or temporary) for cultivation of wheat followed by summer legume and direct seeded rice (instead of transplanted). Beds improve input use efficiency (water, fertilizer, weeding, etc.) for all crops grown on it and can reduce damage caused to legumes by water logging.
- Spreading the present cultivated areas of pulses, soybean, cotton, maize, sugarcane, and sunflower in targeted northern and northwestern districts of the Indian IGP where suitable. This increase in area should be coupled with improved land preparation, seeding, fertilizer application, and crop rotation practices.
- Extending the duration of a crop rotation cycle from two to more seasons so as to introduce legumes in the cropping system for grain and forage.
- Providing a realistic support price for pulse procurement.
- True pricing of water and electricity use for agricultural purposes.
- Penalties and incentives for farmer's for misuse or proper use of irrigation water and electricity including investments in farmers' education.

- Introduction of "boro" or winter rice cultivation where possible and installation of shallow tube wells. In certain states of eastern and northeastern India, large tracts of land remain fallow after the monsoon rice season (e.g., Assam). The cultivation of boro rice due to the installation of shallow tube wells has been promising (Kataki, personal communication). This increased rice production in eastern India will compensate for reduced rice production in northwestern India if its rice-wheat cropping system were to be diversified. Boro rice generally yields approximately 50% more than the monsoon rice due to its longer growing season; however, the quality of the rice grain is considered coarser to the monsoon rice;
- Commercial cultivation of vegetable legumes, e.g., mungbean in uplands;
- Though rainfall in the eastern end of the IGP is one of the highest in the world, water shortages occur during the dry winter months. Water harvesting should be encouraged for use in winter months for increasing legumes and vegetable cultivation in the uplands;
- Access to credit, quality inputs like fertilizers (including micronutrients), seed (including different varieties for different regions), pest control information and tools, and a revamped extension service; and
- The ecological requirements for all crops are well known. Soil and climatic databases should be used and with the aid of GIS and remote sensing, ecological zones suitable for specific cropping systems be identified and farmers should be encouraged to adopt these systems to maximize input use efficiency (Ali and Pande, 1999; Pande et al., 1999; Venkataratnam, 1999). For this approach to be successful, a major effort needs to be undertaken by host institutions of the country.

Will Shifting Cropping Systems Benefit Nutritional Status?

There is now a better understanding of the causes of malnutrition (Smith and Haddad 2000 a and b; UNICEF 1998; WHO, 2000a; ACC/SCN, 2000). A resource for food security, specifically food production, is one of several determinants of the nutritional status of a population group, and hence, the extent of malnutrition. In this context, an appropriate shift in the cereal-cereal cropping system by introduction of legumes is important. Grain legumes store fairly well, therefore, its production, storage, and distribution can also meet the demands of regions within India where its production is not feasible. However, production and storage of perishables like fruits and vegetables is challenging due to limited infrastructure, and hence, local production and marketing is important.

Legumes have been an integral part of Indian agriculture prior to the pre-Green Revolution period. The agronomic advantages of growing legumes are well known, but efforts to reintroduce wide scale legume cultivation for feed and fodder in the IGP has not been very successful in the past-Green Revolution period. In the past, it was argued that per unit land area, cereals yielded the same quantities of protein as legumes, since cereals yielded higher grain per hectare of land compared to the legumes (Lauren et al. 2001). Therefore, the increase in cereal production has met the calorie needs of an ever-growing Indian population, and has to a large extent reduced hunger-related malnutrition (PEM).

However, grain legumes contain, and can therefore, supply several fold higher concentration of vitamins and minerals that are deficient or low in concentration in cereals (Lauren et al. 2001), though the bioavailability of nutrients is an issue. Although legumes produce nutritious grains, nutritious grains it produces, the physiological cost of producing grains for a legume plant is much higher compared to cereals, and therefore, yields lower than cereals. In addition, there are several constraints to growing legumes that includes late planting, extremely dry or wet soils, vulnerability to insects and diseases, and inappropriate varieties. Therefore, higher management skills are required for growing these high-risk legume crops. These skills in a way have slowly been eroded due to the attractiveness of growing rice and wheat between 1970s to 1990s. The gap between farmers and the potential yield for most legume crops is very wide. However, with appropriate management, legume yields can be doubled in the IGP and can supply the essential dietary micronutrients.

CONCLUSION

The shifting of the monoculture of rice and wheat to the rice-wheat cropping system of India during the 1970s have helped meet the calorie needs of the population. However, the percent of malnourished in India, even in the present times, and especially amongst children and women is still very high. Malnutrition often manifests itself as a life cycle from children to the adult stage, thereby reducing productivity. The percent of malnourished between various states in India is highly variable, depending upon many factors. Diversity in the diet to meet the micronutrient intake of foods will enhance the rate of decline in malnutrition, especially micronutrient-related malnutrition amongst population groups in India.

A long-term sustainable approach to induce diversity in diets is to produce enough diverse foods. For this to happen, a second shift in the cropping system needs to happen. Shifting the major cropping system of India, i.e., the rice-wheat system is a feasible and practical option to increase production, supply, and consumption of foods other than cereals. This shift can occur by the targeted diversification of this cropping system with the inclusion of legumes and vegetables, and by ensuring that cereal production meets the demand of the region. Since the infrastructure requirements and managerial skills increase several folds in the order of cereal-based, legume-based, and vegetable cultivation, appropriate government and institutional support is needed to make this shift feasible. A network of national and international institutes in Bangladesh, India, Nepal, and Pakistan through the Rice-Wheat Consortium for the Indo-Gangetic Plains (Reeves, 2001), have been working as partners to introduce diversification in the rice-wheat cropping system. However, these efforts will have to be multiplied several times to have a major impact in the region.

REFERENCES

ACC / SCN. 2000. *Fourth report on the world nutrition situation.* Geneva: ACC / SCN in collaboration with IFPRI. 75 p.

Ali, M., and S. Pande. 1999. Prospects for legumes in the Indo-Gangetic Plain–database requirements. In *GIS analysis of cropping systems,* S. Pande, C. Johansen, J. Lauren, and F.T. Bantilan Jr. (eds). Proceedings of an International Workshop of Databases for GIS Analysis of Cropping Systems in the Asia Region, 18-19 August, 1997, ICRISAT-Patancheru–502 324, Andhra Pradesh, India, Organized by International Crops Research Institute for the Semi-Arid Tropics (ICRISAT) and Cornell University, Ithaca, NY, USA, pp. 53-54.

FAOSTAT. 2000. *Food and Agricultural Organization (FAO) statistical databases,* Rome, Italy: FAO. <http://apps.org/cgi-bin/nph-db.pl>.

FAO. 1995. *FAO digital soil maps of the world and derived soil properties, Version 3.5.* Food and Agricultural Organization of the United Nations, Rome.

FAO. 1997. *Preventing micronutrient malnutrition. A guide to food-based approaches– A manual for policy makers and programme planners.* Prepared by Food and Agriculture Organization of the United Nations and International Life Sciences Institute. ILSI Press.

FAO. 1998. *FAO-Nutrition country profiles: India.* Food and Agricultural Organization of the United Nations, Rome. 33 p.

Hobbs, P., and M. Morris. 1996. *Meeting South Asia's future food requirements from rice-wheat cropping systems: Priority issues facing researchers in the post-green revolution era.* NRG Paper 96-01. Mexico, D.F.: CIMMYT. 46 p.

Kataki, P.K. (ed). 2001a. *The rice-wheat cropping system of South Asia: Trends, constraints, productivity and policy.* Food Products Press, An Imprint of The Haworth Press, Inc., Binghampton, NY, USA. 136 p.

Kataki, P.K. (ed). 2001b. *The rice-wheat cropping system of South Asia: Efficient production Management.* Food Products Press, An Imprint of The Haworth Press, Inc., Binghampton, NY, USA. 305 p.

Kataki, P.K., P. Hobbs, and B. Ahikary. 2001. The rice-wheat cropping system of South Asia: Trends, Constraints, Productivity and Policy–A Prologue. In *The rice-wheat cropping system of South Asia: Efficient production management.* P.K. Kataki (ed.). Food Products Press, An Imprint of The Haworth Press, Inc., Binghampton, NY, USA. pp. 1-26.

Kumar, P., and P.K. Joshi. 2000. *Working with communities to improve nutrition and food security.* March 6-8, 2000, Proceedings of a Conference. CARE India, New Delhi.

Lauren, J., R. Shrestha, M.A. Sattar, and R.L. Yadav. 2001. Legumes and Diversification of the Rice-Wheat Cropping System. In *The rice-wheat cropping system of South Asia: Trends, Constraints, Productivity and Policy.* P.K. Kataki (ed.). Food Products Press, An Imprint of The Haworth Press, Inc., Binghampton, NY, USA. pp. 67-102.

Measham, A.R., and M. Chatterjee. 1999. *Wasting away: The crisis of malnutrition in India.* The International Bank for Reconstruction and Development/The World Bank, Washington, DC. 78 p.

Pande, C. Johansen, J. Lauren, and F.T. Bantilan Jr. (eds). *GIS analysis of cropping systems.* Proceedings of an International Workshop of Databases for GIS Analysis of Cropping Systems in the Asia Region, 18-19 August, 1997, ICRISAT-Patancheru–502 324, Andhra Pradesh, India, Organized by International Crops Research Institute for the Semi-Arid Tropics (ICRISAT) and Cornell University, Ithaca, NY, USA. 158 p.

Paroda, R.S., T. Woodhead, and R.B. Singh (eds). 1994. *Sustainability of rice-wheat production systems in Asia.* RAPA Production 1994/11, 209 p.

Pingali, P., and M. Shah. 2001. Policy re-directions for sustainable resource use: The rice-wheat cropping system of the Indo-Gangetic Plains. In *The rice-wheat cropping system of South Asia: Trends, constraints, productivity and policy.* P.K. Kataki (ed.). Food Products Press, An Imprint of The Haworth Press, Inc., Binghampton, NY, USA. pp. 103-108.

Reeves, T.G. 2001. Foreword. In *The rice-wheat cropping system of South Asia: Trends, constraints, productivity and policy.* P.K. Kataki (ed.). Food Products Press, An Imprint of The Haworth Press, Inc., Binghampton, NY, USA. pp. xvii-xxi.

Sehgal, V. 1999. *Indian agriculture.* Indian Economic Data Research Centre, B-173, Panchvati, Vikaspuri, New Delhi-110018, 600 p.

Smith, L.C., and L. Haddad. 2000a. *Explaining child malnutrition in developing countries.* IFPRI Research Report 111, Washington, DC, USA. International Food Policy Research Institute. 107 p.

Smith, L.C., and L. Haddad. 2000b. *Overcoming child malnutrition in developing countries: Past achievements and future choices.* Food, Agriculture, and the Environment Discussion Paper 30. International Food Policy Research Institute, Washington, DC, USA. 53 p.

UNICEF. 1998. *The state of the world's children 1998.* United Nations Children's Fund, New York, Oxford University Press. 131 p.

Venkataratnam, L. 1999. Use of remote sensing in distribution of environment and crop distribution. In *GIS analysis of cropping* systems, S. Pande, C. Johansen, J. Lauren, and F.T. Bantilan Jr. (eds). Proceedings of an International Workshop of Databases for GIS Analysis of Cropping Systems in the Asia Region, 18-19 August, 1997, ICRISAT-Patancheru–502 324, Andhra Pradesh, India, Organized by International Crops Research Institute for the Semi-Arid Tropics (ICRISAT) and Cornell University, Ithaca, NY, USA, pp. 97-104.

White, J.W., and A. Rodriguez-Aguilar. 2001. An agroclimatic characterization of the Indo-Gangetic Plains. In *The rice-wheat cropping system of South Asia: Trends, constraints, productivity and policy*. P.K. Kataki (ed.). Food Products Press, An Imprint of The Haworth Press, Inc., Binghampton, NY, USA. pp. 53-65.

WHO. 2000a. *Nutrition profile of the WHO South-East Asia region*. World Health Organization, Regional Office for South-East Asia, New Delhi, India. Publication No. SEA-NUT-148. 83 p.

WHO. 2000 b. *WHO global database on child growth and malnutrition*. <www.who.org>.

Yadav, R.L., K. Prasad, and A.K. Singh (eds). 1998. *Predominant cropping systems of India: Technologies and strategies*. Modipuram, Meerut, India, Project Directorate for Cropping Systems Research, 237 p.

Nutritional and Economic Benefits
of Enhanced Vegetable Production
and Consumption

M. Ali
Abedullah

SUMMARY. Vegetables are a major source of dietary micronutrients, but abiotic and biotic constraints limit vegetable production and consumption in Asia. Per capita vegetable consumption in Asia is far below the required level to satisfy the recommended dietary micronutrient intakes. Empirical evidence and discussion in this article show that enhanced vegetable production and consumption in Asia can play a catalytic role in the overall economic development by improving the nutritional status, learning capabilities and managerial capacities of farmers, generating incomes and jobs in both the farm and non-farm sectors, and improving resource use efficiency in agriculture. Rapid urbanization, higher incomes, and greater awareness amongst consumers and producers to diversify their food and production systems have increased the demand for vegetables in Asia. To realize this potential demand, especially during the off-season of vegetable production, trade-oriented and production enhancement strategies are suggested in this article. The trade-oriented

---

M. Ali is Socio-Economist, Asian Vegetable Research and Development Center, P.O. Box 42, Shanhua, Tainan, Taiwan 741, Republic of China (E-mail: mubarik@netra.avrdc.org.tw).

Dr. Abedullah is currently working as Assistant Research Fellow in Institut für Agrarökonomie und Verfahrenstechnik, Universität Rostock, Justus-von-Liebig-Weg 6, 18051 Rostock, Germany (E-mail: abedullah@yahoo.com).

[Haworth co-indexing entry note]: "Nutritional and Economic Benefits of Enhanced Vegetable Production and Consumption." Ali, M., and Abedullah. Co-published simultaneously in *Journal of Crop Production* (Food Products Press, an imprint of The Haworth Press, Inc.) Vol. 6, No. 1/2 (#11/12), 2002, pp. 145-176; and: *Food Systems for Improved Human Nutrition: Linking Agriculture, Nutrition, and Productivity* (ed: Palit K. Kataki, and Suresh Chandra Babu) Food Products Press, an imprint of The Haworth Press, Inc., 2002, pp. 145-176. Single or multiple copies of this article are available for a fee from The Haworth Document Delivery Service [1-800-HAWORTH, 9:00 a.m. - 5:00 p.m. (EST). E-mail address: getinfo@haworthpressinc.com].

policies can help link the favorable vegetable producing areas with consumption centers, and production oriented policies can overcome the biotic and abiotic constraints of vegetable production by developing economically viable, socially acceptable, and environmentally friendly technologies. Both the strategies require government support and increased allocation of research funds and manpower for vegetable cultivation. Government policies to stabilize vegetable production and trade, can mitigate the risk inherit in vegetable production. *[Article copies available for a fee from The Haworth Document Delivery Service: 1-800-HAWORTH. E-mail address: <getinfo@haworthpressinc.com> Website: <http://www. HaworthPress.com> © 2002 by The Haworth Press, Inc. All rights reserved.]*

KEYWORDS. Food systems, nutrition, nutritive value, production, consumption, vegetables

INTRODUCTION

This article analyzes the relationship between vegetable production and overall socioeconomic development. Vegetable production induces agricultural businesses in the rural economy, and generates employment and incomes (Figure 1). Growers learn to manage multiple cropping systems and to deliver quality products in a timely fashion by participating in and experiencing contractual arrangements and sophisticated marketing systems. The managerial skills acquired by operating a successful vegetable production system are the very skills required in running any commercial businesses, and act as a catalyst for socioeconomic development. Furthermore, vegetable production balances the diet by enhancing the supply of essential micronutrients. Increasing vegetable supplies reduces its prices and increases its consumption, thereby improving the health, learning capabilities, and working capacity of the population. All these factors enhance the working efficiency and facilitate and stimulate socioeconomic development.

Empirical studies have established a positive relationship between vegetable consumption and good health indicators. For example, Bouis and Novenario-Reese (1991) established a negative relationship between vegetable consumption and its prices, and a positive relationship between vegetable prices and morbidity rates. Similarly, increased consumption of micronutrient-rich foods from home gardens increased vitamin A availability in Bangladesh and resulted in lower incidences of blindness in children (Yusuf and Islam 1994). Many studies have quantified a negative relationship between cancer and vegetable consumption in relatively affluent societies (Bueno-de-Mesquita et al. 1991; Shibata et al. 1992; Jedrychowshi et al. 1992; Hirayama 1995; Yu et al.

FIGURE 1. Vegetable production and socioeconomic development.

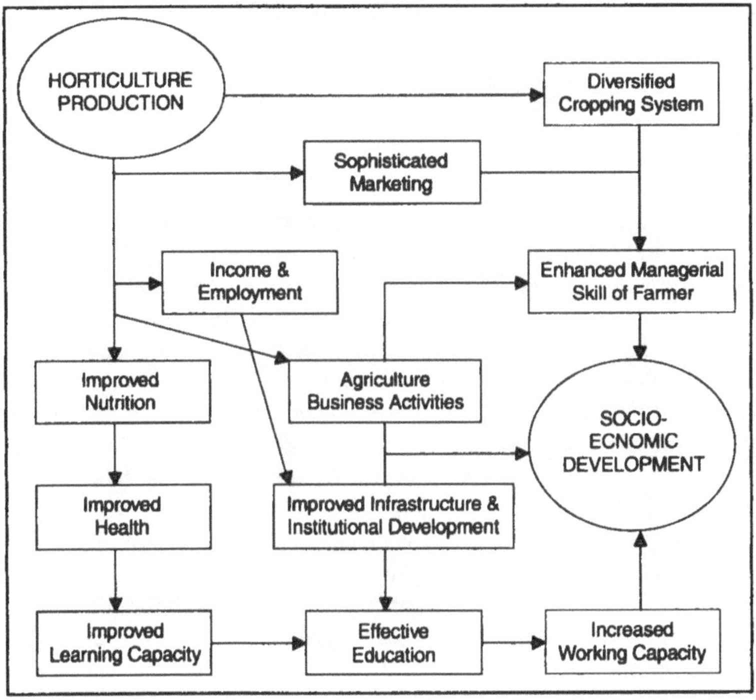

1995). Improvement in health undoubtedly comes through nutritional and economic well-being. Earlier studies, however, lacked a comprehensive discussion on the benefits from the expanded vegetable sector.

This article furnishes empirical evidence on the economic and nutritional benefits from enhanced vegetable production and consumption and explains the potential and constraints of expanding these benefits to a larger scale. The focus of these discussions is primarily on Asia, largely because of the lack of access of the author to relevant data from other regions. However, many of the conclusions arrived at are also relevant to other regions of the world. The sequence of the discussion in this article is as follows: the current status of vegetable production, consumption, and availability in Asia; empirical evidence of the important role of vegetables in food expenditure, micronutrient availability, and food diversification; economic efficiency of vegetables in supplying individual as well as overall nutrients in the diet; the role of increased vegetable cultivation on improving income, employment, and resource use efficiency; the potentials and constraints of expanding the benefits of vegetable cultivation; and, the possible solutions for overcoming these constraints. Finally, selective examples of enhanced vegetable production and consumption from a few countries in Asia are presented.

CURRENT STATUS OF VEGETABLES IN ASIA

Per Capita Availability and Prices

Vegetables are a rich source of essential micronutrients (especially, vitamins, iron, and calcium) and generally have high fiber content (Table 1). Production and supply (and therefore availability) of vegetables influence their consumption. However, per capita vegetable availability in many developing countries is far below the recommended level with respect to adequate micronutrient intake through vegetable consumption (Figure 2). Similar conclusions were arrived at, from the analysis of average vegetable consumption data taken from the household consumption surveys conducted by the National Bureaus of different countries (Ali, 2000). Moreover, per capita vegetable availability in most developing regions of Asia remained almost stagnant during the 1980s and early 1990s (Figure 3), a time when cereal production was on the rise. The rise in real vegetable prices during the 1980s and 1990s in most developing countries of Asia (Figure 4) raises serious concerns about the future increases in vegetable consumption. Increase in its real prices, however, did not induce vegetable production to make a significant impact on per capita consumption due to serious constraints on increasing vegetable production and consumption.

Seasonality

The average annual vegetable supply data actually masks the more serious problem of year-round vegetable availability. Due to seasonality in vegetable supply, its deficiency is more acute during specific times of the year. For example, in Taipei City, which is one of the most developed markets of Asia, the average monthly availability index decreases 20% (Figure 5) in September (end of summer) compared to that in January (end of winter). In less developed markets of Asia, as in Dhaka, Bangladesh, the implications of seasonal vegetable availability is more serious (Figure 5A). Vegetable prices rise 50% (in September) and 35% (in October) in Taiwan and Bangladesh, respectively, compared to prices in January for both the countries (Figure 5B). Therefore, seasonality in both the production and prices of vegetables induces acute off-season micronutrient deficiency problems, which is not depicted by the yearly average vegetable production and consumption data.

TABLE 1. Nutrient Density per 100 g of Edible Portion of Selected Vegetables and Other Food Items.

Food group/ commodity	Energy (kcal)	Protein (g)	Fiber (g)	Vitamin A (RE)	Vitamin B₁ (mg)	Vitamin B₂ (mg)	Vitamin C (mg)	Niacin (mg)	Calcium (mg)	Iron (mg)
Vegetables										
Carrot	33	1.0	0.8	8782	0.03	0.04	4	0.70	26	0.4
Radish	19	0.7	0.5	0	0.01	0.02	16	0.36	24	0.2
Onion	39	1.0	0.5	0	0.03	0.01	5	0.38	24	0.3
Garlic	33	2.6	1.2	276	0.04	0.06	37	0.64	75	2.0
Pak choi	12	1.0	0.4	225	0.02	0.04	38	0.48	101	1.3
Common cabbage	22	1.1	0.5	5	0.02	0.02	31	0.29	49	0.3
Chinese cabbage	11	1.0	0.4	5	0.01	0.02	18	0.37	38	0.4
Mustard	18	0.8	0.5	64	0.01	0.05	33	0.48	94	1.3
Kale	26	2.4	0.8	718	0.00	0.01	-	0.18	238	1.9
Kangkong	24	1.4	0.8	378	0.01	0.10	14	0.70	78	1.5
Amaranth	15	1.8	0.5	180	0.03	0.06	13	0.34	131	4.1
Spinach	20	1.9	0.7	581	0.05	0.07	8	0.46	70	1.9
Eggplant	23	1.2	0.8	3	0.06	0.03	5	1.08	16	0.4
Sweet pepper	21	0.7	0.8	31	0.03	0.03	80	0.68	9	0.3
Chili	58	2.1	4.3	352	0.16	0.14	134	2.00	15	7.0
Tomato	25	0.9	0.6	83	0.02	0.02	21	0.59	10	0.3
Vegetable soybean	125	14.0	2.4	18	0.34	0.09	16	1.00	38	2.5
Cereals										
Wheat	362	13.9	2.2	0	0.42	0.09	10	5.78	9	4.0
Corn	65	2.2	0.5	1	0.04	0.05	4	0.83	1	0.4
Rice	353	7.0	0.2	0	0.10	0.03	-	0.70	6	0.2
Meat										
Beef	331	14.8	-	32	0.05	0.13	0.0	2.83	5	2.3
Mutton	198	18.8	-	14	0.09	0.27	-	3.10	8	0.6
Chicken	160	15.7	-	17	0.03	0.10	18	4.00	3	0.8
Seafood										
Fish	127	10.8	-	37	0.06	0.09	0.5	2.54	34	0.6

Adapted from Food Industry Research and Development Institute and Pintung University of Science and Technology (1998).

FIGURE 2. Vegetable availability (kg/capita/annum) in selected Asian countries during 1993.

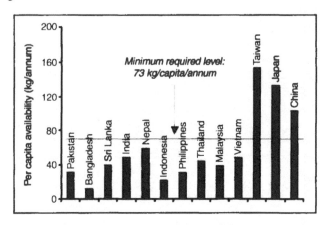

FIGURE 3. Regional trends in per capita vegetable availability in Asia, 1981-93.

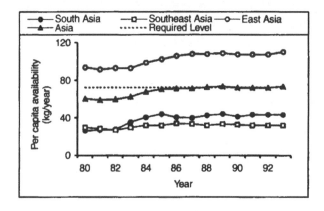

Annual Fluctuation

Generally, the year-to-year total production fluctuates more for vegetables than for cereals (Table 2). This fluctuation is because of the lack of government support programs to stabilize vegetable production compared to that of cereals. As a result, consumption of vegetables, and hence, micronutrient availability, varies considerably between similar seasons of different years. For example, Bouis and Novenario-Reese (1991) found that vitamins A and C adequacy ratios in the Philippines dropped from 1.95 and 1.46, respectively, in the first round of a household survey carried out in August 1984, to 0.71 and 0.53 in the fourth round carried out exactly one year later.

FIGURE 4. Deflated average vegetable prices in Asia during 1980-93.

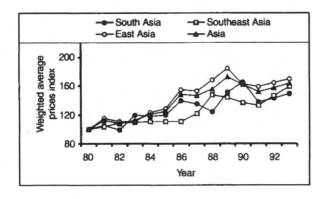

FIGURE 5. Seasonality in vegetable availability and prices in Dhaka (Bangladesh) and Taipei (Taiwan) markets.

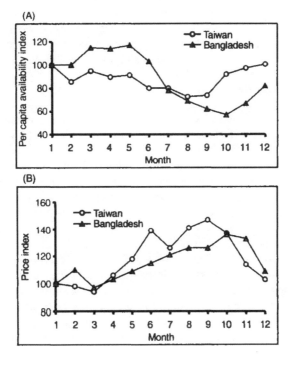

TABLE 2. Detrended Coefficient of Variation (CV) in Area, Production, and Yield of Vegetables and Cereals During 1980-93.

Region	Detrended CV in vegetables (%)			Detrended CV in cereals (%)		
	Area	Yield	Production	Area	Yield	Production
South Asia	9.69	10.40	8.17	2.08	3.73	3.82
Southeast Asia	14.51	11.09	5.37	2.35	2.46	2.86
East Asia	4.05	5.37	4.43	1.89	3.90	4.17
Asia	2.83	2.35	3.05	1.46	1.59	2.85

Adapted from Ali (2000).

ROLE IN FOOD EXPENDITURE, NUTRIENT AVAILABILITY AND FOOD DIVERSITY

Budget Share

The budget share (percentage of the total food expenditure) allocated to vegetables varies considerably between countries and for regions within a country. For example, the share-allocation to vegetables is 22% of the food budget in Taiwan but only 5% in Indonesia. In other developing countries of Asia, the food budget expenditure on vegetables ranges between 9-15%. Variations in the budget share of vegetables were higher across regions within a country than for income groups within a region (Ali, 2000).

Nutrient Availability

Household consumption surveys conducted by the socioeconomic unit of the Asian Vegetable Research and Development Center (AVRDC) for selected Asian countries suggested that nutrient deficiencies (except calcium) and vegetable consumption were closely related (Table 3).[1] For example, vegetable consumption in the Philippines, Cambodia, and Bangladesh was less than the minimum required level, and consequently, the availability of vitamins A, B_1, and B_2 in these countries were deficient. Bangladesh and Cambodia foods were also deficient in niacin (availability was less than the lower recommended range). It appeared that the availability of iron from foods in these countries (except in Cambodia) was close to the recommended level; but most of the iron in their food was from rice that has very low bioavailability. Vegetable consumption was slightly higher than the minimum required level in South Vietnam; therefore, vitamin A supply was sufficient, although vitamins B_1 and B_2, niacin, and iron could be considered deficient. In Taiwan, vegetable consumption was sufficient; therefore, all other micronutrients except calcium were above the recommended level.

Estimates of nutrient availability suggested that food energy consumption in all the countries were similar and higher than the lower recommended range (Table 3). Where seasonal consumption data were available (only in the Philippines and Taiwan), seasonality in micronutrient availability was also related to the seasonality in vegetable supply and consumption.

Despite low consumption of vegetables, they are the major sources of vitamins A, C, and B$_2$. They also provide a significant portion of iron, calcium, and vitamin B$_1$ (Table 4). Therefore, of the micronutrients available from diets, a majority comes from vegetables, and increasing vegetable supply is the natural solution to tackling micronutrient deficiencies.

TABLE 3. Daily Vegetable and Nutrient Consumption in Selected Asian Countries.

Item (unit)	Recommended level[1]	Country				
		South Vietnam	Cambodia	Philippines	Taiwan	Bangladesh
Vegetables (g)	200	239	170	106	460	126
Energy (Kcal)	1800-2400	1919	1914	2187	1929	2006
Protein (g)	45-63	69	68	39	81	67
Calcium (mg)	800-1200	514	455	533	594	330
Iron (mg)	10-15	12	9	12	16	13
Vitamin A (IU)	4200-5000	4812	2818	3530	9907	2620
Vitamin C (mg)	50-70	81	53	75	239	62
Vitamin B$_1$ (mg)	1.0-1.5	1.0	0.8	1.2	1.5	0.5
Vitamin B$_2$ (mg)	1.2-1.8	0.7	0.5	1.2	1.2	0.7
Niacin (mg)	13-20	13	12	28	17	12

[1]Recommended levels of nutrients were taken from Food and Nutrition Board (1989). These levels are average for males and females above the age of 10 years.
Source: Unpublished survey data of the Socioeconomic Unit, AVRDC.

TABLE 4. Contribution of Vegetables (%) in Supplying Nutrients in Selected Countries of Asia.

Nutrient	South Vietnam	Cambodia	Philippines	Taiwan	Bangladesh
Calories	2.5	1.9	5.1	5.6	5.5
Protein	6.5	4.0	8.4	10.7	9.8
Calcium	25.9	16.9	36.6	36.9	29.4
Iron	24.3	20.1	27.6	35.1	23.7
Vitamin A	80.6	58.7	60.5	75	78.1
Vitamin C	81.2	73.4	82.1	47.4	63.4
Vitamin B$_1$	16.8	14.8	15.1	17.7	21.5
Vitamin B$_2$	34.9	20.4	18.6	31.7	22.4
Niacin	9.4	6.2	7.2	16.2	9.4

Source: Unpublished survey data of the Socioeconomic Unit, AVRDC.

Diversification of Diet

Diversity in the diet, measured as the number of different foods consumed in one day, is an important criterion to judge the quality of food consumed. Vegetables are a major source of diversification of food. For example, in South Vietnam, Laos, Cambodia, Philippines, Taiwan and Bangladesh, an average family consumes 12, 11, 11, 20, 21, and 14 different food items daily, respectively, and vegetables were a major source of food diversification (Table 5).

Diversification in vegetable diets[2] increases over time, perhaps influenced by the increase in incomes, as in Taiwan (Figure 6). The differences in vegetable food diversification in the diets of Philippines and Taiwan (Figure 7) may be due to the difference in incomes and cultures. This trend implies that higher incomes create diversified demand for vegetables, and different cultures have different levels of diversity in vegetable production. In a given culture, diversification in the diet increases with the level of expenditure on food and with the presence of home garden, but decreases if the head lady of the house is employed (Ali et al. 2000).

ECONOMIC NUTRITIVE EFFICIENCY OF VEGETABLES

Why should vegetables be part of a Food Systems approach to improve micronutrient availability to humans? Vegetables are the most economical source of micronutrients and of overall nutrient supply. In this section, comparisons are made on the cost of individual nutrients from different food

TABLE 5. Average Number of Food Items Consumed Daily by Food Group in Selected Countries of Asia.

Food group	South Vietnam	Laos	Cambodia	Philippines	Taiwan	Bangladesh
Cereals	1.6	1.0	1.0	2.0	2.3	2.0
Vegetables	3.6	5.1	3.2	4.9	6.9	5.9
Fruits	0.5	1.3	0.5	1.0	2.1	0.3
Meat	0.9	1.0	0.7	2.0	1.9	0.2
Seafood	0.8	1.1	1.8	4.0	1.8	0.8
Egg and milk	0.4	0.3	0.3	1.9	1.9	0.6
Others[1]	4.1	1.1	3.4	4.0	4.1	4.4
Total	11.9	10.9	10.9	19.8	21.0	14.2

[1]"Others" includes sugar, drinks, salt, oils, etc.
Source: Unpublished survey data of the Socioeconomic Unit, AVRDC.

FIGURE 6. Trends in the diversity of vegetable consumption in Taiwan.

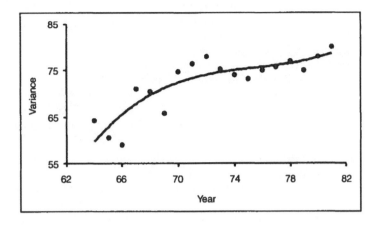

FIGURE 7. Differences in the diversity of vegetable consumption in Taiwan and the Philippines.

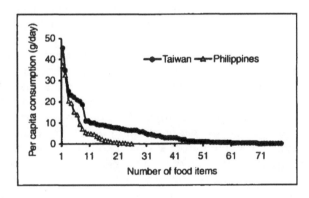

groups followed by an estimate of the economic efficiency of food commodities and of groups of commodities in supplying all nutrients important for health in the diet.

Relative Nutrient Cost

The relative nutrient cost ($/unit of nutrient) of an individual nutrient is the ratio of the total expenditure made by the community on all the commodities containing the nutrient, divided by the nutrient supply from the consumption of those commodities. The relative nutrient costs of nine nutrients important for health were estimated from the household consumption survey data collected by the socioeconomic unit of AVRDC, and reported for South Vietnam and Bangladesh in Table 6. The nutrient costs of vitamins, iron, and calcium are lowest when sourced from vegetables.[3]

Economic Nutritive Efficiency of Vegetables

Vegetables may be an economically efficient source of one nutrient, but may be inefficient of others. However, the economic efficiency of supplying all nutrients important for health depends upon the dollar value of all nutrients present in vegetables (henceforth termed as "relative nutritive value") compared to the price paid for the commodity. The relative nutritive value ($/100 g) of a commodity is the value of all nutrients present in the commodity evaluated at the respective nutrient cost estimated from the whole diet ($/unit of nutrient) divided by the number of nutrients considered. The economic nutritive efficiency is the ratio of the relative nutritive value ($/100 g) and the market price of the commodity ($/100 g). A nutritive efficiency greater than one for a commodity suggests that its nutritive value is higher than its cost, and vice versa if the efficiency is less than one (see Ali and Tsou, 2000 for more details).

The nutritive efficiency of vegetables is always greater than one, implying that the value of nutrition from vegetables is higher than the price consumers they payed for them. However, the relative ranking of nutritive efficiency of vegetables varies across countries. It was highest in South Vietnam and Bangladesh, second after cereal in the Philippines and Cambodia, and third after cereals and eggs and milk in Taiwan (Table 7). Therefore, the nutritive efficiency of vegetables greater than one implies that reallocation of food budget from other food items having nutritive efficiency less than one to vegetables would improve the dollar value of nutrition of the whole diet without any added cost. Such substitution from any other commodity becomes even more profitable if nutritive efficiency of the vegetable is highest.

However, for reallocation of the food budget to vegetables, individual vegetables with high nutritive efficiency need to be identified for each region. Normally, nutritive efficiency of less-used and indigenous-in-nature leafy vegetables is the highest. For example, amaranth, sauropus, sweet potato leaves, kangkong, and Indian spinach have highest nutritive efficiency in South Vietnam, while the efficiency is highest for stringbean tops, Chinese mustard, Pak-choi, carrot, and sweet potato leaves in the Philippines (Table 8).

IMPACT OF VEGETABLE CULTIVATION

To characterize vegetable farmers and to analyze the impact of vegetable cultivation on employment, income, nutrition, and other development related

TABLE 6. Nutrient Cost (US$/unit) from Different Food Sources in South Vietnam and Bangladesh.

Nutrient/country	Calories (kcal)	Protein (g)	Calcium (mg)	Iron (mg)	Vitamin A (IU)	Vitamin B_1 (mg)	Vitamin B_2 (mg)	Niacin (mg)	Vitamin C (mg)
South Vietnam									
Cereal	0.11	4.75	1.09	43.18	1.58	320.83	943.04	21.09	2.41
Vegetable	0.81	8.70	0.28	13.41	0.01	231.19	148.96	30.23	0.56
Fruit	0.85	53.03	2.73	25.03	0.07	1105.93	1353.07	154.35	2.38
Meat	0.64	9.05	19.32	76.52	0.35	571.33	959.61	46.44	-
Seafood	1.19	6.36	0.47	123.66	2.21	2418.99	992.03	59.74	152.29
Milk and egg	0.36	10.22	1.49	48.23	0.08	894.93	419.07	958.21	80.21
Bangladesh									
Cereals	0.09	4.51	2.57	36.32	0.52	376.50	499.78	15.11	1.52
Vegetable	0.23	3.52	0.39	10.43	0.02	208.70	172.36	24.16	0.70
Fruit	0.53	37.96	1.69	41.20	0.03	1116.64	475.82	88.10	2.07
Meat	0.62	3.12	3.46	16.19	0.58	2679.56	551.22	28.26	-
Seafood	1.18	8.73	0.67	99.97	3.82	5993.78	2122.36	80.72	7.87
Milk and egg	0.73	12.33	0.59	109.06	0.10	1055.96	283.02	613.62	24.46

Source: Unpublished survey data of the Socioeconomic Unit, AVRDC.

TABLE 7. Nutritive Efficiency of Major Food Groups in Selected Countries of Asia.

Food group	South Vietnam	Cambodia	Philippines	Taiwan	Bangladesh
Cereal	1.25	2.2	1.64	2.21	1.1
Meat	0.52	0.3	0.72	0.96	0.7
Seafood	0.64	0.7	0.39	0.65	0.5
Vegetable and pulses	2.38	1.4	1.42	1.18	2.2
Fruit	0.54	1.1	0.45	0.54	0.5
Egg and milk	0.66	0.8	1.02	1.88	0.6
Others	1.58	1.6	0.53	0.79	.1.5
Whole diet	1.02	1.03	1.01	1.03	1.0

Source: Unpublished survey data of the Socioeconomic Unit, AVRDC.

parameters, production and consumption surveys were analyzed in selected Asian countries.[4] These surveys provide opportunities to understand the economic role of vegetables by comparing cereal and vegetable production and vegetable and non-vegetable farmers.

Who Are the Vegetable Farmers?

It is normally perceived that only rich farmers grow vegetables, but empirical evidence refutes this perception. In terms of resource endowment, vegetable farmers are not rich to start. They have a family size and house area of a typical farming community. Vegetable and non-vegetable farms are similar in the farm soil types, land preparation methods practiced by farmers, percent of water pumps owned, and percent of vegetable area irrigated. On the contrary, there are indications that vegetable farmers are resource poor as their average farm size is smaller compared to non-vegetable farmers in most cases.

However, vegetable farmers are more educated (Table 9), have a better understanding of markets as they earn higher off-farm incomes, and commit appropriate investments to make their land suitable for vegetable cultivation (e.g., their lands are better drained).

Employment

Vegetable cultivation demands more labor (Table 10) compared to field crops, such as cereals. It is estimated that on average converting a hectare of rice to vegetable cultivation in one season, generates one year-round job.

TABLE 8. Nutritive Efficiency of Major Food Commodities in Selected Countries of Asia.

Food group	South Vietnam	Cambodia	Philippines	Taiwan	Bangladesh
Rice	1.995	2.191	1.718	2.137	1.039
Pork	0.620	0.263	0.765	1.018	-
Beef	0.214	0.272	0.411	0.639	1.280
Chicken	0.347	0.336	1.097	0.423	0.335
Fish	0.645	0.685	0.395	0.566	0.454
Egg	0.696	0.777	0.973	2.345	0.509
Milk	0.431	-	1.087	1.096	0.581
Corn	0.280	0.322	0.287	1.169	0.781
Potato	0.729	0.462	0.797	0.587	0.675
Carrots	2.702	2.164	1.776	2.900	2.273
Onion	0.737	0.250	0.373	0.485	0.530
Garlic	0.562	0.432	0.295	0.620	0.361
Pak-choi	1.622	1.451	1.764	1.240	1.180
Chinese mustard	2.001	3.074	-	2.653	1.893
Kangkong	4.476	2.889	-	2.497	2.988
Cabbage	1.725	1.116	0.699	1.034	3.526
Chinese cabbage	-	1.880	1.113	0.961	-
Lettuce	-	1.944	-	1.466	-
English Spinach	-	-	2.099	3.150	6.487
Cauliflower	1.762	0.776	1.008	0.819	1.407
Pepper	2.132	1.074	1.428	1.004	2.077
Mungbean	-	6.284	2.450	1.271	1.669
Eggplant	0.982	0.488	0.674	0.575	1.033
Tomato	1.584	1.849	0.811	0.524	1.869
Pineapple	0.402	0.513	0.248	0.666	-
Orange	0.382	0.262	0.151	1.098	0.207
Mango	0.298	0.408	0.518	0.561	0.419
Soybean	-	6.386	1.472	3.669	1.605
Lady's finger	3.885	-	0.741	1.404	2.175
Horse radish	-	-	4.856	-	0.869
Jute leaves	2.816	-	5.629	-	2.360
Amaranth	11.865	13.750	-	3.483	8.605
Sauropus	9.072	-	-	-	-
Sweet potato leave	6.966	-	4.437	3.440	-
Indian spinach	4.410	-	-	2.960	8.116
Basil	-	-	-	4.850	5.42
Turmeric	-	-	-	-	6.633

Source: Estimated from the unpublished survey data of the Socioeconomic Unit, AVRDC.

A large number of laborers used for vegetable cultivation are hired. Family labor becomes engaged in critical decision-making processes of production and marketing and the hired labor is used for routine vegetable production activities such as input application, weeding and harvesting. Hiring of labor becomes essential because timeliness of operation is critical to vegetable production, and often the number of family laborers is not sufficient to undertake

TABLE 9. Difference in Vegetable and Non-Vegetable Farmers in Selected Characteristics in Selected Countries of Asia.

Character	South Vietnam	Laos	Cambodia	Bangladesh
Larger family size	No	No	No	No
Bigger house size	No	No	No	No
Higher percentage of farmers owning water pumps	No	No	No	No
Higher percentage of Irrigated land	No	No	No	Yes
Higher percentage of light soils	No	No	No	Yes
Higher percentage of land plowed by tractor	No	No	No	No
Smaller farm size	Yes	Yes	Yes	Yes
Better education of household head	Yes	Yes	Yes	Yes
Higher off-farm income	Yes	-	Yes	Yes
Higher percentage of good drained land	Yes	Yes	No	Yes

Note: "Yes" implies that the difference in the parameter values between vegetable and non-vegetable farmers is consistent with the statement, and the difference is statistically significant. "No" implies that the difference is either opposite to the statement and significantly different or it is not significant at least at the 10% level.
"-" implies information is not available.
Source: Estimated from the unpublished survey data of the Socioeconomic Unit, AVRDC.

TABLE 10. Labor and Non-Labor Input Use and Cash Cost in Vegetables and Cereals in Selected Countries of Asia.

Input/Crop	South Vietnam	Laos	Cambodia	Bangladesh
		Labor (day/ha)		
Vegetables	297	223	437	338
Cereals	111	100	81	133
		Fertilizer (kg/ha)		
Vegetables	534	91	148	276
Cereals	197	75	46	113
		Manure (t/ha)		
Vegetables	7.6	1.3	1.7	5.0
Cereals	1.8	0.3	0.3	1.4
		Pesticide (No. of spray)		
Vegetables	7.9	0.5	6.2	6.5
Cereals	4.1	0.1	0.6	1.3
		Irrigation (No.)		
Vegetables	31	21	50	3.3
Cereals	7	1	4	2.0
		Cash cost (US$/ha)		
Vegetables	625	134	388	428
Cereals	249	65	77	143

Source: Estimated from the unpublished survey data of the Socioeconomic Unit, AVRDC.

all tasks of production. For example in Taiwan, on an average 25% of the total labor used in vegetable production is hired compared to 6% for cereal production. This difference in the percentage of hired laborers used is more for commercial compared to subsistence vegetable production. As an implication of this, higher proportion of hired laborers increases the demand for liquidity in vegetable production.

Moreover, vegetable farms engage more labor from vulnerable population groups, like women. For example in Taiwan, 61% of the labor used for vegetable production were women, but for cereals it was 48%. Similar conclusions were made from studies in Guatemala (Braun et al. 1989).

Agriculture Business Activities and Multiplier Effect

Vegetable cultivation requires more purchased inputs such as fertilizers, pesticides, and irrigation water, which also obligate more liquidity in hand (Table 10). This ultimately translates into higher demand for agricultural business activities, i.e., more loans are required to finance vegetable production, and more fertilizer and pesticide sales shops are needed.

In developing countries, most vegetables (except from home-garden) are commercially produced for the market. The expansion in vegetable production creates substantial demand for marketing activities. As vegetables have shorter shelf life compared to cereal crops, sophisticated marketing infrastructure, such as better roads, storage facilities, etc., are essential. Once such infrastructure is established, the efficiency of the whole marketing system improves.

Commercial production creates a higher multiplier effect for a given increase in vegetable production, compared to the same increase in cereals. Through a hypothetical example,[5] the same worth of initial increase in income for both sectors was shown to create a multiplier effect of 3 in vegetables and less than 2 in cereals. This is because vegetables sell more outputs to other sectors thereby generating higher incomes for other sectors.

Economic Efficiency

Lower agricultural productivity in developing countries is due to the lower economic efficiency of its production system. Therefore, economic efficiency of production systems is an important criterion to judge the economic viability of different crops and hence to compare the role of different crops in uplifting productivity of the agricultural sector. Economic efficiency can be defined in terms of individual input (i.e., input-use efficiency or partial productivity) or overall inputs employed (i.e., output efficiency). First, partial productivity of fertilizer, labor, and irrigation are compared between vegetable and rice production on vegetable growing farms. The partial productivity is measured as:

Partial productivity of an input =
(Gross revenue − Variable cost)/Quantity of the input

In estimating the partial productivity of variable inputs (e.g., labor or water), cost of only that input is considered as variable, while costs of all other inputs are fixed.

The partial productivity of fertilizer, labor, and water are significantly higher for vegetable than for rice cultivation (Table 11). This high productivity implies that shifting resources from rice to vegetable cultivation will improve the overall economic efficiencies of the resources engaged in crop production, which will generate additional incomes for farmers from these given resources. That is why net returns per ha of land and benefit-cost ratio is much higher in vegetables than in cereals.

Output efficiency of two groups can be compared in terms of net return, unit output costs or benefit-cost ratio, or technical efficiency defined as production at the given level of input use. Here output efficiency of rice production is compared between vegetable and non-vegetable farmers (Table 12). Although rice yield was not different, total cost of producing similar yields was significantly lower on vegetable farms than on non-vegetable farms. Therefore, net return and the benefit-cost ratio significantly increased while the unit cost of rice production decreased on vegetable farms compared to non-vegetable farms (Table 12).

It can be argued that higher output efficiency of vegetable farms may be due to the differences in the farm size, education, irrigation status, and input use. The production function analysis of the combined data sets for the three Indo-China countries suggests that technical efficiency in rice production was

Table 11. Resource Use Efficiency in Vegetables versus Rice Cultivation in Selected Countries of Asia.

Crop/Input	South Vietnam	Laos	Cambodia	Bangladesh
Land (US$/ha)				
Vegetables	1151	696	452	553
Cereals	120	80	48	30
Labor (US$/labor day)				
Vegetables	7.7	5.9	3.8	4.4
Cereals	4.1	1.6	2.0	1.4
Irrigation (% return on irrigation cost)				
Vegetables	21	11	8	65
Cereals	15	42	21	40
Benefit-Cost ratio (%)				
Vegetables	106	170	96	81
Cereals	43	54	53	13

Source: Estimated from the unpublished survey data of the Socioeconomic Unit, AVRDC.

TABLE 12. Economics of Cereal Cultivation on Vegetables versus Non-Vegetable Farms in Selected Countries of Asia.

Type of farm/parameter	South Vietnam	Laos	Cambodia	Bangladesh
Yield (t/ha)				
Vegetable farm	4.8	2.4	2.2	2.1
Non-vegetable farm	4.6	2.5	2.3	2.1
Total cost (US$/ha)				
Vegetables farm	430 (56)	247 (24)	184 (42)	196
Non-vegetable farm	448 (60)	302 (29)	209 (37)	244
Net-return (US$/ha)				
Vegetables farm	137	84	52	86
Non-vegetable farm	87	64	24	39
Benefit/cost ratio (US4/100US$)				
Vegetables farm	49	54	55	44
Non-vegetable farm	31	54	40	16
Unit output cost (US$/t)				
Vegetables farm	102	107	96	93
Non-vegetable farm	106	119	96	116

Source: Estimated from the unpublished survey data of the Socioeconomic Unit, AVRDC.
Note: The figures in parenthesis are percentage share of cash costs in the total cost.

20% higher on vegetable compared to non-vegetable farms. This implies higher rice production even after controlling for the effect of input use in production and for the differences in education, farm size and irrigation status of the two groups.[6]

Vegetable cultivation improves output efficiency of other crops. This improvement is due to the improvement in the managerial capacity of vegetable farmers, as they learn production processes and understand agriculture markets. Vegetable farmers must experience and learn these skills, as profitability in vegetables is highly sensitive to climatic, biological, and economic environments. Once farmers learn these capabilities, they can apply them to other crops.

Income

Shifting from cereal to vegetable cultivation improves resource use efficiency. It also improves output efficiencies from other agricultural production systems. This improved efficiency results in higher overall farm incomes (Table 13). Though vegetable farmers own smaller physical assets, especially land, their earnings from crop cultivation are higher compared to that of non-vegetable farmers. By adding these earnings to the off-farm incomes, the earning difference between the vegetable and non-vegetable farms become wider, favoring the former.

TABLE 13. Farm Income (US$/family/year) on Vegetable versus Non-Vegetable Farms in Selected Countries of Asia.

Type of farm/income source	South Vietnam	Laos	Cambodia
Vegetable farm	1467	311	191
Income from cereals	59	32	40
Income from vegetables	1093	274	87
Income from other crops	5	5	9
Off-farm income	310	-	55
Non-vegetable farm	488	75	88
Income from cereals	176	27	66
Income from vegetables	-	-	-
Income from other crops	59	48	2
Off-farm income	253	-	20

"-" implies information is not available, or not applicable
Source: Estimated from the unpublished survey data of the Socioeconomic Unit, AVRDC.

Sustainability of the Cropping System

Intensive vegetable production practices in the uplands may have sustainability problems, but vegetables grown as part of a cropping system can help break the pathogen cycle of a cereal-cereal rotation. For example, in Pakistan Punjab, a one percent increase in the concentration of vegetables will increase the total factor productivity of the crop production system by about 0.14% (Ali 2001). Integrating cultivation of leguminous vegetables (e.g., mungbean and soybean) in a cereal-cereal cropping system will improve the productivity, profitability, and sustainability of the cereal-cereal system (Ali et al. 1997).

Vegetable Cultivation and Micronutrient Availability

Higher incomes earned by the vegetable-farm households improve the quantity and quality of their diet vegetable farmers spends on and consumes more food, especially vegetables (Table 14). This diversity enhances micronutrient availability of farm families (Table 15) and improves their health. The household consumption survey data from India suggests that vegetable farmers spend significantly less on medicines and have higher probability of sending their children to school compared to non-vegetable farmers.

POTENTIALS, CONSTRAINTS, POSSIBILITIES AND LIMITATIONS ON EXPANSION

Potentials

Vegetable cultivation has several advantages: nutritional, economic, sustainability, and diversity. However, production can only be increased if consumers

TABLE 14. Effect of Vegetable Cultivation on Food Consumption.

Type of farm/parameter	South Vietnam	Laos	Cambodia	Bangladesh
Expenditure on food (US$/capita/day)				
Vegetable farmers	0.400	0.479	0.360	0.317
Non-vegetable farmers	0.320	0.397	0.318	0.293
Vegetable consumption (g/capita/day)				
Vegetable farmers	254	194	178	180
Non-vegetable farmers	220	159	152	120
Expenditure on vegetables (US$/capita/day)				
Vegetable farmers	0.040	0.073	0.042	0.049
Non-vegetable farmers	0.030	0.057	0.034	0.035

Source: Estimated from the unpublished survey data of the Socioeconomic Unit, AVRDC.

accept higher supplies. In the context of these advantages, what is the scope of expanding vegetable production and supplies? Are vegetables preferred commodities for people such that consumption increases as they are made economically affordable through higher incomes or lower prices?, or, are they inferior commodities implying consumption will reduce as incomes rise or prices fall? Review of vegetable demand literature suggests that vegetables demand and consumption are responsive to incomes and prices. The demand elasticity of price ranges between −0.2 and −0.8, with an average of −0.6. Average income elasticity is around 0.40 with wide variations across species and regions (Ali, 2000). These elasticities imply that people consume more vegetables when economically affordable.

On the other hand, rapid economic growth, urbanization, and awareness of the advantages of diversifying the cereal-based diet have created strong demand for diversifying the cereal-cereal production system. Declining cereal prices, shortage of water due to deteriorating irrigation infrastructure, reduced profitability of irrigation investment (Rosegrant and Pingali 1994), and/or competing water demand for domestic use are driving farmers to replace cereals, especially rice, with more efficient water-utilizing crops like vegetables.

To what extent can vegetables diversify the existing cereal-cereal system? Wide variations in the proportion of vegetable to cereal area suggest both the limits and potential for such diversification. Vegetable area can be as high as one third of the total cereal area in Taiwan and South Korea and one fourth in Japan, but as low as 2%-6% in most of the South and Southeast Asian countries (Ali, 2000). This variation is mainly due to economic conditions like input and output prices, (especially output prices), labor wage, rental rates of machines, price of inorganic fertilizer access to markets and information regarding input output prices, risk-covering policies, and physical factors such as climate, irrigation, erosion, drainage, soil, and topography.

TABLE 15. Micronutrient Availability on Vegetable versus Non-Vegetable Farm Families in Selected Countries of Asia.

Nutrient	Unit	South Vietnam		Laos		Cambodia		Bangladesh	
		Vegetable	Non-Vegetable	Vegetable	Non-Vegetable	Vegetable	Non-Vegetable	Vegetable	Non-Vegetable
Calories	(kcal)	1940	2008	2013	1838	1815	1807	1995	2029
Protein	(g)	68	68	71	62	65	61	68	61
Calcium	(mg)	537	522	334	272	447	378	332	295
Iron	(mg)	11.6	9.9	10.1	7.9	8.2	6.4	13.4	11.7
Vitamin A	(IU)	5095	4020	3272	1812	2705	2419	2708	2027
Vitamin B_1	(mg)	0.95	0.90	0.87	0.75	0.72	0.69	0.55	0.51
Vitamin B_2	(mg)	0.70	0.60	0.63	0.52	0.48	0.46	0.67	0.61
Niacin	(mg)	13	13	16	14	11	11	12	12
Vitamin C	(mg)	84	60	65	42	53	32	67	50

Source: Estimated from the unpublished survey data of the Socioeconomic Unit, AVRDC.

Constraints

Despite the potential for increasing vegetable production and consumption, the supply- and demand-side scenario for vegetables can impose severe constraints. The supply-side constraints can be divided into two groups: production and marketing (Ali and Tsou, 1997).

Production Constraints

Production constraints can be biotic, abiotic, management, or institutional. Abiotic stresses, like high temperature especially at night (Peet and Willits, 1993), and flooding (Midmore and Poudel, 1996). Biotic stresses, especially during the summer months, result in high yield losses, creating high production risk environment and seasonality in.

The farmers' desire to avoid risks coupled with the lack of pest control information and technical skills lead to excessive use of chemicals, resulting in higher production but also, health and environmental costs for both farmers and consumers. Thus, vegetable production is restricted only to those farms that can afford these costs and bear production and marketing risks. Institutional constraints such as insufficient and untimely input supplies including credit and seed, poor coverage and quality of extension services, and labor shortages during critical times especially when cereal and vegetable cultivations overlap may be significant production constraints in some countries.

Fine soils with little aeration and poor drainage sometimes impede the diversification of rice-based systems. For example, in Batac, Philippines, about 90% of the coarse soils are under vegetables and about 75% of fine soils are under rice cultivation (Mirjam, 1997).

Vegetable cultivation is very sensitive to both excessive and a shortage of water supplies. Therefore, vegetables are mostly grown on the irrigated part of the farm. Lack of irrigation facility on the farm, irregular water supply from public canals, or finances to build irrigation structure usually impedes vegetable cultivation.

Marketing Constraints

These include poor shelf life of vegetables combined with inadequate marketing, storage, packaging, and grading facilities, wide seasonal and annual fluctuations in vegetable prices, lack of information among producers on price developments and on consumer preferences for different attributes of vegetables, and poorly developed transportation facilities.

Demand Constraints

The availability of vegetables at affordable prices, lack of information on the importance of micronutrients, and the role of vegetables in supplying micronutrients seasonal availability, and localized social taboos against some vegetables are major constraints on the demand side.

Solutions and Possibilities

As the price elasticity of vegetables is generally higher than income elasticity, reducing prices through technological innovations has a greater impact on consumption than through economic development. Moreover, increased income can only generate additional demand. Unless such demand is fulfilled through additional supplies, it simply results in higher prices.

It should be noted that income elasticities of demand is expected to concentrate more during the off-season as vegetables are relatively abundant during the peak supply period. This scenario combined with the fact that most Asian cities are located in the lowland tropics creates a high demand for summer production technologies.

Technologies to overcome environmental stresses for vegetable cultivation are available and depending upon vegetable prices and physical factors that affect costs, harsh environments can be ameliorated. For example, vegetable farmers on the periphery of Bangkok build and regularly maintain ditch and dike systems called sorjan to manage flooding in vegetable fields (Sritunga, 1975). Similar systems are used to grow year-round vegetables in China (Plucknett et al. 1981) and Indonesia (Pingali, 1992). Technologies such as hydroponics are also available for the tropics (AVRDC, 1995). Planting chili on raised (40 cm vs. 20 cm) and narrow (1.0 m vs. 1.5 m) beds can improve plant survival and total fruit yield in the rainy season (AVRDC, 1992). Grafting of tomato on eggplant rootstocks improves its survival in flooding and enhances yield many fold. Combining raised beds, fruit set hormones, and simple plastic rain shelters can increase tomato yields three folds (AVRDC, 1993).

Poor internal drainage (e.g., in heavy soils) may not be a major obstacle to overall expansion of vegetable cultivation, if economically viable technologies, knowledge, and expertise to improve drainage are available. In upcountry Banderawaela, Sri Lanka, where external drainage is good due to slope of the land, vegetable-farmers apply 10-20 tons of manure to every crop and change the topsoils every 3-4 years. A similar situation exists in the Cameron Highlands of Malaysia.

Cheap mechanical power made available through contractual arrangement of machines partly alleviates constraints due to labor shortages and improves farmers' ability to bring large areas under vegetable cultivation. Other operations such as weeding and insect monitoring can be combined with chemical use for integrated pest management. Growing of determinate vegetable varieties, which can be harvested once or a few times, can partly alleviate the constraints on harvesting indeterminate varieties.

Introduction of modern vegetable technologies along with government policy and support programs for summer vegetable production has been a sustainable strategy to increase vegetable production and reduce seasonality. In Taiwan for example, introduction of summer tomato varieties by AVRDC has reduced seasonality in tomato prices, especially during the summer months of August-November (Figure 8).

Most Asian countries have highland areas where environmental conditions are favorable for vegetable-cultivation when it is very hot and humid in the lowlands. For example, summer vegetable supply for Bangkok mainly comes from Chiang Mai, for Manila from Baguio, and for Kuala Lumpur from the Cameron Highlands. Maintaining good trade and transportation links with these areas within a country can reduce seasonality in vegetable supply.

Limitations to Overcoming Constraints

Although technological solutions are available to overcome vegetable production constraints, these solutions are expensive to install, operate, and maintain, and require very good management skills. Therefore, adoption of these practices and solutions are economically viable only in a limited economic environment when vegetable supplies are extremely limited and prices are quite high.

Market access for upland vegetable producers, where favorable environment normally exists for summer vegetable cultivation compared to the lowlands is often difficult and costly (Midmore et al., 1996). Despite recent

FIGURE 8. Reduction in seasonal tomato prices at the retail level in Taiwan.

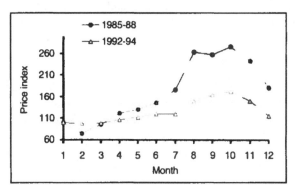

improvements in the supply of vegetables from these areas, such sources satisfy only a small proportion of the potential summer-vegetable demand; therefore, seasonality of vegetable production and availability remains a big issue.

The managerial skills required for vegetable production is the most binding constraint towards diversification of the cereal-based production system into vegetables. Vegetables are management intensive crops and their profits are responsive to the timeliness of management operations. Adjusting production decisions to marketing potential is the major skill required, which is usually lacking in the uneducated and ill-informed farmers of developing countries.

As discussed earlier, vegetable production is input sensitive; consequently, it entails higher operational costs than cereals. To manage this constraint, informal arrangements such as obligatory sale of output to commission agents who finance inputs, are quite common in Asia. The cost of financing is expected to decline as financial institutions develop in the near future; however, high financial requirements combined with high risk will continue to be a major constraint in vegetable cultivation.

During the dry season in irrigated lowlands, it is relatively easy to switch to vegetable crops. However, entire irrigation structures (water flow-rate at the head, irrigation canals, channels and drainage, field slope, etc.) sometimes need to be rehabilitated to make rice fields suitable for vegetable cultivation. This rehabilitation requires additional investment, which is economical only if consumers can afford to pay higher prices for vegetables.

SUCCESSFUL EXAMPLES OF VEGETABLE EXPANSION

There have been marginal improvements in diversifying Asian cereal based systems as the proportion of vegetable area to cereal area increased from 3.6% in 1980 to 7.2% in 2000. The increase is more prominent in China, mainly because vegetable area has been expanding and cereal area has been reducing. Similar phenomena were observed, although with less intensity, in Taiwan, Japan, and South Korea. Small increases in the share of vegetable area over cereal area occurred in South Asia, while this ratio remains almost stagnant for Southeast Asia (Ali, 2001).

There has been a significant improvement in vegetable production value as a proportion of cereal production value. In Asia, as a whole, the proportion has almost doubled from 17% in 1980 to 30% in 1993. The change is pervasive all over Asia (Figure 9). This change is mainly the result of increasing relative price of vegetables to cereals and some increase in vegetable production in China and India. A few country specific examples are discussed in the following paragraphs.

FIGURE 9. Trends in the proportion of the value of vegetables to cereal in Asia.

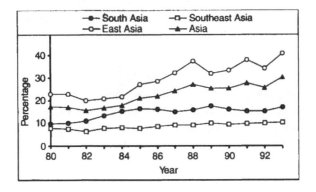

Bangladesh

From 1990 to 1999, per capita availability of farm produced vegetables (excluding home-garden supplies) in Bangladesh increased by 18% from 34 g to 40 g. During this period, new vegetable production technologies were introduced through a collaborative vegetable development project. In addition, farm housewives were part of a vegetable awareness-training schedule. Farmers adopting new vegetable production technologies produced 38% higher vegetable yields on an average compared to farmers who did not. The economic efficiency in input use, especially of land, labor, and water employed for vegetable cultivation improved by 65%, 40%, and 12%, respectively. Overall farm income of vegetable farmers increased by about 10% and generated about US$ 8.8 million to producers in terms of income from vegetable production and consumers because of greater vegetable availability at lower prices. Vegetable consumption and micronutrient availability on adopter farm families were also significantly higher than at non-vegetable and non-adopter vegetable farm families (Ali and Hau, 2001).

The AVRDC in collaboration with an NGO, Hellen Keller International, promoted a specially designed home garden (16 m^2) to provide nutrient-rich vegetables over most of the year to Bangladesh families. Per capita vegetable consumption significantly increased among the home-garden adopter families compared to non home-garden adopter families. There was an increased consumption of micronutrient-rich foods, especially provitamin A, which reduced the likelihood of vitamin A deficiencies. Consequently, higher consumption of vegetables lowered the incidence of blindness and improved the weight and height of children (AVRDC, 1994).

Pakistan

The adoption of high yielding, short-duration, yellow mosaic virus resistant mungbean varieties in the cereal-based system in Pakistan lead to 55% yield increase, four-fold income, and 25% reduction in unit cost. Wheat productivity in the wheat-mungbean rotation increased by 19% compared to wheat-wheat or wheat in rotation with other crops. Mungbean production in the country increased from 32,000 t in 1981 to 80,000 t in 1999. The expansion of mungbean cultivation in the fallow-wheat rotation expanded the sustainability advantage of the leguminous crop on a larger wheat area. Therefore, increase in wheat productivity in the country was highest in the mungbean growing areas. This technological innovation generated about US$20 millions annually, which was distributed almost equally between producers and consumers (Ali et al., 1997).

Thailand

Asparagus cultivation in Thailand started in 1985 with training of farmers by AVRDC and distribution of seed by a private company in Taiwan. Within a few years, asparagus replaced 3000 ha of rice area. This replacement generated about US$ 20 million of annual income to producers, created 19,500 additional jobs, and prompted new agricultural business activities in the area (AVRDC, 1998).

CONCLUSIONS

This article highlighted the nutritional and economic benefits of vegetable production and consumption. Vegetables are a dense and the most economical source of micronutrients and minerals. They are a major source of vitamins, iron, and calcium, and contribute to diversity in the diet. In fact, the economic efficiency of vegetables in supplying overall nutrient is one of the highest among all the food groups, and the highest for the leafy vegetable type. Vegetable cultivation generates income, employment, and may help to maintain the sustainability of resources engaged in agricultural production. Vegetable farmers consume a healthier diet than non-vegetable farmers. Engaging in vegetable production improves the learning and managerial capacity of farmers, which is an essential input to overall economic growth.

Despite these advantages, vegetable availability is far below the minimum required level in most developing countries of Asia. In addition, vegetable production is highly seasonal and annual production is highly unstable. A stage, however, has been set for the rapid expansion of vegetable production, which currently is insufficient to meet minimal per capita vegetable intake requirements. Increased incomes, population growth, and urbanization have created additional demand for vegetables. On the other hand, the needs to diversify production, to recuperate the sustainability of cereal-cereal system, and improve water use efficiency are the factors that have generated additional opportunities for vegetable cultivation to expand. These forces are reinforced by consumer demand for a diversified diet.

Both production- and trade-oriented strategies should be used to overcome shortages and seasonality of vegetable supplies. Production-oriented strategies should focus on developing high-yielding stress-tolerant varieties and management technologies so that more farmers can produce more vegetables at lower per-unit costs without damaging the environment and maintaining long-term resource productivity. Although many technologies are available to ameliorate stresses and reduce production risks, they are expensive, can be environmentally unfriendly, and adoption is limited. Making these technologies economically viable and more environmentally friendly for a wider range of environments is a continuing challenge to vegetable researchers.

Trade-oriented strategies should promote national and international trade in vegetables, taking advantage of higher production and lower costs in favorable vegetable growing areas. The success of such strategies is most likely for long and medium storage life crops and would require a sufficiently developed marketing system to allow cheap and rapid transport of vegetables with minimal storage losses. Such strategies should look more towards favorable regions within the country, as import is relatively expensive for developing economies. For this purpose, favorable vegetable growing regions need to be identified and trade should be promoted with these regions. However, trade oriented policies are likely to be successful only in cases where vegetables have less localized preferences.

Successful production of adequate good quality vegetables leads to good consumers' health, more jobs, diversified and higher incomes to producers, long-term sustainability of the agriculture resource base, and overall development of the economy. With current vegetable production technologies, the area under vegetables in South and Southeast Asia needs to be tripled to make per capita vegetable availability equal to that of East Asia. This expansion would require 14 million additional hectares for vegetable cultivation. On the assumption that this area increase for vegetable production would occur by replacing cereal producing areas, and that each hectare of vegetable production will create a minimum of one year-round job when such a substitution is made, this will generate an additional 14 million jobs. Based on current yields, there will be an additional vegetable output of 128 million tones. An additional 14 million jobs are expected for post-harvest handling of this output. With the present average value of vegetables at US$300 per ton, an additional US$ 37 billion in income for poor Asian farmers is expected. A similar income will be generated for the middlemen who will haul this output to the consumer.

However, a minimum level of farmers' education and managerial-skill development, field-market linking infrastructure, and favorable government policies to encourage and stabilize vegetable production are required. Under this scenario, technological innovation can act as a catalyst to expand vegetable production. The enhanced management capabilities of vegetable-growing farmers will be a key in the rapid socioeconomic development of the whole economy.

NOTES

1. These surveys were conducted in 3-5 provinces/districts of Cambodia, Laos, South Vietnam, and Bangladesh during 1998-2000. Provinces/districts with the largest vegetable cultivated areas were selected in these countries. In addition, consumption surveys were also conducted in the Philippines (Central Luzon area) and Taiwan (across the country). In all of these surveys, the data was recorded per meal and per family basis using recall method. Data was recorded on: the names and quantities of all food items consumed in the three meals within the preceding 24 hrs at the time of the survey; food price, number of people participating in each meal; and the source of the food. Except in Taiwan, both vegetable and non-vegetable farmers were included in the sample for comparison purposes. Vegetable and non-vegetable farmers were randomly selected from the main vegetable growing villages of each 3-5 provinces/districts. The sample ranged 49-114 depending upon the size of the province/district and availability of vegetable farmers.

2. Changes in diversity in the diet were measured as the percentage deviation in the number of vegetables consumed from an average number of vegetables consumed during 1964-81.

3. Nutrient cost can be estimated from all food commodities containing a particular nutrient in the whole diet, or from food items in each food group. In this case, it was estimated separately for each food group.

4. The production and consumption surveys were linked in South Vietnam, Laos, Cambodia, and Bangladesh. The operation of consumption surveys is explained in footnote 1. The production surveys include farmers' characterization, input quantities and costs of all inputs, and yield and return from all crops grown during the year completed just before the survey.

5. This example assumes 90% of the vegetable and 30% of the cereal output sold in market. Similarly, 40% of the inputs in vegetables compared to 50% in cereals are assumed to be have been purchased.

6. The production function included quantities of seed, fertilizer, farm manure, labor, and irrigation status (irrigated field = 1, and zero otherwise) as independent variables. To control for selectivity bias in vegetable farmers, another farm-characteristic equation was specified where farmer type (vegetable farmer = 1, and zero otherwise) was dependent on the level of education, farm size, and irrigation status. The form of production function specified was translog, and the farm-characteristic equation was in log linear form. Both equations were estimated simultaneously using the two stage least square method.

REFERENCES

Ali, M. (ed.) 2000. Dynamics of vegetable production, distribution, and consumption in Asia. AVRDC publication no. 00-498, Shanhua, Tainan, Taiwan, 470p.

Ali, M. 2001. Diversification with Vegetables to Improve Competitiveness in Asia, In Agricultural Diversification and International Competitiveness. Asian Productivity Organization, Tokyo.

Ali, M., and V.T. Hau. 2001. Economic and nutritional impact of AVRDC/USAID/ BARRI project in Bangladesh, AVRDC publication, Shanhua, Tainan.

Ali, M., and S.C.S. Tsou. 1997. Combating micronutrient deficiencies through vegetables–a neglected food frontier in Asia. Food Policy, 22(1), pp. 17-38.

Ali, M., and S.C.S. Tsou. 2000. The integrated research approach of the Asian Vegetable Research and Development Center (AVRDC) to enhance micronutrient availability, Food and Nutrition Journal, 21 (4), pp. 472-482.

Ali, M., I.A. Malik, H.M. Sabir, and B. Ahmad. 1997. The mungbean green revolution in Pakistan. AVRDC, Technical Bulletin No. 24, Shanhua, Tainan, Taiwan, 66p.

Ali, M., S.N. Wu, and M.H. Wu. 2000. Valuing the net nutritive gain of policy interventions: An application to Taiwan household survey data, AVRDC, Shanhua, Taiwan.

AVRDC (Asian Vegetable Research and Development Center). 1992. AVRDC 1991 progress reports. AVRDC, Shanhua, Tainan, Taiwan.

AVRDC (Asian Vegetable Research and Development Center). 1993. AVRDC 1992 progress reports. AVRDC, Shanhua, Tainan, Taiwan.

AVRDC (Asian Vegetable Research and Development Center). 1994. Annual progress report for 1993. AVRDC, Shanhua, Tainan, Taiwan.

AVRDC (Asian Vegetable Research and Development Center). 1995. AVRDC 1994 progress reports. AVRDC, Shanhua, Tainan, Taiwan.

AVRDC (Asian Vegetable Research and Development Center). 1998. AVRDC report 1997. AVRDC, Shanhua, Tainan, Taiwan.

Bouis, H.E., M.J. Novenario-Reese. 1991. The determinants of household-level demand for micronutrients: An analysis for Philippine farm households. International Food Policy Research Institute, Washington, DC. 84p.

Braun J.V., D. Hotchkiss, and M. Immink. 1989. Nontraditional export crops in Guatemala, effects on production, income, and nutrition. Research Report 73. International Food Policy Research Institute and Institute of Nutrition of Central America and Panama, Washington, DC, 99p.

Bueno-de-Mesquita, H.B., P. Misonneuve, S. Runia, and C.J. Moerman. 1991. Intake of foods and nutrients and cancer of the exocrine pancreas: A population-based case-control study in the Netherlands. International Journal of Cancer, 48(4), pp. 540-549.

Food and Nutrition Board (1989). Recommended Dietary Allowances, 10th edition, National Academy Press, Washington, DC.

Food Industry Research and Development Institute and Pintung University of Science and Technology. 1998. Food composition table in Taiwan area. Public Health Division, Executive Yuan. Taipei, 471p.

Hirayama, T. 1995. Green-yellow vegetables for human health with special reference to cancer prevention. Journal of Japanese Society for Horticultural Science, 63, pp. 965-974.

Jedrychowshi, B.W., H. Boeing, T. Popiela, J. Wahrendrof, B. Tobiasz-Adamczyk, and J. Kuling. 1992. Dietary practices in households as risk factors for stomach cancer: A familial study in Poland. European Journal of Cancer Prevention, 1(4), pp. 297-304.

Midmore, D.J., and D.D. Poudel. 1996. Asian vegetable production systems for the future. Agricultural Systems, 50 (1), pp. 51-64.

Midmore, D.J., H.G.P. Jansen, R.G. Dumsday, A.A. Azami, D.D. Poudel, S. Valasayya, J. Huang, M.M. Radzali. N. Fuad, A.B. Samah, A.R. Syed, and A. Nazlin. 1996. Technical and economic aspects of sustainable production practices among vegetable growers in the Cameron highlands, Malaysia. Technical Bulletin No. 23. AVRDC, Shanhua, Tainan, Taiwan, 64p.

Mirjam, W. 1997. A comparative agronomic and socioeconomic study of rice and rice-vegetables farms in Ilocos Norte, Philippines. MS thesis, Wageningen Agricultural University, Wageningen, p. 30+26 pages of un-numbered annex.

Peet, M.M., and D.H. Willits. 1993. Evaluating high night temperature effects on tomato, In Kuo, C.G. (ed.) Adoption of food crops to temperature and water stress. AVRDC, pp. 175-187, Tainan, Taiwan.

Pingali, P.L. 1992. Diversifying Asian rice-farming systems: A deterministic paradigm. In Barghouti, S., Garbux, L. and Umali, D. (Eds.), Trends in agricultural diversification: Regional perspectives. World Bank Technical Paper no. 180, The World Bank, Washington, DC, pp. 107-126.

Plucknett, D.L., R.F. Jr. Chandler, and T.M. Mc Calla. 1981. Fertilization of vegetables. In Plucknett, D.L., and Beemer, H.L. Jr. (Eds.), Vegetable farming systems in China. Boulder, Colorado, Westview Press, pp. 39-44.

Rosegrant, M.W., and P.L. Pingali. 1994. Policies and technologies for rice productivity growth in Asia. Journal of International Development, 6(6), pp. 665-688.

Shibata, A., A. Paganini-Hill, R.K. Ross, M.C. Yu, and B.E. Henderson. 1992. Dietary beta-carotene, cigarette smoking, and lung cancer in men. Cancer Causes and Control, 3(3), pp. 207-214.

Sritunga, S. 1975. The intensive ditch and dike method for vegetables cultivation in Thailand. MSc Thesis, Nueva Ecija, Central Luzon State University, Philippines, 108p.

Yu, M.W., H.H. Hseih, W.H. Pan, C.S. Yang, and C.J. Chen. 1995. Vegetable consumption, serum retinol level, and risk of hepatocellular carcinoma. Cancer Research, 55(6), pp. 1301-1305.

Yusuf, H.K.M., and N.M. Islam. 1994. Improvement of nightblindness situation through simple nutrition education intervention with the parents. Ecology of Food and Nutrition, 31(3-4), pp. 247-256.

Agroforestry Systems
for Food and Nutrition Security–
Potentials, Pathways
and Policy Research Needs

S. C. Babu
V. Rhoe

SUMMARY. Food insecurity and malnutrition continue to be the most daunting development challenges in most developing countries. Increases in the productivity of cereal grain crops have helped many developing countries achieve self-sufficiency in meeting the energy requirements, but malnutrition still exist. Agroforestry–growing useful tree crops with annual crops–could provide a solution to food security micronutrient malnutrition. The paper develops a conceptual framework for identifying pathways of how agroforestry systems can contribute to nutrition security and its potential as a food-based nutrition intervention. Furthermore, a theoretical framework for studying the interactions of agroforestry and nutrition security is developed. Finally, policy implications and research needs are identified. *[Article copies available for a fee from The Haworth Document Delivery Service: 1-800-HAWORTH. E-mail address: <getinfo@haworthpressinc.com> Website: <http://www.HaworthPress.com> © 2002 by The Haworth Press, Inc. All rights reserved.]*

S. C. Babu is Senior Research Fellow and Senior Training Advisor, IFPRI, 2033 K Street, N.W., Washington, DC 20006 (E-mail: s.babu@cgiar.org).

V. Rhoe is Senior Research Assistant, IFPRI, 2033 K Street, N.W., Washington, DC 20006 (E-mail: v.rhoe@cgiar.org).

[Haworth co-indexing entry note]: "Agroforestry Systems for Food and Nutrition Security–Potentials, Pathways and Policy Research Needs." Babu, S. C., and V. Rhoe. Co-published simultaneously in *Journal of Crop Production* (Food Products Press, an imprint of The Haworth Press, Inc.) Vol. 6, No. 1/2 (#11/12), 2002, pp. 177-192; and: *Food Systems for Improved Human Nutrition: Linking Agriculture, Nutrition, and Productivity* (ed: Palit K. Kataki, and Suresh Chandra Babu) Food Products Press, an imprint of The Haworth Press, Inc., 2002, pp. 177-192. Single or multiple copies of this article are available for a fee from The Haworth Document Delivery Service [1-800-HAWORTH, 9:00 a.m. - 5:00 p.m. (EST). E-mail address: getinfo@haworthpressinc.com].

177

KEYWORDS. Agroforestry policy, agroforestry systems, dynamic optimization, food-based intervention, food security, nutrition security

INTRODUCTION

Food insecurity and malnutrition continue to be the most daunting development challenges in most developing countries. Worldwide, about 800 million people are affected by the lack of adequate food, 160 million preschool children are malnourished, and about 2 billion people suffer from anemia (FAO, 1999; ACC/SCN-IFPRI, 2000). Increases in the productivity of cereal grain crops have helped many developing countries achieve self-sufficiency in meeting the energy requirements at least at the national level. Yet, poor adoption of production technologies, frequent droughts, and poor food and nutrition policies continue to contribute to household food insecurity and child malnutrition. Furthermore, micronutrient malnutrition such as vitamin A deficiency, iron deficiency, and iodine deficiency disorders remain unabated in many developing countries. Recent developments in food-based approaches, in terms of designing appropriate farming systems and nutritionally balanced diets show some promise in addressing the micronutrient malnutrition (Babu, 2001; Ruel and Levin 2001).

Designing an appropriate agroforestry system that incorporates trees, animals, and annual crops to meet the household nutritional requirement is one such approach (Babu and Rajasekaran, 1991; Babu, Hallam, and Rajasekaran, 1994). There are two major pathways to food and nutrition security through agroforestry. The first increases the availability of nutrients to people through tree crops that supply fruits and vegetables, and the second increases the availability of food either by improving crop yields through the application of green leaf manures or by improving livestock productivity by providing fodder (Babu, Hallam, and Rajasekaran, 1995; Rajasekaran, Warren, and Babu, 1994). While there are some studies that analyze the food security and nutritional contribution of agroforestry systems (FAO, 1989; Longhurst, 1987), there has only been a few rigorous studies directed towards assessing the constraints and challenges faced by farmers in using the tree component of the agroforestry system as a potential source of food and nutrients.

The purpose of this paper is to develop a conceptual framework for identifying pathways of agroforestry systems that contribute to nutrition security and to develop a theoretical framework for studying the interactions of agroforestry and nutrition security. The pathways to the contribution of agroforestry to nutrition security are identified next. Then, the potential of agroforestry as a food-based nutrition intervention is presented. Subsequently, the contribution of various components of agroforestry to the dynamics of household food security of smallholder farms is developed in a growth theoretic framework. Policy implications and research needs are then identified, and finally there are concluding remarks.

PATHWAYS OF AGROFORESTRY CONTRIBUTION TO RURAL NUTRITION

It is useful to trace the pathways through which agroforestry can contribute to food security and nutrition. Understanding the agroforestry-income-consumption-food-nutrition security linkages is important for identifying, analyzing, and rectifying the constraints and challenges in maximizing the benefits of agroforestry systems for food and nutrition security. Figure 1 presents a conceptual framework for studying the agroforestry-nutrition security linkages. Adoption of an agroforestry system as a food-based strategy depends on several underlying factors. First, land availability to grow tree crops is an important determinant of agroforestry farming system. Second, land tenure policies that do not facilitate private ownership of land may reduce the investment on land improvement because the benefits may not accrue to the occupant in the long run. Third, the opportunity cost of growing trees in place of annual food crops could be higher, particularly in irrigated and high-potential farming areas. Fourth, labor market factors such as high rural wages and low supply of agricultural laborers may encourage the transfer to tree crops thus facilitating the shift from monocropping to agroforestry.

Farming systems that face poor soil fertility provide incentives for adoption of agroforestry for green manures and tree-crop-soil interaction. In areas where the contribution of livestock to cattle manure is low, agroforestry remains the main source of soil nutrients. Given the high cost of chemical fertilizer inputs and poor availability in remote areas, agroforestry can play an important role. Finally, the demographic factors within the household such as availability of household labor, land ownership, and knowledge of the household head may determine the adoption of agroforestry.

The tree components of the agroforestry system can contribute to increased food availability at the household level through four major pathways. First, the contribution of fodder supplement can increase the productivity of livestock. Higher productivity can result in greater food availability and/or higher incomes. Second, green leaf manure harvested and ploughed *in situ* and tree-crop-soil interaction can increase the soil fertility and result in improved productivity of food and non-food crops. Higher soil fertility is likely to increase the food/cash crop productivity and household income that will, in turn, contribute to food availability. Third, fruits and vegetables harvested from the tree component of agroforestry will directly contribute to improved dietary quality and micronutrient consumption, and indirectly, contribute through the sale of

FIGURE 1. Agroforestry and food nutrition security linkages. [Based on Smith and Haddad (2000), UNICEF (1998), and Babu and Mthindi (1994)]

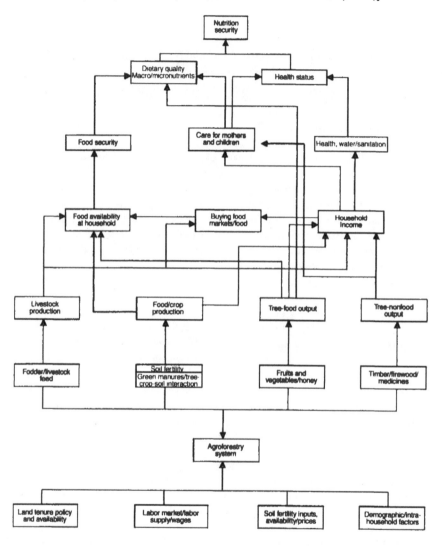

these items to the market for income in order to purchase food. Finally, the non-food tree outputs such as timber for housing and firewood for fuel contribute to income that can be used to acquire food. Indirectly, availability of fuel wood from tree components may also contribute to nutrition security–by reducing the search for fuel wood which could increase time availability for child care (Filmer and Pritchett, 2001). Presumably, the increased cash income from non-food products can increase the resources spent on child care and health care of household members. This cash income along with food availability, can contribute to nutrition security if additianol income is used to purchase nutritious food products.

While the conceptual framework provides potential pathways, the final benefit from agroforestry to nutrition security will depend on several socioeconomic, institutional, and policy factors. In the next section, what we already know about these four pathways to nutrition security will be discussed.

AGROFORESTRY AS FOOD-BASED INTERVENTION

Agroforestry can be defined as a system of farming in which trees, animals, and annual crops are strategically planted and grown to maximize output through various interactions of the system components (Nair, 1990). Agroforestry interventions can contribute to food and nutrition security in several different ways. Agroforestry interventions can ensure food availability, strengthen access to food and nutrients in rural areas, and play a complementary role in utilization by increasing the quality of the diet. Increased production of non-food agroforestry outputs can improve income, which in turn, can improve household food consumption. Additional benefits from agroforestry that support increasing food and nutrition security include increasing the available time of household members and the productivity of existing crops. Well-designed agroforestry systems can also increase the diversity of food consumed. It is well known that benefits can be higher when the increased income from food-based interventions is spent on food and nutrition-related consumption. Four conditions need to be met in order to increase the food and nutritional benefits of agroforestry as a food-based intervention: the additional income generated by agroforestry is earned and controlled by women; the stream of income from agroforestry is regular and frequent, even if the absolute amounts are small; the income is in-kind primarily in the form of food; and nutrition and health education is provided (Fanta, 2001).

Once these conditions are met, the four pathways in which agroforestry can improve nutrition security can be followed. The first method in which nutrition security can be enhanced is through the consumption of food produced by trees (seeds, stems, tubers, leaves, mushrooms, sap, and nectar). For example, in Nigeria, some of the rural population consumes non-conventional leaf vegetables, which contains a variety of minerals–calcium, iron, zinc, and manganese. The six leaves studied–*Amaranthus spinosus*, *Adansonia digitata*, *Moringa oleifera*, *Adansonia digitata*, *Cassia tora*, and *Colocasia esculenta*–have a higher level of calcium than common vegetables (Barminas, Carles, and Emmanuel, 1998), which may reduce a number of micronutrient deficiencies. Another case study showed that several edible wild plants in Niger contain more antioxidant than potatoes and spinach. Although antioxidants contain anticancer properties, most people only ate these plants in time of food insufficiency. Therefore, more research is needed to learn how to entice people to consume these foods.

Another method that may achieve nutritional security is through the selling of non-food tree products. Selling non-food tree products such as medicines and timber can increase the income of the household (Ogden, 1996), which then can be used to purchase high nutrient food products, health care, and/or child care. For example, the *Vitellaria paradoxa* tree produces oil that is used in many expensive cosmetics, facial creams, and soaps. Agroforestry farmers can sell this scarce oil in order to generate income (ICRAF, 1997) that may be used to purchase needed goods. Although timber products have established markets, the commercialization of non-timber products is impeded by organizational and structural problems, therefore, local people have received limited welfare gains from the sale of these items (Tshiamala-Tshibangu and Ndjigba, 1999). For that reason, policy research is needed to improve the efficiency of these markets.

The third method is through soil fertility benefits from green manure and tree-crop-soil interaction. In Eastern Zambia, ICRAF researchers and their counterparts have developed an agroforestry system that enhances soils fertility, which increases crop yields. This alternative method requires *Sesbania sesban* trees to be planted, and then clear felled. The twigs and leaves are then mixed with the soil. This process has resulted in at least the doubling of maize yields (Kwesiga, 1999). Moreover, nitrogen-fixing trees can improve soil fertility through the colonization of root nodules, which fixes atmospheric nitrogen, therefore, enhancing the soil's fertility (Uchimura, 1994). Although agroforestry enhances soil fertility, it has been shown that crops only absorb 20% of the nutrients that agroforestry species release during the crop season (Palm, 1995). Thus, the choice of the tree component may determine the level of soil fertility benefits from agroforestry.

The last method in which nutrition security can be enhanced is through fodder. For example, the *Samanea saman* (Merr) tree could be used in a silvopastoral system for cattle because it produces palatable pods that can be used for feed during the dry season (Durr, 2001). This fodder will sustain the life and health of the farmer's livestock, and therefore, livestock production will be sustained and income generated. Furthermore, supplementing *Imperata* grasslands with legumes has increased production of fodder on smallholder farms (Calub, Anwarhan, and Roder, 1996).

While there are several potential benefits of agroforestry towards nutrition security, it is not clear what would be the optimal level of tree planting that will generate sustainable food and nutrition security. Designing studies to evaluate the nutritional benefits of agroforestry require as a first step theoretical exposition of the dynamic contributions of agroforestry. In the next section, a growth-theoretical framework for analyzing the conditions under which agroforestry could be used as a direct food and nutrition intervention is developed.

A DYNAMIC MODEL FOR OPTIMIZING FOOD CONSUMPTION FROM AGROFORESTRY

Considering the fruits and vegetables from the tree component of agroforestry systems could be considered as a stock of food to be depleted over a certain period of time for analyzing household food security issues (Phillips and Taylor, 1990; Nuppaneu, 1991). Several paradigms could be used in modeling the contributions of agroforestry systems to household food security. Considering the simultaneous decisions of household production and consumption, the food from agroforestry could be modeled along with the stochastic production of agricultural staples under the agricultural household model framework (Roe and Graham-Thomas, 1986). Alternatively, the provision of fruits and vegetables from the tree component of an agroforestry system could be treated as insurance for attaining a certain level of food security in the presence of fluctuations in the of field crops production (Phillips and Taylor, 1990). Yet, another way is to model the food consumed from agroforestry systems is as a problem of optimal use of food stock from agroforestry (Babu, 1992). The general model presented here is based on an optimal-control model developed earlier for optimizing the consumption of foods from seasonal production[1] (Babu, Hallam, and Rajasekaran, 1994). Consider a food security index function $C(Q)$, which is depended on the production of food from the tree component Q. While food security also depends on other foods, for simplicity they are not explicitly included in this function. For any function $f(x)$, f_x is the first derivative and f_{xx} is the second derivative of f with respect to x, it is assumed that $C_Q > 0$ and $C_{QQ} < 0$ for concavity of the function C. The growth of food stocks (x) from the tree component is given by

$$\dot{x} = [f(x) - \mu x - Q] \qquad (1)$$

Where μ is the rate at which food waste and other waste occur when food is not harvested in time. The flow of food from trees is given by the production function $f(x)$. This function is assumed to be increasing and strictly concave. The food security from the consumption of food from the tree component of agroforestry is maximized with the discount rate δ, using the following dynamic objective function.

$$\int_{t=0}^{\infty} C(Q)e^{-\delta t}\, dt \qquad (2)$$

Forming the Hamiltonian function to apply the maximum principle, the optimization problem becomes (Chiang, 1992);

$$H_t = e^{-\delta t} C(Q) + \phi[f(x) - \mu x - Q] \qquad (3)$$

Where ϕ is the co-state variable associated with the growth of food stock. By maximizing the food security function C, subject to the constraint (Equation 1), one could choose the optimal levels of consumption of food from agroforestry (Q), the stock of food on the trees (x) and the opportunity cost of the growth constraint of the food stock, ϕ. To obtain qualitative inferences in the absence of specific functional forms of C and f, the Hamiltonian is differentiated with respect to x and Q. However, the presence of the discount rate δ, generally adds to the complexity of the derivatives and the manipulation of results for further intuition. Thus, the Hamiltonian function is made into a current-value Hamiltonian ($\tilde{H}$) (Chiang, 1992);

$$\tilde{H} = He^{-\delta t} = C(Q) + \theta[f(x) - \mu x - Q] \qquad (4)$$

Where $\theta = \phi e^{-\delta t}$ interpreted as the current-value Lagrange multiplier. The first order conditions are:

$$\tilde{H}_Q = C_Q - \theta = 0 \qquad (5)$$

$$\tilde{H}_\theta = f(x) - \mu x - Q = \dot{x} \qquad (6)$$

$$-\tilde{H}_x = \dot{\theta} = -\theta[f_x - \mu] + \delta\theta \qquad (7)$$

Given the specific functional forms, Equations 5-7 could be used to solve for Q, x and θ. Equation 5 states that at the optimum, the marginal increase in food security due to increases in tree food consumption should be equal to the shadow price of tree food stock. Equations 6 and 7 provide two differential equations involving the variables x and θ. However, to analyze the dynamic relationship between the stock of food from agroforestry and household food security, it may be easier to work with equations involving Q and x.

Differentiating (Equation 5) with respect to time, we have

$$\dot{\theta} = C_{QQ}\dot{Q} \qquad (8)$$

Using Equation 8 in Equation 7 along with Equation 5 we have,

$$-\dot{Q} = \frac{C_Q}{C_{QQ}} [f_x - (\mu + \delta)] \tag{9}$$

To understand the qualitative relationships in determining optimal use of food from agroforestry, a phrase diagram (Dixit, 1990) could be drawn in Q and x space using Equations (6) and (9).

The equations which define the curves $\dot{x} = 0$ and $\dot{Q} = 0$ are given by

$$Q = f(x) - \mu x \text{ at } \dot{x} = 0 \tag{10}$$

and

$$f_x = \mu + \delta \text{ at } \dot{Q} = 0 \tag{11}$$

The curve for $\dot{x} = 0$ is shown as a concave curve in $x - Q$ space in Figure 2. Q is expressed on this curve as the difference between $f(x)$ and μx. The curve expressed by $\dot{Q} = 0$ (Equation 11) requires that the slope of $f(x)$ should be equal to, $\mu + \delta$, which is a constant. This constant corresponds to a unique value of x at $\bar{x}$. The curve for $\dot{Q} = 0$ is shown as a vertical line at $\bar{x}$ in Figure 2. The steady-state values of the stock of food (x) in the tree component of an agroforestry system and the level of consumption of food (Q) is determined by the intersection of the two curves at point E. These values are distinct from the values, x^* and Q^* at which the curve, $\dot{x} = 0$ has the maximum value at point S. This is because at S the derivative of $\partial Q/\partial x$ is equal to zero and f_x is equal to μ. The value of x corresponding to this slope denoted by x^* is larger, and lies right of $\bar{x}$.

To analyze the phase diagram for the starting values of the initial stock of food $(x_{(0)})$ and the initial consumption level of food $(Q_{(0)})$ from agroforestry, which would result in steady-state levels of these variables, equations (Equation 6) and (Equation 9) are partially differentiated.

$$\frac{\partial \dot{x}}{\partial Q} = -1 \leq 0 \tag{12}$$

and

$$\frac{\partial \dot{Q}}{\partial x} = \frac{-C_Q}{C_{QQ}} f_{xx} \leq 0 \tag{13}$$

FIGURE 2. Steady-state food security from agroforestry.

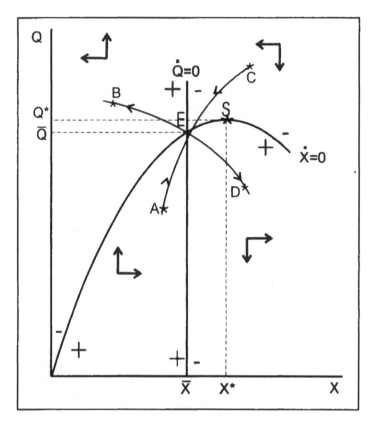

By the concavity properties of the food security index function C (Q) and $f(x)$, the sign of values at the right hand side of the above equations are negative. It could be inferred from Equation 12 that as the consumption of food from the tree component of agroforestry increases the growth rate of its stock should decrease and be negative by the same amount. Prior to achieving this negative growth rate, the food stock should have a positive and zero growth rates. Thus, as consumption increases, the stock, x, should increase below the curve $\dot{x} = 0$, and decrease above the curve. From Equation 13, it could be noted that as the stock of food increases the growth of consumption decreases which means prior to achieving this negative growth rate, the consumption of food should have the states of positive and zero growth rates. These movements are represented by the positive (+) and negative (−) signs next to the curves that split the Qx space into four quadrants. The arrowheads drawn in each quadrant reflect the nature of these movements.

According to these arrowheads, the movement of a particular combination of initial values of food stock from the tree component and the associated consumption level could be traced towards achieving the steady-state equilibrium levels [$\overline{Q}$, $\overline{x}$] at point E. The intertemporal values of such equilibrium is shown to be a saddle-point and are unique. Thus, to achieve the steady-state level of food security through agroforestry, it is necessary to start at levels of Q and x that lead to point E. This means that given the initial stock of x at period $t = 0$, the corresponding level of consumption (Q) must lie on the path that will attain the steady-state. One such combination is shown at a point A in Figure 2.

The model results also indicate that unless the initial levels of stock of food and consumption are on steady-state path, the use of food from agroforestry to achieve household food security will not be sustainable; either stocks will increase continuously accompanied by decreasing levels of consumption–a situation which is typical when the food is overproduced coinciding with a food surplus season–or stocks will decrease continuously with increasing levels of consumption–a situation which arises when limited number of trees providing food along with exhaustion of food stock in a short period of time due to drought or famine. Thus to attain a long run sustainable use of agroforestry systems for household food security, their design should be based on the requirements of food from agroforestry and the optimal number of trees in an agroforestry system which would meet this requirement.

To better understand the dynamics of Figure 2, we will provide several examples to explain the direction of the arrows. At point A, the stock of food is to the left of $\dot{Q} = 0$ and the consumption of food is below $\dot{x} = 0$; therefore, both the stock and consumption of food are below their equilibrium value. The following scenario should assist in understanding the movements of these two variables. A developing country is experiencing a drought so food stocks are low and people can only consume what is available. As the drought begins to subside, production increases, and therefore, the stock of food increase. Since people were consuming less than they need or desired, their consumption level will increase. Both the stock and consumption of food will continue to increase until they are satisfied (equilibrium level). At point B, both the stock and consumption of food are falling. Instead of the drought subsiding, it continues. Now the stock of food is shrinking, and therefore, people must decrease their consumption of food.

At point C, the consumption of food is above $\dot{x} = 0$ and the stock of food is to the right $\dot{Q} = 0$. Ultimately, both of these will decrease. Imagine, the supply of food was in excess of demand, and then a flood destroyed part of the remaining crop. The supply of food still exists but this supply is shrinking and therefore, prices are rising. People will reduce their consumption of food until an equilibrium level is reached.

At point D, the stock of food is growing, but the food needs of the population have been satisfied, therefore, people are no longer increasing their consumption of food.

The theoretical exposition presented above is an attempt to capture the dynamic nature of the multiseasonal contribution of food from the tree component of agroforestry and its interaction with annual food crops. Several implications for policy research could be derived from the results of the model. Some of them are presented in the next section.

POLICY IMPLICATIONS FOR DESIGNING AGROFORESTRY SYSTEMS FOR FOOD AND NUTRITION SECURITY

Introduction of agroforestry as a food-based nutrition intervention requires several considerations. The adoption of agroforestry crucially depends on land availability. Unless surplus land is available that can be spared for tree planting, short-term profit from annual crops may discourage farmers from investing for the long-run benefits of agroforestry. Benefits of agroforestry in terms of food security and nutrition may accrue to the family more when the system is chosen and operated by women. However, this depends on the nature of agroforestry in terms of labor-increasing or labor reducing technology. Agroforestry requires a high level of labor during the planting and establishment stage of the tree component; however, given the stream of benefits that come from little or no labor inputs in subsequent stages, the initial labor investment becomes worthwhile. A major determinant of the nutritional impact of agroforestry would be how the additional income generated will be controlled and spent. There is, as in any other new crop production system, a better chance of additional income being spent on nutrition if this income is received or controlled by women.

Agroforestry has a better chance of contributing to food security and nutrition if it reduces the seasonal variability in the supply and the price of basic food crops. Thus, the design of agroforestry systems to achieve household security should consider the seasonality of agroforestry food production, food consumption habits, and productivity of various fruit bearing tree species in order for the system to attain long-run sustainable equilibrium levels of agroforestry food. Such an approach would require an interdisciplinary team of scientists representing the fields of horticulture, forestry, nutrition, as well as social sciences.

The adoption of agroforestry among smallholder farmers currently faces the challenge of short-run benefits from monocropping, which seems higher than the long-run benefits of an agroforestry system. This challenge is particularly so when the land available for crop production is scarce due to increased population pressure. Procedures for valuation of land should include the food security contribution of tree species as one of the criteria. Furthermore, agroforestry extension systems should consider the importance of recording and comparing the values of land based on food security contribution at regular intervals. This procedure requires collaboration of agronomists, extensionists, and land husbandry specialists.

Further research is needed to incorporate the stochastic nature of production (Larson, 1992) of both field crops and tree components due to rainfall variations in dryland farming systems. Farmers' behavior in choosing a specific combination of components in an agroforestry system to meet the household food security and nutritional requirements should be studied with respect to their attitude towards risk and uncertainty in order to provide better information and feedback to biological researchers (Babu and Rajasekaran, 1991).

The food tree component of an agroforestry system is also a form of stored value. Depending on the use of its output, it could be considered a liquid asset along with the livestock component. This liquid asset contributes to household food security both directly by harvesting food stock from trees and indirectly by selling the tree products for purchase of foods. Thus, the nature of the farmers' liquidity preference would influence the adoption and the mixture (food and nonfood) of agroforestry system components.

The adoption of agroforestry may have an impact on biodiversity when the farmers, who traditionally followed bushfallow cultivation, adopt agroforestry with a single tree component. For instance, such a change in the farming system would reduce multi-species farming to a multi-purpose (single species) tree farming. Implications of such a change on a regional basis should be fully understood in developing agroforestry technologies. This single species tree farming also has implications for wild food availability, and hence, food security at the household level.

CONCLUDING REMARKS

Food and nutrition insecurity continue to threaten a large share of the population, particularly in rural parts of developing countries in Asia and sub-Saharan Africa. Food-based interventions to reduce macro- and micronutrient malnutrition have shown great promise. In this article, we have identified agroforestry as one such intervention. Evaluation of food-based interventions for their contribution to increased food and nutrition security remains grossly inadequate; therefore, measuring the nutritional contribution of agroforestry systems is essential. While agroforestry has a large potential to contribute to food and nutrition security, several factors must be addressed for increasing its benefits. Matching the design of agroforestry with specific nutritional problems is important. This matching will require documenting and making inventory of nutrition-oriented agroforestry systems for various agro-ecological regions. Analysis and screening of appropriate tree components for their nutritive values must be undertaken. Appropriate cultivation practices must be developed along with proper extension methods for disseminating agroforestry technology. Furthermore, research is needed in evaluating the introduction of tree components for its benefits towards changes in the consumption patterns and nutritional improvements.

NOTE

1. This model is a theoretical exposition of the dynamics of the system.

REFERENCES

ACC/SCN-IFPRI. 2000. *Nutrition Throughout the Life Cycle.* 4th Report on The World Nutrition Situation. Geneva: ACC/SCN in collaboration with IFPRI.

Babu, S. C. 1992. *Agroforestry Ecosystems, Technological Change and Optimal Use of Green Manures–Policy Implications for Designing Research Strategies.* Mimeo. Joint IFPRI/UNICEF Food Security Programme, Bunda College of Agriculture, Malawi.

Babu, S. C., A. Hallam, and B. Rajasekaran. 1994. *Agroforestry and Household Food Security Interaction: Implications for Multi-Disciplinary Research Policy.* Paper presented at the International Association of Agricultural Economists Conference in Harare, Zimbabawe.

Babu, S. C. and B. Rajasekaran. 1991. Agroforestry, Attitude Towards Risk, and Nutrient Availability; A Case Study of South India Farming Systems. *Agroforestry Systems.* 15: 1-15.

Babu, S. C. and G.B. Mthindi. 1994. Household Food Security and Nutrition Monitoring. *Food Policy.* 19 (3): 272-284.

Babu, S. C., A. Hallam, and B. Rajasekaran. 1995. Dynamic Modeling of Agroforestry and Soil Fertility Interactions: Implications for Multi-Disciplinary Research Policy. *Agricultural Economic.* 13: 125-135.

Babu, S. C. 2001. *Food Policy and Nutrition Security in Asia-Strategies and Policy Options.* Washington, DC: International Food Policy Research Institute.

Barminas, J. T., M. Carles and D. Emmanuel. 1998. Mineral Composition of Non-Conventional Leafy Vegetables. *Plant Foods for Human Nutrition,* 53 (1): 29:36.

Cook, J. A., D. J. VanderJagt, A. Dasgupta, G. Mounkaila, R. S. Glew, W. Blackwell, and R. H. Glew. 1998. Use of the Trolox assay to estimate the antioxidant content of seventeen edible wild plants in Niger. *Life Sciences.* 63(2): 106-110.

Calub, A. D., H. Anwarhan, H., and W. Roder. 1996. Livestock Production Systems for Imperata Grasslands. *Agroforestry Systems.* 36(1/3): 121-128.

Chiang, A. 1992. *Elements of Dynamic Optimization.* London: McGraw-Hill.

Dixit, A. K. 1990. *Optimization in Economic Theory,* Second Edition. Oxford: Oxford University Press.

Durr, P. A. 2001. The Biology, Ecology and Agroforestry Potential of the Raintree, *Samanea saman* (Jacq.) Merr. *Agroforestry Systems.* 51(3): 223-237.

FAO (Food and Agriculture Organization). 1989. *Forestry and Food Security.* FAO Forestry Paper No. 90. Rome: Food and Agriculture Organization of the United Nations.

FAO (Food and Agriculture Organization), 1999. *The State of Food Insecurity in the World–1999.* Rome: Food and Agricultural Organization of the United Nations.

Fanta (Food and Nutrition Technical Assistance Project). 2001. *Improving the Nutrition Impacts of Agriculture Interventions: Strategy and Policy Brief.* Food and Nutrition Technical Assistance Project. Academy for Educational Development, Washington, DC. <http://www.fantaproject.org> Update March 2001.

Filmer, D. and L. Pritchett. 2002. Environmental Degradation and the Demand for Children: Searching for the Vicious Circle. *Environmental and Development Economics.* 7(1): 123-146.

ICRAF (International Center for Research in Agroforestry). 1997. *Mali Trees for Food Security.* <http://www.worldbank.org/html/cgiar/newsletter/june97/9icraf.html>. Updated June 1997 (accessed May 11, 2001).

Kwesiga, F. 1999. *Improved Fallows for Sustainable Food Security in Eastern Zambia.* Transactions of the Zimbabwe Scientific Association. Conference Paper Supplement. pp. 72-83.

Larson, B. 1992. Principles of Stochastic Dynamic Optimization in Resource Management: The Continuous-Time Case. *Agricultural Economics.* 7(2): 91-107.

Longhurst, R. 1987. *Household Food Security, Tree Planting, and the Poor: The Case of Gujaret.* Social Forestry Network Paper 5d. London: Overseas Development Institute.

Nair, P. K. R. 1990. *The Prospects for Agroforestry in the Tropics.* World Bank Technical Paper No. 131. Washington, DC: World Bank.

Nuppaneu, S. 1991. *Optimal Control Model for Household Food Security.* Mimeo. University of Zimbabwe, Harare.

Ogden, C. L. 1996. *Considering Nutrition in National Forestry Programmes.* <http://www.fao.org/docrep/W216E/w2167e00.htm> accessed 5/15/01.

Palm, C. A. 1995. Contribution of Agroforestry Trees to Nutrient Requirements of Intercropped Plants. *Agroforestry System.* 30(1/2): 105-124.

Phillips, T. and Taylor, D. 1990. Optimal Control of Food Security: A Conceptual Framework. *American Journal of Agricultural Economics.* 72(5): 1304-1310.

Rajasekaran, B., M. Warren, and S. C. Babu. 1994. Farmer Participatory Approach to Increase Fodder Security Through Agroforestry Systems. *Agriculture and Human Values.* 11(1): 1-9.

Roe, T. and T. Graham-Thomas. 1986. Yield Risk in a Dynamic Model of the Agricultural Household. In I. J. Singh, L. Squire, and J. Strauss (eds.) *Agricultural Household Models.* Baltimore: Johns Hopkins University Press.

Ruel, M. T. and C. E. Levin. 2001. *Assessing the Potential for Food-Based Strategies to Reduce Vitamin A and Iron Deficiencies: A Review of Recent Evidence.* International Food Policy Research Institute, MOST, and the USAID Micronutrient Project.

Smith, L. C., and L. Haddad. 2000. *Explaining Child Malnutrition in Developing Countries*. IFPRI Research Report 111, Washington, DC, USA. International Food Policy Research Institute. 107p.

Tshiamala-Tshibangu, N. and J. D. Ndjigba. 1999. Use of Non-Wood Forest Products in Cameroon: A Forest Project in Mount Koupe. *Tropicultura*. 2(16/17): 70-79.

Uchimura, E. 1994. *Role and Effective Use of Nitrogen-Fixing Trees in Agroforestry Systems*. JIRCAS International Symposium Series (Japan). No. 1: 78-84.

UNICEF. 1998. *The State of the World's Children 1998*. United Nations Children's Fund, New York, Osford University Press. 131p.

Quality Protein Maize:
Overcoming the Hurdles

S. K. Vasal

SUMMARY. Quality Protein Maize (QPM), a nutritionally enhanced maize, was developed by researchers from CIMMYT using too genetic systems–opaque-2 and genetic modifiers. The use of these two genetic systems overcame the highly complex problems that were inherent in the original soft endosperm opaques. This review describes the ever-evolving breeding options and strategies for the development of QPM with examples from the CIMMYT maize program, where much of the research and practical breeding work has been done. The soft endosperm opaque-2 materials developed earlier had poor agronomic performances and lacked producer and consumer acceptance. To overcome these constraints, subsequent research explored various options, with and without high lysine mutants. Like other institutions, CIMMYT researchers tried and critically examined the merits and demerits of different strategies. Of all the strategies available, the selection for modified kernels in which CIMMYT scientists had gained information, experience, and confidence seemed viable. To implement this strategy, modified opaque-2 donor stocks were built and were subsequently used for expanding the QPM developmental efforts. A large volume of QPM germplasm was developed using different breeding options, which were later merged and reorganized into a fixed number of pools and populations to permit working in homozygous opaque-2 genetic backgrounds. The development of QPM hybrids was the next turning point in the mid-80s. During

S. K. Vasal is Distinguished Scientist and Maize Breeder (and co-recipient of the World Food Prize, 2000), CIMMYT, Apdo Postal 6-641, 06600 Mexico, D.F., Mexico (E-mail: s.vasal@cgiar.org).

[Haworth co-indexing entry note]: "Quality Protein Maize: Overcoming the Hurdles." Vasal, S. K. Co-published simultaneously in *Journal of Crop Production* (Food Products Press, an imprint of The Haworth Press, Inc.) Vol. 6, No. 1/2 (#11/12), 2002, pp. 193-227; and: *Food Systems for Improved Human Nutrition: Linking Agriculture, Nutrition, and Productivity* (ed: Palit K. Kataki, and Suresh Chandra Babu) Food Products Press, an imprint of The Haworth Press, Inc., 2002, pp. 193-227. Single or multiple copies of this article are available for a fee from The Haworth Document Delivery Service [1-800-HAWORTH, 9:00 a.m. - 5:00 p.m. (EST). E-mail address: getinfo@haworthpressinc.com].

the QPM developmental process, serious problems inherent in the op-aques were circumvented and since then, rapid progress has been made. There is a renewed interest in QPM and several countries have recently released QPM varieties and hybrids. To further accelerate the QPM de-velopmental process, to enhance its popularity amongst nations and its farmers, and to meet future challenges, innovative ideas and the tools of biotechnology will be needed. *[Article copies available for a fee from The Haworth Document Delivery Service: 1-800-HAWORTH. E-mail address: <getinfo@haworthpressinc.com> Website: <http://www.HaworthPress.com> © 2002 by The Haworth Press, Inc. All rights reserved.]*

KEYWORDS. Quality protein maize, opaque-2 gene, modified kernels, breeding options, strategies, soft opaques, tryptophan, lysine

INTRODUCTION

Maize (*Zea mays* L.) is one of the three major cereal crops and its share of the total world grain production is substantial and significant. Its worldwide economic importance is due to its trade as a food, feed, and an industrial grain crop. The total area under maize has fluctuated at around 130 million hectares with a total production of 574 million tons (Ito, 1998). A large portion (66.8%) of the global maize produced is utilized as animal feed. The use of maize for direct human consumption has remained stable at around 100 million tons per year for the past decade. In approximately 20 developing countries, maize is a staple food crop and meets the protein and calorie requirements of its human population. Unfortunately, maize protein is of poor nutritional quality as it is deficient in two essential amino acids, lysine and tryptophan, which the hu-man body cannot synthesize and thus has to be supplemented. Improving the nutritional quality of staple food crops including maize is, therefore, a noble goal. This strategy is particularly important for cereal crops as benefits can reach hundreds of millions of people rapidly, without changing the traditional food habits of the consumers.

Biochemists discovered the nutritionally deficient characteristics of maize about 90 years ago. Yet, research initiatives to remedy the deficiency traits of maize had to wait for almost 50 years until the discovery of high lysine mutant opaque-2 (o_2) maize (Mertz et al. 1964) by distinguished Purdue scientists that paved the way for its genetic manipulation. However, this mutant maize had several inherent problems related to storage, pest damage, appearances of its kernels, and agronomic performance. This review discusses the general but pertinent aspects of high quality protein research and the breeding strategies employed to circumvent problems of a complex nature that enabled the development of the QPM germplasm.

NUTRITIONAL AND BIOCHEMICAL CHARACTERIZATION OF NORMAL MAIZE

The germ and the endosperm constitute the two most important parts of a maize kernel. They vary in size and their relative contribution to the quantity and the quality of protein. Depending upon the type of maize, the germ and the endosperm may contribute 8-10% and 80-85% of the kernel's weight, respectively, while the pericarp and the aleurone layer contributes to the rest of the kernel's weight. The germ protein is superior to the endosperm protein in both its quantity and quality. The corn endosperm protein consists of four fractions (Osborne 1897): the water-soluble albumins (3%), salt soluble globulins (3%), alcohol soluble zein or prolamine (60%), and alkali soluble glutelin (34%). In contrast, the germ protein is predominantly in the form of albumin (+60%) while containing a relatively small alcohol soluble fraction (Schnieder 1955; Tsai 1979; Wall and Paulis 1978). These protein fractions vary in their lysine content. In general albumins, globulins, and glutelin are quite rich in their lysine content (> 2 g/100 g protein) compared to the very low levels in the prolamine fraction (0.01%). This fraction is, therefore, nutritionally deficient and cannot support the growth of rats (Osborne and Mendel 1914a, b). The poor nutritional quality of the endosperm protein results from the high proportion of prolamine (zein) fraction (Table 1), which is practically devoid of lysine. Lysine in maize is considered to be the first limiting amino acid and tryptophan the second. The unfavorable amino acid composition, especially of lysine and tryptophan, reduces the protein value of ordinary maize for monogastric animals and humans as they cannot synthesize these amino acids.

HIGH QUALITY PROTEIN MUTANTS

In the absence of specific genes and gene combinations, the genetic manipulation and breeding of high quality protein varieties and hybrids of maize was not possible. In the mid-sixties, the discovery of the first mutant allele opaque-2,

TABLE 1. Protein Fractions in the Endosperm of Normal and Opaque-2 Maize.

Protein fraction	Normal	Opaque-2
Albumins	3.2	13.2
Globulins	1.5	3.9
Prolamine	47.2	22.8
Glutelin	35.1	50.0

which has twice (o_2) the levels of lysine and tryptophan compared to normal maize, paved the way for such breeding efforts (Mertz, Bates, and Nelson 1964). The search for newer and better mutants has continueds. Following the discovery of the opaque-2 mutant, another mutant allele floury-2 (fl2) with similar effects was identified (Nelson et al. 1965). Additional mutants that have been identified are: opaque-7 (McWhirter 1971); opaque-6 (Ma and Nelson 1975), floury-3 (Ma and Nelson 1975), mucronate (Salamini et al. 1983), and defective endosperm B30 (Salamini et al. 1979). Mutants with a high lysine and high zein content have also been reported (Nelson 1981). Two such mutants are opaque 7749 and opaque-11. Unfortunately, none of the new mutants offered any real advantage over the opaque-2; therefore, the main focus of CIMMYT's work on quality protein maize has involved an intensive use of the o_2 gene. Double mutant combinations of o_2 fl_2 (Nelson 1969) and su_2 o_2 (Paez 1973; Glover et al. 1975; Vasal et al. 1980) have also been developed and studied. Initially, these combinations generated great interest as they produced translucent kernels, however, the results in different genetic backgrounds were not the same. Several research programs around the world that have tried these combinations have had limited successes. More detailed information on these double mutant combinations can be found in some earlier CIMMYT publications (Vasal 1994; Bjarnason and Vasal 1992).

Changes in the Amino Acid Profile

Of the mutants described in the previous section, the o_2 and fl_2 mutants have been studied the most for their biochemical effects and alterations in their amino acid profile. Both these mutants have higher levels of lysine and tryptophan, the two most limiting amino acids in the endosperm protein of normal maize. Compared to normal maize, these mutants also have a higher histidine, arginine, and aspartic acid, and glycine levels, but have lower glutamic acid, alanine, and leucine levels. A notable reduction in leucine is desirable for a more favorable leucine-isoleucine ratio, which in turn helps to liberate more tryptophan for niacin biosynthesis. The level of methionine is also higher in mutants such as fl_2, o_7, and o_6.

Alterations in Protein Fractions

The introduction of o_2 or other mutant alleles into normal maize alters the relative amounts of the maize endosperm protein four fractions (Table 1). The prolamine or zein fraction is drastically reduced by almost 50% with a concomitant increase in the relative amounts of other fractions such as albumins, globulins, and glutelin that are rich in their lysine contents. It is, therefore, apparent that o_2 and other high lysine mutants increase their levels of lysine and tryptophan by suppressing the synthesis of lysine-deficient prolamine fraction.

The mutant alleles are located on different chromosomes; on chromosome 7 in the o_2, on chromosome 4 in the fl_2, on chromosome 10 in the o_7, on chromosome 8 in the fl_3, and on chromosome 7 in the $De\text{-}B_{30}$. Most mutants are recessive and express their effects on zein synthesis only when present in their homozygous states. The fl_2 and fl_3 are semi-dominant and their effect on protein quality and kernel opacity depends upon the dosage of the recessive alleles in the triploid endosperm. Mutant genotypes have several features in common: a reduced zein fraction, soft chalky endosperm texture, and are deficient in their ability to accumulate sufficient dry matter.

MAJOR DRAWBACKS AND SOME KEY PROBLEMS

The commonly observed association in crops of secondary or pleiotropic effects is a negative influence on its agronomic performances concurrently with the drastic but desirable effects of its major genes, also holds true for the o_2 and other mutants. The opaque-2 conversions of the normal counterparts, in general, have an adverse affect in its agronomic performances (Alexander 1966, Lambert et al. 1969; Harpstead 1969; Sreeramulu and Bauman 1970; Gevers 1972; Sriwatanapongse et al. 1974; Singh and Asnani 1975; Bauman 1975; Vasal 1975; Vasal et al. 1980, 1984; Glover and Mertz 1987; Glover 1988; Villegas et al. 1992).

For both the OPVs and the hybrids of the original soft endosperm opaque-2 materials, reduction in yield is its most serious drawback. On an average, the yield is 10-15% less, depending upon the genetic background of the materials. However, genetic background effects with a higher or lower than average yield value have also been observed. An inherent early cessation and reduced dry matter accumulation is the major reason for this yield difference. The reduction in yield is also reflected by the reduced kernel weight and density. The second major problem is the unattractive kernel phenotype. The conversions change the kernels to a dull and soft chalky appearance, not acceptable to the producers and consumers accustomed to the normal hard, shiny, flinty grains. Loose packing of starch granules, air spaces, and an amorphous protein matrix are possible reasons for the formation of such kernel phenotypes. Apart from the soft phenotype of the yellow maize, its color intensity is also reduced. Kernel phenotype is of particular concern especially for farmers in developing countries.

Physiological drying of the converted materials is also adversely affected. At harvest, the kernels retain more moisture and post-harvest kernel drying is very slow. A thicker pericarp, hydrophilic compounds, and higher potassium content are possible reasons interfering with the faster drying of the mutant kernels. The tendencies for the mutant kernels to retain moisture longer also result in its higher incidences and greater vulnerability to the ear rot causing pathogens. In regions experiencing low and cold temperatures, the soft opaques also suffer from reduced germination and poor stand establishment. The soft floury o_2 kernels are also subject to kernel cracking, and therefore, to varying degree of losses during the process of its mechanical harvesting. The post-harvest losses are also substantial due to the greater damage caused by the stored grain pests. The aforementioned drawbacks vary in magnitude for different regions of the world, but were considered sufficiently difficult, inter-related, complex, and viewed with serious concerns that changed the optimism and high hopes of developing nutritious maize of the mid-sixties and early-seventies to deep disappointment and frustration. A reduced interest in nutritious maize breeding efforts coupled with a decline in funding source, forced many programs and institutions to have either less involvement or to completely abandon QPM research activities with some exceptions.

The genetic effects of o_2 differ in different genetic backgrounds and even within the same background, especially when populations are structured on a family basis. Differential genetic background effects can play a magnificent role in the selection and development of superior desirable genotypes. Innovative strategies and approaches are sometimes needed to manipulate them to a breeder's advantage.

BREEDING STRATEGIES
FOR DEVELOPING QUALITY PROTEIN MAIZE GERMPLASM

Early efforts at CIMMYT and elsewhere were directed towards developing soft chalky opaque-2 varieties and hybrids. Conversion of normal endosperm OPVs and inbreds to standard soft opaque-2 phenotype was attempted on a worldwide basis using a straightforward standard backcrossing procedure. In some instances, the conversion program was slightly modified to gain time either by skipping segregating generation or identifying plants that carried o_2 allele in heterozygous condition. A wide array of opaque-2 varieties and hybrids were developed using this approach. It may also be pointed out that the conversion process was greatly facilitated by the opaque-2 phenotype that served as a useful marker in selecting opaque-2 kernels during the segregating generations. The story with the opaque-2 hybrids was not very different. Inbred lines entering into a particular hybrid combination were converted to opaque-2 in developing an opaque-2 hybrid version of its normal counterpart. Thus, conversion efforts all around the world resulted in the development of a large number of soft endosperm opaque-2 varieties and hybrids, but unfortunately, most of them suffered from problems described earlier. The backcross programs did not help to remedy problems that were often encountered in soft opaque-2 materials. In addition to the conversion programs, a few breeding programs at different institutions developed broad-based opaque-2 populations and synthetics using different procedures and approaches (Dudley et al. 1975; Singh et al. 1977; Motto et al. 1978; Vasal et al. 1982). A detailed discussion of various procedures used by different breeders can be found in a review article published by Vasal (1994).

The population improvement efforts in soft opaque-2 materials have been rather limited. CIMMYT has used full-sib recurrent selection and modified half-sib procedure to improve some soft opaque-2 populations such as Texpeno opaque-2, CIMMYT opaque-2, and Composites I, J, and K (Vasal 1994). Others have also used recurrent selection procedures. A modified ear-to-row procedure was used in Iowa Super Stiff Stalk synthetic (BSSS-o_2) and synthetic disease-oil (DO-o_2) developed at the University of Illinois. Two cycles of selection conducted in these materials increased the lysine yield by 8-14%, most of the progress resulting from an increase in grain yield (Dudley et al. 1975). Full-sib and selfed-progeny selection procedures have also been proposed and used by other research workers (St. Martin et al. 1982; Zorilla and Crane 1982).

With time, the problems confronting the soft opaque-2 materials were well recognized and understood, and maize breeders started exploring new ideas, approaches, and criteria's that could remedy at least some of the most serious problems in the soft opaque-2 materials. Most of the selection criteria emphasized the need for selection of improved kernel hardness, but by different ways. The light transmission and opacity score methods were suggested by Paez et al. (1969). This method involved the selection of modified opaques with different degrees of translucent or vitreous kernels using an illuminated glass screen, not necessarily associated with better kernel weight and density. The method being rather simple with no costs involved, except for the time needed to select the desired kernel types. Improvement in kernel hardness of soft opaques could also be determined by the kernel shearing strength (Loesch et al. 1977). Kernel shearing strength is a mechanical procedure that measures kernel hardness with accuracy and precision. A shear press is used for this purpose requiring an optimal sample size of 10 grams per measurement. Heritability estimates for two groups of 100 s_2 families of BSBB o_2/o_2 were 0.77 and 0.88 suggesting that the selection for kernel hardness in these synthetics would be effective. Since opaque-2 kernels have little mechanical strength and fracture easily, this procedure potentially could help improve kernel hardness and reduce kernel breakage. Establishing optimal values for mechanical methods of measuring kernel hardness will help determine the important agronomic and protein quality traits as well as test hypothesis and relationships between grain quality, protein quality, disease and insect response, and germination percentage in opaque-2 maize. Although small amounts of kernels are needed to measure kernel hardness, its principal disadvantage is its relatively higher cost and otherwise limited usefulness in a conventional maize-breeding program.

Increasing kernel density has also been suggested as a way to improve kernel hardness (Motto et al. 1978; Wessel-Beaver et al. 1984). Wessel-Beaver et al. (1984) used two methods of volumetric measurements to determine kernel density: water displacement and cage methods. Other methods used have been selection for relative kernel mass, visual screening, and selection for translucent/modified opaque-2 kernels (Gevers 1992). Selection of kernels using both relative kernel mass (RKM) and translucence are expected to accelerate the accumulation of genetic modifiers (Gevers 1992). This procedure should help bring about a close resemblance of opaques to normal kernel phenotype in terms of hardness and translucence with a minimal decline in its lysine content.

Since kernel phenotype of soft opaques has been a major hurdle in it'gaining acceptance, CIMMYT breeders have routinely used light transmission method as a strategy for improving kernel appearance and circumventing other problems considered important.

DEVELOPMENT OF HARD ENDOSPERM OPAQUE-2 MAIZE AT CIMMYT

The phenotypic and agronomic limitations of soft opaque-2 maize varieties and hybrids were the major reasons for its poor acceptance, even though the kernels were of improved nutritional value. CIMMYT breeders experimented with several alternative approaches for overcoming these constraints. Unfortunately, many of the suggested approaches failed to produce satisfactory results (Vasal 1994). Coupled with reduced funding, de-emphasis or abandonment of research efforts partially or completely by many Institutes, and lack of alternative and innovative approaches, breeding efforts aimed at developing nutritionally improved opaque-2 cultivars that could compete with normal maize cultivars, therefore, suffering a setback since the mid-1970s. Fortunately, the few research institutes that relentlessly continued their research activities to overcome the constraints of developing competitive nutritious maize were International Center on Maize and Wheat Improvement (CIMMYT), Crows Hybrid Seed Co., USA; and the South African Maize Program at the University of Natal. More recently, research institutes that have revived their interest in QPM are Texas A&M University, USA and the national agriculture programs of China, Brazil, India, Ghana, and Sasakawa Global 2000 Maize Project in Africa.

As discussed earlier, for many developing countries the problems of low yield and unacceptable seed quality traits associated with the soft opaque-2 grain texture were its major constraints. It was therefore necessary to increase the grain yield and develop a strategy to modify soft opaque-2 kernel appearance that was indistinguishable from the normal maize. Paez et al. (1969) published the first research note that provided such a hope. This note suggested the selection of modified opaques for improving kernel phenotype without sacrificing protein quality. Following such an important discovery, Dr. J. H. Lonnquist, then Director of the Maize Program, CIMMYT and a visiting scientist, Dr. V. L. Asnani, from India also initiated an exploratory research effort at CIMMYT in 1969. This research found the presence of partially modified opaque-2 kernels in different opaque-2 converted varieties. Initially, the selected ears were handled on an ear-to-row basis. Kernels with different degrees of modifications were concurrently sorted and their behavior studied in the following generations. The protein qualities of different modified classes were also monitored during this process. As this strategy began to show promise, this small effort grew into a full-fledged research program by the mid-1970s. By then CIMMYT's maize breeders had accumulated sufficient information and gained confidence that this approach, in addition to modifying kernel phenotype, could help overcome other problems affecting standard soft opaque-2 genotypes. The timely funding by the UNDP Global Project to CIMMYT helped accelerate the development of the hard endosperm opaque-2 maize. As the name implies, this modified maize had o_2 recessive allele to boost its protein quality and had a modified kernel appearance resembling the normal endosperm maize genotypes. The Director of the Maize Program, Dr. E. W. Sprague and CIMMYT maize breeders named this special maize as Quality Protein Maize (QPM). The success of QPM was due to breeders and biochemists working as part of an interdisciplinary team. The sequence of events that led to the development of this maize is quite interesting and will be discussed later. As is apparent, the strategy was to look desperately for genetic variation for kernel modification from soft opaque-2 cultivars that were developed mostly through the conversion programs. In this context, the development of soft o_2 genotypes was, therefore, not a wasteful effort. It was only from these materials that the modified opaques were selected.

BEGINNING OF A COMBINED TWO GENETIC SYSTEM APPROACH

The first phase of this project was tedious, and at times, disappointing and frustrating. Looking for genetic variations in partially modified kernels of soft opaques was a desperate strategy. As promises of this new approach grew into a reality, efforts were made to identify genetic variation for modified kernels in practically all-genetic backgrounds in which o_2 allele had been successfully introduced. This exercise involved selection of the so-called modified opaques from all opaque-2 breeding activities at CIMMYT. Partially modified ears were selected from the ongoing opaque-2 conversion programs, populations, and composites undergoing improvement, opaque-2 population crosses and the seed increases of opaque-2 materials for international testing and from other types of o_2 trials. As expected, the frequency of such ears was quite low. Fortunately, since CIMMYT breeders were handling numerous populations, several ears were selected. This initial effort also helped breeders to identify genetic backgrounds exhibiting a higher frequency of modified opaque-2 ears. Though varying numbers of modified ears were identified from different genetic backgrounds, some populations were particularly interesting for their contribution of modified ears: Ant. Ver. 181 o_2 × Venzuela-1 opaque-2, Thai opaque-2 composite, Composite K, CIMMYT opaque-2 composite, PD (MS)6–Gr. Am., and PD (MS)6-Eto-Cuba-Pop. Crist.1. Of great interest, was the cross population of Ant. Ver 181 o_2 × Venzuela-1 opaque-2 that showed an unusually high frequency of modified ears when grown in a yield trial. Good-looking ears from all the replications were selected and modified kernels sorted from each ear, and subsequently used for recombination to develop the first modified opaque-2 population. The occurrence of an unexpectedly high frequency of modified ears from this particular population cross encouraged CIMMYT breeders to demonstrate the value of this strategy and for expediting the progress of selection and development of QPM germplasm with desired kernel characteristics. This chance event renewed the enthusiasm and hopes of developing competitive QPM germplasm.

Development of Modified Phenotype Opaque-2 Donor Stocks

When selection for vitreous opaques was initiated, the need to develop donor stocks with modified kernel phenotypes having good quality protein was realized. Good donor stocks were needed to facilitate the conversion of normal materials to QPM as rapidly as possible. Based on the genetic variations encountered in different materials and the continuing selection for modified kernels in individually selected modified ears, two possible approaches were considered to develop appropriate QPM donor stocks: intrapopulation selection for kernel modification and synthesis of hard endosperm opaque-2 families.

Intrapopulation Selection for Kernel Modification

This approach required cyclic selection of modified kernels with an acceptable level of protein quality. Before widely adopting this strategy, it was imperative to choose appropriate opaque-2 populations having modified ears in relatively higher frequencies. Four tropical populations and one highland population that met this criterion were Composite K, Ver. 181-Ant.gpo. o_2 × Venzuela-1 opaque-2, Thai opaque-2 Composite, PD(MS)6H.E. o_2, and Composite 1. Controlled pollinations using full-sib selection procedure were used in four tropical populations. The breeding process involved selection of superior families followed by the selection of the best plants in these superior families for pollination. Plant to plant crosses were attempted to develop full-sibs. Only families with a good protein quality were used for pollination. At harvest, good-looking modified ears were selected and later sorted individually for modified kernels that were then used for planting the next season's crop. Simultaneously, samples of 10 kernels were analyzed for protein quality. At least 3 to 4 cycles of selections were required, before such materials exhibited an acceptable level of kernel modification to be used as donor stocks. The half-sib approach employed for Composite 1 was quite similar to the modified ear-to-row approach used by Lonnquist (1964). The procedure required planting half-sib families in an isolated half-sib recombination block using a ratio of 2 female: 1 male. At harvest, selections of modified ears were made between and within families. The modified kernels selected from each ear were analyzed before planting the crop for the next season. This procedure enabled the recombination and generation of new families. In addition, two cycles of selection in one year became possible. The QPM pools that were developed subsequently were also subjected to this selection procedure.

Synthesis of Hard Endosperm Opaque-2 Families

The second strategy employed to develop QPM donor stocks involved the use of superior hard endosperm opaque-2 families. These families had been improved for kernel modification either through full-sib or selfed progeny selection for at least 3-4 generations. The yellow families were recombined by controlled pollination to develop yellow hard endosperm opaque-2 composite (Yellow H.E. o_2) (Population 39). Similarly, recombination of the White families resulted in the formation of White H.E. o_2 composite (Population 40). The selection of individual plants in superior families coupled with the selection of good-looking modified ears and kernels continued during and following the recombination process. The families used in the recombination process were not only highly modified, but also had good protein quality.

For both of the above strategies, once the populations were either identified or formed, at least 5-6 additional cycles of selection were needed for achieving good kernel modification. By mid-1974, it was felt that these materials had acquired a reasonably high frequency of genetic modifiers and could, therefore, be used successfully as QPM donor stocks. The stage was thus set for the conversion of normal materials to hard endosperm opaque-2.

EXPANDED QPM DEVELOPMENT EFFORTS AND STRATEGIES

The development of the QPM donor stock provided new hopes for building a wide array of QPM germplasm. The two approaches adopted to achieve this goal were (1) the use of a modified backcrossing-cum-recurrent selection designed to handle the two genetic systems of opaque-2 gene and modifiers effectively and efficiently during the conversion process, and (2) development of genetically broad based QPM gene pools with different adaptations, maturity, grain color and texture.

A Modified Backcrossing-Cum-Recurrent Selection Program

A modified backcross-cum-recurrent selection procedure had to be used to develop a resource base with a wide array of QPM germplasm. To achieve this objective, it was necessary to generate QPM versions of several potentially important normal endosperm maize populations and pools with different adaptations, maturities, grain color, and texture. To initiate this conversion process, one or more QPM donor stocks were used. The intent was to transfer the opaque-2 gene to boost protein quality, modify kernel appearances, and to improve agronomic performances using the polygenically inherited system of genetic modifiers. As one would expect, a standard backcross system would not have been effective, and therefore, a modified procedure was necessary to produce the QPM germplasms of desired kernel characteristics. Therefore, CIMMYT breeders designed an appropriate procedure, by combining the features of both backcrossing and recurrent selection programs. The salient features of this modified scheme are as follows.

- The procedure was adopted in maize populations that were undergoing improvement using full-sib or half-sib progeny based recurrent selection procedures. Thus an improved version/cycle of the recurrent parent was used in each backcross.
- The degree of kernel modification achieved was an important factor that determined the time for attempting the next backcross. The complex inheritance of the opaque-2 modifiers often dictated the advancing of the F2 generation to F3 and beyond to improve upon the frequency of favorable modifiers prior to making the next backcross.
- With this scheme it was possible to work in homozygous o_2 backgrounds essential for accumulating genetic modifiers, but the procedure did slow down the recovery of the recurrent parent genotype.
- This procedure also laid emphasis on the selection for modified kernels in every generation, in addition to other traits. The backcrossed families were handled separately as a subgroup for a generation or two before being merged with families homozygous for the opaque-2 gene and being improved continuously every generation through recurrent FS selection.
- Selection for stable modifiers became necessary, provided families were evaluated at another location in one season and recombined during the following season.

- After each backcross, it was not necessary to start all over again. Therefore, the research efforts used in accumulating modifiers were not lost.
- The scheme also permitted accumulation of other modifiers controlling kernel weight and density. This control required selection in segregating generation of only those backcrossed families exhibiting no difference in kernel weight between the opaques and normals.
- During the recombination process, each family was crossed with several other families in a full-sib manner. Families having a common parent were planted along side each other in the following season. This procedure allowed researchers to study the behavior of each family for their ability to transmit the hard endosperm opaque-2 trait to other families.
- At any stage during the conversion process, if the materials performed satisfactorily, their seed was increased and used for various types of breeding activities including evaluation trials.

It is important to mention that during the conversion process, emphasis was laid on attributes (both plant and seeds) that resulted in the improvement of materials for yield, kernel appearance, reduced ear rot incidence, and rapid kernel drying characteristics. A number of potentially useful normal maize populations and pools were converted to H.E. o_2 types using the above procedure. Compared to their normal counterparts, some of the QPM populations performed competitively for yield and other agronomic traits (Table 2). Additionally, the modified kernels had better stability over different environments. During the conversion process, continuous monitoring of protein quality ensured that these new materials had the quantity and quality of protein very similar to the soft opaque-2 types.

Development of Genetically Broad-Based
Hard Endosperm Opaque-2 Pools

The conversion process described in the preceding section was used only for a limited number of materials. However, realizing the need for different QPM genotypes around the world, a number of QPM gene pools were also developed. Efforts were made to accumulate genetic modifiers in these pools from as many sources as possible in homozygous opaque-2 backgrounds. These pools were formed in several different ways as described below.

- Genetic mixing of hard endosperm opaque-2 varieties, variety-crosses and of hybrids, if available.
- Genetic mixing of soft endosperm opaque-2 materials followed by selection of genetic modifiers in homozygous opaque-2 genetic backgrounds.

- Crossing of soft opaque-2 varieties with one or more hard endosperm opaque-2 sources followed by selection of genetic modifiers in each cycle of selection.
- Selection of hard endosperm opaque-2 families was started independently for each of the several opaque-2 populations. Continuous selection in these families was practiced by growing either selfed progenies in each generation or through some form of mild inbreeding procedure involving plant-to-plant crosses. Few generations between and within ear selection for modified opaque-2 kernels involving the families exhibiting good modified appearances were recombined either by controlled pollination procedures or in a half-sib isolation block using varying male to female ratios. The subsequent generations of the QPM pools so formed were then handled by the same procedure.
- Crosses of normal maize varieties to one or more H.E. o_2 donor stocks were also developed. The F_1 crosses so developed were advanced to the F_2 generation by selfing or sib-mating procedures. Advancing in a half-sib recombination block or by planting as a balanced bulk in isolation could also advance the F_1 crosses to F_2. Segregating ears not showing soft opaque-2 kernels were preferentially selected. The selected ears were shelled individually and the hard endosperm opaque-2 segregates were sorted carefully. Partially modified kernels that were sure to carry the homozygous o_2 allele were preferred over nearly normal looking kernels at least in the segregating generations to avoid the possibility of selecting some heterozygous normal kernels. The selected segregates were planted either as a bulk in isolation or on a family basis in a half-sib recombination block in isolation. Selection of modified ears and modified kernels in each ear was continued for at least 3-4 cycles to accumulate favorable modifiers.
- QPM pools formed via one of the above-mentioned ways had a mixed kernel texture. Selection for good modifiers continued at least in several of the initial cycles. Once good progress was achieved for kernel modification, the flints and dents were split into two pools with specific kernel textures.
- Normal inbreds were crossed to one or more hard endosperm opaque-2 sources and the F_1 crosses were advanced to F_2 by selfing. Hard endosperm opaque-2 segregates were selected from selfed progenies and then recombined to develop a hard endosperm opaque-2 pool.
- Inbred based QPM germplasm was also used to develop the QPM pools. The QPM pools so developed were extremely useful for the hybrid program due to the higher probability of extracting superior QPM lines.

TABLE 2. Comparisons of Normal and QPM Versions for Yield and Other Agronomic Traits.

Material	Yield in tons/ha		QPM as	Ear height (cm)		Days 50% silking		Ear rots (%)	
	Normal	QPM	% of normal	Normal	QPM	Normal	QPM	Normal	QPM
Tuxpeno 1	6.19	6.15	99.4	111	110	61	60	2.2	5.4
Mix.1 Col. Gpo.1xEto	6.12	5.68	92.9	107	105	60	58	2.9	4.5
Mezcla Amarilla	5.43	5.24	96.4	103	106	58	58	2.9	5.7
Amarillo Dentado	5.35	5.23	97.7	125	110	61	57	2.5	3.2
Tuxpeno Caribe	6.39	5.90	92.3	117	115	61	58	2.5	4.2
Ant.Rep. Dominicana	5.35	5.08	94.9	100	112	56	57	2.3	3.7
La Posta	6.47	5.90	91.2	131	122	62	59	3.1	4.0

QPM POOLS DEVELOPED

Using some of the procedures described above, the CIMMYT maize program was able to develop a large number of QPM pools with tropical and subtropical adaptations and different grain colors and textures. A few highland QPM pools have also been developed, but because of the longer cropping cycle and only one season per year, the progress has been rather slow compared to the tropical and subtropical pools. A total of seven hard endosperm opaque-2 tropical and 6 subtropical pools were developed and improved continuously using a modified half-sib improvement selection procedure. The important characteristics of these QPM pools have been listed in Table 3.

Handling of QPM Pools

Once the QPM pools were developed and thoroughly recombined in at least 3-4 cycles of recombination, they were uniformly handled using the same breeding procedure.

- All QPM gene pools were improved using a half-sib family structure. The half-sib (HS) families were planted in a HS recombination block with a preferred male to female ratio of 1:2. The pools were planted sufficiently away from normals to prevent contamination by normal pollen.
- Enough families (400-500) were handled in each pool to perpetuate a substantially large population size of 8000 to 9000 plants.
- The use of half-sib selection system permitted the completion of one cycle of selection per season or two cycles per year.
- Protein quality was monitored continuously and at the desired stages of each cycle of selection, 10-15 kernels of each family were analyzed. The quality of the segregates that were planted and subjected to analysis were

similar so as to reduce selection bias. The families that registered poor protein quality were rejected either before planting or before harvesting, depending upon the availability of the data.

- A balanced male composite was constituted from only those families exhibiting acceptable quality protein levels. It was, therefore, important to analyze the families for protein quality before planting, to prevent inferior families from entering into the male composite.
- Detasselling undesirable tall and diseased plants either before or during the flowering time helped in the selection of superior plants in male rows.
- Between and within family selection was practiced in each pool to maintain ± 500 families. Strong selection pressure was discouraged to prevent depletion or a loss of useful genes or traits necessary for maintaining future progress and providing a better opportunity for recombination among linked genes.
- The QPM gene pools were treated open-ended to permit introgression of new germplasm.
- To make rapid progress, modifications for the handling of the QPM gene pools were introduced. All selected ears at harvest did not have to enter into the male composite, therefore, ears saved at harvest could be grouped either as males or females depending upon the family from which they were selected. All ears selected in the previous cycle were entered as female families. The male composite, however, was formed from only those ears designated as males at harvest time.
- Initially, all QPM gene pools were handled at only one location. With an improvement in this process, some pressure was exercised for stability of kernel modification by planting families in at least two locations.
- Genetic improvement in QPM pools was monitored continually for grain yield and other traits of particular interest. To monitor two or more rows of each cycle of selection with or without replication were planted at the end of each pool.

Use of Partial Contamination Technique in Pools

To select for better kernel weight and density in QPM pools, a partial contamination technique was used at least in some tropical QPM gene pools. In white QPM pools, planting 15-20% of the hills in the male rows with a normal yellow endosperm material contaminated 15-20% of the kernels in each ear. The rest of the hills in the male rows were planted with the white QPM pool. At harvest both yellow and white kernels formed in each ear. Since the yellow kernels resulted from the contamination by normal pollens, they were heterozygous for the opaque-2 gene. The selected ears were shelled individually and

TABLE 3. QPM Gene Pools and Their Characteristics.

QPM pool number	Adaptation	Maturity	Seed color	Seed texture
Pool 15 QPM	Tropical	Early	White	Flint-Dent
Pool 17 QPM	Tropical	Early	Yellow	Flint
Pool 18 QPM	Tropical	Early	Yellow	Dent
Pool 23 QPM	Tropical	Late	White	Flint
Pool 24 QPM	Tropical	Late	White	Dent
Pool 25 QPM	Tropical	Late	Yellow	Flint
Pool 26 QPM	Tropical	Late	Yellow	Dent
Pool 27 QPM	Subtropical	Early	White	Flint-Dent
Pool 29 QPM	Subtropical	Early	Yellow	Flint-Dent
Pool 31 QPM	Subtropical	Intermediate	White	Flint
Pool 32 QPM	Subtropical	Intermediate	White	Dent
Pool 33 QPM	Subtropical	Intermediate	Yellow	Flint
Pool 34 QPM	Subtropical	Intermediate	Yellow	Dent

the kernels sorted for grain color. An equal number of white and yellow kernels from the same ear were compared for kernel weight. For planting the next season crop, only those ears where the QPM kernels had a kernel weight comparable to the normal kernels were selected. The same procedure could be used for the yellow H.E. o_2 materials, but one would need to select for a different kind of seed marker (perhaps purple) in the normal endosperm for exhibiting a clearcut influence or xenia effect on the F1 contaminated kernels. The contamination technique was, therefore, an excellent method for accumulating favorable genetic modifiers for kernel weight and density (Table 4).

The half-sib procedure used at CIMMYT has been a simple, effective, and practical strategy for improving the QPM pools for yield and seed quality traits. The procedure allows for the recombination and generation of new families for the next cycle of the same season. Handling a large number of families and plants using this procedure permitted the integrated selection against a wide array of complex inter-related undesirable traits without drastically affecting the population size and protein quality attributes. The QPM gene pools developed at CIMMYT not only serve as a reservoir for useful genes for further selection, but could also be put to use in several other ways. An elite fraction of good families could be selected from a QPM pool for a more intensive selection process. In addition, such QPM pools can serve as excellent donor stocks for hard endosperm modified opaques. Superior families from a given QPM pool can also be introgressed into a corresponding QPM population already undergoing population improvement. The QPM pools can also serve as a source for extracting QPM lines for developing QPM hybrids. Since most of the QPM gene pools have not been subjected to selfed progeny selection pro-

TABLE 4. 100 Kernel Weight Comparison of Normal and Opaque-2 Kernels from Partially Contaminated Ears with Normal Yellow Pollen.

Material	No. of ears sampled	100 kernel wt. (g)		Difference (g)	Difference (%)
		Normals	Opaques*		
White O_2 B.U. Pool (Flint)	825	29.22	27.42	1.80**	5.83
White O_2 B.U. Pool (Dent)	795	27.19	25.31	1.87**	5.53

* Includes soft and modified opaques.
** Significant at P = 0.01.

cedures, one may expect a low frequency of good lines surviving the inbreeding effects.

REORGANIZATION OF QPM GERMPLASM AND NEW THRUSTS IN GERMPLASM MANAGEMENT STRATEGY

Beginning in 1970, the CIMMYT maize program has perhaps carried out the world's largest quality protein maize program. Earlier research efforts focused on devising research strategies and procedures for overcoming the complex problems of the opaque-2 materials. The breeding and selection strategies used by the CIMMYT maize breeders were carefully chosen after exploring several options. It would have been difficult and perhaps impossible to solve every problem individually. The combined use of opaque-2 gene in conjunction with modifiers facilitated tackling all problems simultaneously. As explained in the foregoing sections, using different methodologies, CIMMYT maize breeders were quite successful in developing a whole array of broadbased QPM germplasm. This development was accomplished within a relatively short time span of no more than 8 years. The total QPM germplasm developed during this period was quite voluminous and could not be handled in an effective and efficient manner through systematic breeding efforts. The merging and reorganization of QPM germplasm was, therefore, necessary to reduce the total volume to a level that could be managed efficiently. The merging process began in 1978 and continued for almost two years. The factors considered important during the merging of QPM germplasm were: adaptation, maturity, grain color, genetic, and phenotypic similarity. All types of QPM germplasm including those developed by the conversion program were included in the merging process. For materials resulting from the conversion program, it was felt that sufficient backcrosses had already been made to the recurrent parent and perhaps little would be gained by pursuing additional backcrosses. A faster progress could perhaps be expected by improving some of these versions directly through cyclic recurrent selection schemes. Since most of the QPM germplasm had been developed at one site in Mexico, an important consideration for CIMMYT breeders was that the future efforts in QPM germplasm management should emphasize higher yield, dependability, and stable kernel modification in varied environments.

Therefore, the available QPM germplasm was merged into pools and populations with adaptation and kernel characteristics most widely needed for use in developing countries. CIMMYT maize breeders also relied tremendously on the information and past experiences of the international maize testing program. Since both the early and late maturing germplasm are in great demand in many developing countries, a decision was made to merge germplasm types that would belong either to the early or late maturity groups. Countries needing intermediate maturing maize germplasm could either cross early and late or modify the maturity to meet specific requirement. Based on the available information, seven tropical and six subtropical QPM gene pools were formed. These are listed in Table 3 along with some important characteristics. In addition to the QPM gene pools, ten advanced and new QPM populations were developed. Six of these populations were tropical and four were subtropical in their adaptation. The number, name, and some of the important attributes of these populations are described in Table 5. Some of these populations were improved through international progeny testing trials for yield, adaptation, seed quality traits, and other important agronomic attributes. The procedures for handling these populations have been described in earlier publications (Vasal et al. 1982, 1984). As part of the population improvement program, some site specific and across site narrow genetic base experimental varieties were also developed to facilitate and encourage the use of these materials in regions where the performance and acceptability of QPM as human food or animal feed have been good.

TABLE 5. QPM Populations and Their Characteristics.

Population number	Name	Adaptation	Maturity	Seed color	Seed texture
61	Early Yellow Flint QPM	Tropical	Early	Yellow	Flint
62	White Flint QPM	Tropical	Late	White	Flint-semiflint
63	Blanco Dentado-1 QPM	Tropical	Late	White	Dent
64	Blanco Dentado-2 QPM	Tropical	Late	White	Dent
65	Yellow Flint QPM	Tropical	Late	Yellow	Flint
66	Yellow Dent QPM	Tropical	Late	Yellow	Dent
67	Templado Blanco Cristalino QPM	Subtrop.	Interm.	White	Flint
68	Templado Blanco Dentado QPM	Subtrop.	Interm.	White	Dent
69	Templado Amarillo QPM	Subtrop.	Interm.	Yellow	Flint
70	Templado Amarillo Dent QPM	Subtrop.	Interm.	Yellow	Dent

The merging and reorganization of the QPM germplasm into a manageable number of pools and populations helped create a focus on the future strategies of its management. All QPM germplasm from this point on was managed in homozygous opaque-2 backgrounds. This merging accelerated the progress towards rapid accumulation of favorable modifiers for kernel modification and kernel weight and density. Working in homozygous opaque-2 backgrounds was also advantageous as it reduced the errors occurring due to misclass-ification and selection of normal kernels during the segregating generations. Moreover, when materials are handled in homozygous opaque-2 backgrounds, one can select normal looking modified kernels with certainty.

RESULTS AND PROGRESS

This section will briefly discuss the results and the progress made in solving the problems affecting the opaques and in developing QPM germplasm. The information presented herein will cover mostly CIMMYT's experience in QPM research.

Overcoming Problems

Several problems associated with the opaque-2 germplasm prevented the large-scale use of such germplasm worldwide. Recognizing the importance of overcoming these problems, CIMMYT scientists prioritized their research activities towards solving these problems, without which the cultivars with improved nutritional value would never gain acceptance amongst the farmers of the developing and developed world. The procedures and strategies used at CIMMYT have produced encouraging results both in solving these problems and more importantly, in developing a wide array of QPM germplasm adapted to tropical and subtropical environments for the developing world. CIMMYT QPM populations will also serve as important donor sources for modifying genes for temperate maize breeding programs.

Improvement in Kernel Phenotype

A major breakthrough has been made in modifying the phenotype of soft opaques to a more normal looking phenotype with a shiny and acceptable appearance. Kernel modification in all QPM germplasm has improved continuously with a concomitant decrease in within ear variability for this trait. There is scope for further improvement and this process will continue to be challenging in the future. Only a fraction of the total available data at CIMMYT will be presented to highlight the progress made on various aspects of kernel modification.

- The number of soft opaque-2 ears has reduced dramatically over the years (Figure 1). In fact it is hard to find a completely soft opaque-2 ear in any of the CIMMYT QPM germplasm. Figure 1 shows a decrease in the percentage of soft ears in different cycles of selection of tropical and subtropical QPM gene pools, respectively.
- Progress towards acceptable kernel modifications has been tremendous in practically all QPM germplasm (Table 6). Figure 1 also shows very clearly that kernel modification has improved continuously in different cycles of selection of QPM gene pools.
- The frequency of different kernel modification classes has been changing consistently over the cycles (Figure 2). A general trend observed in tropical and subtropical QPM gene pools is presented in Figure 3. The soft opaque-2 kernel with a score of 5 has practically disappeared. The frequency of kernels with a score of 4 has decreased continuously over the cycles. Kernels with a score of 3 have varying trends both in the tropical and subtropical QPM gene pools. More importantly the figure shows an encouraging upward trend in the frequency of kernel scores 1 and 2.
- Within ear variation for kernel modification still exists practically in all QPM germplasm. The results presented in Table 7, however, shows a clear reduction in within ear variability as indicated by the decrease in the standard deviation with the progress in the cycles of selection.

The above data clearly demonstrate the improvements that have been made in the kernel modification scores over different cycles of selection. Enough within-ear genetic variability for kernels still exists; therefore, there is a continuing need for future efforts to improve this trait. Therefore, a shift from non-inbred family based selection schemes to selfed progeny selection schemes for accelerating the rapid accumulation of genetic modifiers controlling kernel modification in QPM cultivars is needed.

Reducing Yield Gap

The opaque-2 system is considered genetically defective in its ability to accumulate dry matter in its grain. The grain yield recovery of the recurrent parent in o_2 counterparts was not satisfactory, despite the number of backcrosses realized in converting any given material. It was, therefore, envisioned from the beginning that no single approach would help rectify this serious problem. Thus a series of strategies singly and in combination were deployed to narrow down and reduce the yield gap.

FIGURE 1. Improvement in kernel modifications of QPM germplasm through different cycles of selection.

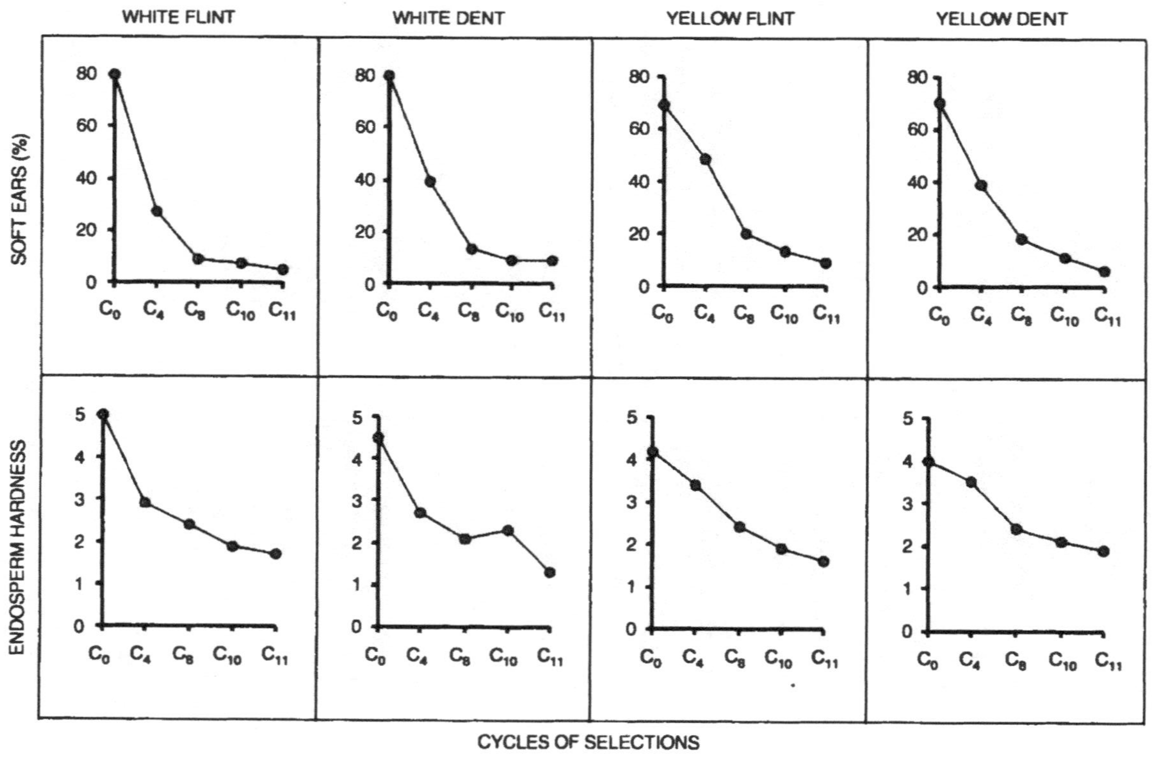

TABLE 6. Improvement in Kernel Modification During Different Cycles of Selection.

Material	Kernel modification[*]			L.S.D (.05)
	C_0	C_4	C_9	
Temperate × Trop. H.E.o_2 (Flint)	3.1	2.6	2.1	0.26
Temperate × Trop. H.E.o_2 (Dent)	3.0	2.5	2.2	2.20
Blanco Cristalino H.E.o_2	3.7	2.8	2.3	0.20
Amarillo Dentado H.E.o_2	3.2	2.6	2.4	0.43

[*] Rating scale 1-5 (1– Completely vitreous, 5–Completely soft).

FIGURE 2. Changes in the frequency of kernel modification classes through different cycles of selection.

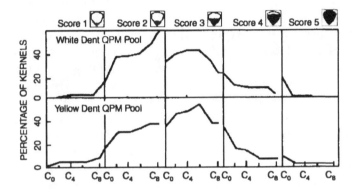

- Exploitation of the differences in the kernel weight of the normal and opaques in the segregating generations.
- Recurrent selection for yield and continuous accumulation of genetic modifiers for better kernel weight and density.
- Indirect field criteria, such as rejection of ears with open row spacing especially during the process of selection for hard endosperm did help improve the performance of QPM for yield.
- Conscious introduction of breeding schemes and switching over to appropriate strategies when needed, to help overcome the yield barrier.
- Shifting the emphasis from a backcross procedure to working with homozygous o_2 background for faster accumulation of genetic modifiers for kernel hardness, weight, and density.
- Exploiting the genetic background effects and materials where yield differences were not so pronounced.
- Improving yield performances by developing hybrid-oriented source germplasm and exploitation of yield heterosis.

- Indirectly improving yield by minimizing losses resulting from ear rot causing pathogens and stored grain pests.
- Adopting partial contamination techniques by using pollens from normal materials to select and accumulate favorable modifiers for kernel weight and the degree of kernel modification.
- Improving the kernel phenotype to resemble the normal phenotype also accounts for the reduction in the yield gap.

The data collected over the years from several international QPM trials that had non-opaque or normal entries as checks convincingly show that the yield gap between QPM and normal has practically disappeared (Figure 3). Cycles of selection studies also showed an improvement in yield and other traits including kernel modification scores (Table 8). Similar or near similar genetic background comparisons between normal and QPM have provided useful and encouraging information (Table 2). Though small differences existed for some genotypes, by in large, most QPM genotypes were quite competitive in their performances. Yield comparisons between the best QPM versus the best normal as well as results from some on-farm trials also showed little or no differences (Bjarnason and Vasal 1992). Exciting results have been observed with QPM hybrid trials tested nationally and internationally (Vasal 1994; Bjarnason and Vasal 1992; Cordova 2000). As can be seen from the more recent data, some of the best QPM hybrids have outperformed the best normal checks included in such trials (Tables 9 and 10). The superior performances of the QPM hybrids in recent years have led national programs in Mexico, Brazil, Guatemala, Honduras, EL Salvador, China, India, Vietnam, and others to release QPM hybrids.

FIGURE 3. Improvement in the yield of QPM compared to the normal germplasm during the QPM developmental process.

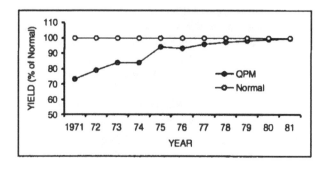

TABLE 7. Mean Kernel Modification Score, Standard Deviation, Range and Weinberg Constant Values of Different Cycles of Selection in Yellow QPM Grown in 1978.

Cycle	Mean kernel modification score[a]	Standard deviation	Range	Weinberg constant
C_1	3.7	1.07	2.9–4.8	1.60
C_4	2.9	0.92	2.3–3.7	1.57
C_7	2.3	0.81	1.6–3.2	1.29
C_9	2.2	0.91	1.2–3.5	1.23

[a] Rating scale 1 to 5 (1–Completely modified; 5–Completely soft).

TABLE 8. Comparisons of Original and Latest Cycle of Selection in Two QPM Gene Pools.

Material	Cycle	Yield (kg/ha)	Days to flower	Plant height (cm)	Soft ears (%)	Ear aspect[*]	Endosperm[*] modification
Temperate × tropical QPM (Flint)	C_0	4,437	59	212	66	4.0	4.2
	C_{12}	4,920	55	192	4	2.2	1.6
Temperate white QPM	C_0	3,445	55	204	34	3.5	3.7
	C_5	3,669	55	192	10	2.3	1.9

* Rating scale 1-5 : 1–Excellent; 5–Poors.
** Rating scale 1-5 : 1–Completely modified; 5–Completely soft.

Ear Rots and Insect Resistance

Remarkable levels of resistance to ear rot causing pathogens have been achieved for most of the currently available QPM populations and pools (Vasal et al. 1984; Bjarnason and Vasal 1992; Vasal 1994; Vasal 2001) due to several direct and indirect selection factors. While the direct selection (natural and artificial) for ear rot resistance has been practiced, improvements in other traits such as improved kernel phenotype, better drying, reduced influence of temperate germplasm, reduction in the frequency of alleles causing pericarp splitting and perhaps conscious selection for better husk cover, has helped reduce ear rot incidence. Moreover, in superior performing QPM hybrids, the ear rot scores have not been different from the better performing normal checks (Vasal 1994). Selection during inbreeding generations for inbred line development has also helped improvement of this trait.

Compared to normal kernels, soft opaques suffer more damages due to the stored grain pests, especially the maize weevil, *Sitophilus zeamais* (Ortega et

TABLE 9. Performance of Superior Tropical QPM Hybrids Across 41 Locations in Latin America and Asia, 1999-2000.

Pedigree	Grain yield (tons/ha)	Ear rot (%)	Silking (%)	Ear modification[*]	Tryptophan
(CML-141 × CML-144)	6.40	5.5	55	1.6	0.088
(CML-141 × CML-144) CML-142	6.29	6.2	55	1.7	0.081
(CML-142 × CML-146)	6.28	6.3	55	2.2	0.100
(CML-142 × CML-150)	6.20	7.8	55	2.0	0.089
(CML-142 × CML-150) CML-176	6.08	7.5	55	2.0	0.086
(CLQ-6203 × CML-150)	5.80	7.2	55	2.3	0.090
(CML-144 × CML-159) CML-176	5.64	6.0	56	1.7	0.094
(CML-144 × CML-159) (RE)	5.93	5.9	56	1.9	0.093
LOCAL CHECK-1	5.95	7.6	55	1.9	0.050

[*] Rating scale 1-5; 1–Completely hard, 5–Completely soft.

TABLE 10. Performance of Selected Superior Hybrids Across 15 Locations in Mexico, Central America, and Venezuela.

Pedigree	Grain yield (tons/ha)	Ear rot (%)	Silking (%)	Ear modification[*]	Tryptophan
CML-141 × CML-144	6.29	3.5	51	1.7	0.088
(CML-142 X CML-150) × CML-176	5.99	4.5	51	1.6	0.086
(CLQ-6203 X CML-150) × CML-176	5.98	4.7	51	1.7	0.084
CML-142 × CML-146	5.96	4.9	51	1.9	0.100
(CML-141 X CML-144) × CML-142	6.00	5.7	51	1.5	0.080
NH991	6.01	4.2	51	1.8	0.050
LOCAL CHECK-1	5.38	5.1	51	2.0	0.050

[*] Rating scale 1-5; 1–Completely hard, 5–Completely soft.

al. 1975; Gupta et al. 1970). It is a common observation at CIMMYT that the QPM suffers from less stored grain pests' damage. Though there may be other reasons for the reduced damage to QPM, it is believed that improved kernel phenotype has helped reduce this damage.

Moisture Content at Harvest

Higher grain moisture content at harvest is no longer a problem for QPMs (Vasal et al. 1984). Improved kernel phenotype, better dry matter accumulation, and visual selection for faster drying ears has contributed to improved drying abilities of QPMs.

Maintenance of Protein Quality

Protein quality was continuously monitored during all stages of the selection process. The major drawback of the genetic modifier approach was the differential decline in protein quality for some genotypes, as one selected for modified phenotype. Monitoring the protein quality was, therefore, strictly pursued with the excellent support of the protein quality laboratory at CIMMYT. Protein analyses were done in a rapid, efficient, and timely fashion. Reduction in protein quality upon selection for modifiers did slow down the breeding progress, but through continuous rejection of families with poor protein quality the breeders were able to maintain acceptable protein quality levels in the QPM germplasm. Most QPM pools (Table 11) and populations have acceptable levels of protein quality. Information from selection studies shows the same trend (Table 12). Different versions (normal, soft, and modified) of the same material showed that the soft and modified opaques were superior in their protein quality compared to the normal versions and differences between soft and modified opaques were negligible (Tables 13 and 14).

QPM HYBRID DEVELOPMENT

For the development of QPM hybrids, both the opaque-2 gene and the modifying gene complex that provides the normal looking kernel appearances are

TABLE 11. Percent Protein, Tryptophan, and Lysine in the Whole Grain of QPM Pools.

QPM gene pool	Protein (%)	Tryptophan in protein (%)	Lysine in protein (%)	Quality index*
Pool 15 QPM	9.1	0.94	4.2	4.6
Pool 17 QPM	8.9	1.04	4.5	4.5
Pool 18 QPM	9.9	0.93	4.0	4.6
Pool 23 QPM	9.1	1.03	3.8	4.2
Pool 24 QPM	9.4	0.92	3.8	4.0
Pool 25 QPM	9.8	0.94	4.0	4.0
Pool 26 QPM	9.5	0.90	4.1	4.3
Pool 27 QPM	9.5	1.05	4.2	4.8
Pool 29 QPM	9.2	1.06	4.3	4.8
Pool 31 QPM	10.2	0.96	4.1	4.5
Pool 32 QPM	8.9	1.04	4.2	4.5
Pool 33 QPM	9.3	1.05	-	4.2
Pool 34 QPM	9.1	1.10	4.1	4.5

* Quality index is calculated by dividing DBC by percent protein.

TABLE 12. Protein, Tryptophan, and Lysine in Different Cycles of Selection of Three QPM Materials (endosperm analysis).

Material	Cycle	Protein (%)	Tryptophan in protein (%)	Lysine in protein (%)	Quality index*
Yellow fling QPM	C_0	8.0	0.78	2.90	3.2
	C_6	8.0	0.75	2.90	3.2
PD (MS)6 QPM	C_0	8.5	0.78	2.50	2.8
	C_4	8.8	0.78	2.60	3.0
Temperature × tropical QPM	C_0	8.0	0.66	3.20	3.2
	C_8	8.0	0.68	2.90	3.2

* Quality index is calculated by dividing DBC by percent protein.

TABLE 13. Protein, Lysine, and Tryptophan Content in Endosperm of Normal, Soft Opaque-2 and Modified Opaque-2.

Version type	Protein (%)	Tryptophan in protein (%)	Lysine in protein (%)
Normal	9.20	0.40	2.00
Soft opaque	8.00	1.00	3.80
Modified opaque	9.93	0.85	3.40

TABLE 14. Protein Fractionation of Normal, Soft Opaque, and Hard Endosperm Opaque-2 Versions of Tuxpeno-1.

Fraction	Tuxpeno normal	Tuxpeno soft opaque-2	Tuxpeno H.E.o$_2$
I (Albumins + Globulins)	6.2	20.6	15.5
II (Zein)	39.2	8.1	10.4
III (Zein-like)	19.7	10.7	16.2
IV (Glutelin-like)	13.6	18.5	21.4
V (Glutelins)	22.4	42.5	36.6

involved. Due to an earlier emphasis on the development and improvement of its pools and population, yield heterosis in QPM could not be exploited until the mid-80s. Hybrid-related activities were initiated in normal and QPM germplasms in early 1985. The QPM hybrid development program had distinct advantages over the OPV QPM germplasm (Vasal 1986, 1987). These advantages include: (1) providing opportunities for yield enhancement through exploitation of yield heterosis, (2) maintain seed purity of inbred progenitors for agronomic and quality traits such as protein quality and kernel modification, (3) increasing efficiency and cost effectiveness due to reduced dependency on laboratory facilities for protein quality, (4) developing hybrids with a greater appeal, as the hybrids with good QPM lines had greater uniformity and stability for kernel phenotype, (5) overcoming stress related problems more efficiently and effectively, (6) increasing market acceptability, and (7) enhancing the development of the private seed industry.

As with the beginning of any hybrid development program, a complete knowledge of the combining ability and heterosis amongst the available germplasm is absolutely necessary. For the CIMMYT maize program, this information was generated for the subtropical (Vasal et al. 1993a) and tropical QPM materials (Vasal et al. 1993b) in two separate diallel studies. Considering the broad nature of the QPM germplasm, the high-parent heterosis was not very striking in either of the two studies. Populations 62, 63, and 37 in tropical QPM germplasm showed a significant and positive GCA effects for yield, and pool 23 QPM, pool 25 QPM, populations 62, 64, and 65 had negative GCA effects for kernel modification. The negative values for kernel modification were considered desirable. Based on the results of these studies, the tropical QPM materials considered most desirable for hybrid work were populations 62, 63, and 65. The information from subtropical diallel studies revealed that materials most useful for hybrid work were populations 68 and 69 and pools 32 QPM and 34 QPM. More detailed information on hybrid-related activities can be found in some earlier CIMMYT publications.

The QPM developed inbreds at CIMMYT has primarily involved QPM germplasm sources developed at CIMMYT. Recycling among good elite inbreds has been initiated and new sources of inbreds will be generated from these QPM pedigree populations. The maize program has also converted a few elite normal inbreds to QPM. The CIMMYT program has already announced the availability of 55 QPM inbreds to public and private researchers worldwide. The development and testing of hybrids has greatly expanded during the past 3-4 years. Several countries in Central and South America, Asia, and Africa have released QPM hybrids mostly based on CIMMYT QPM germplasm and QPM inbreds. The performances of some of the QPM hybrids during international trials have been quite encouraging and exciting. In some locations, QPM hybrids have even outperformed the normal check entries (Tables 9 and 10).

SOURCES OF QPM GERMPLASM

CIMMYT holds the largest volume of QPM germplasm that has been developed, and research efforts to continuously improve the deficiency traits of the original soft endosperm opaque-2 materials continues. Ten broad based populations are now available that have tropical and subtropical adaptations and are either white or yellow seeded. Except population 61, most of the populations are of full-season maturity. Additionally, 13 QPM gene pools are available with tropical and subtropical adaptations. They vary in their grain color and are either late or early maturity. In addition to the availability of the above-mentioned basic germplasm, several QPM experimental varieties and synthetics have been formed based on data from international progeny testing trials. These have been tested in QPM variety trials and their seed has been made available to interested breeders on request. Two high-oil QPM populations have also been developed and are available to breeders on request. These are white dent H.E. o_2 (HO) and Temperate $\times$ Tropical H.E. o_2 (HO). The oil content in these populations ranges from 6.5% to 7.0%. Many QPM lines have also been developed and 55 of these lines were released and made available to maize researchers worldwide during the early 1990s (Vasal 1993). The seed of the QPM hybrids were also supplied on request for experimental purposes. Moreover, QPM lines and pedigree populations in the process of development and selection will also be made available to our collaborators.

QPM RELEASES AND SOME SUCCESS STORIES

Following the encouraging developments at CIMMYT, QPM activities have been revived in several countries of Central and South America, Asia, and Africa. The Sasakawa Global-2000 program is concentrating its efforts in several countries of Africa. QPM variety Obatanpa is regularly planted over several thousands of hectares in Ghana. Other countries in Africa such as Mali, Burkina Faso, Benin, Ethiopia, Uganda, and Mozambique are growing limited areas of 5000-10,000 hectares of QPM varieties. Several countries in Latin America have shown a renewed interest and have released QPM varieties and hybrids (Table 15). In the past two years, Mexico has released several QPM varieties and a few 3-way and single cross QPM hybrids. Last year, QPM was planted on 40,000 hectares in Mexico. In the next 2-3 years, the area planted to QPM is likely to increase to at least half a million hectares. Other countries in Central and South America such as Guatemala, El Salvador, Nicaragua, Columbia, Venezuela, Peru, and Brazil have also released QPM hybrids and are growing some QPM commercially. All countries are hopeful that the area planted to QPM will increase up to 50,000 hectares by the year 2003. South Africa has maintained interest in QPM and its hybrids are planted on at least 20,000 hectares. In China, interest in QPM has grown tremendously and has full Government support. During 1999 and 2000, QPM hybrids were released and planted in an estimated several hundred thousand hectares in many provinces of China. It is hoped that enough QPM hybrid seed will also be produced to cover approximately half a million hectares by the year 2003. In addition, several provinces in China have active QPM breeding programs for QPM hybrid development. The release of two QPM hybrids during 2001 and the greater resource allocation for QPM work has renewed QPM research interest in India.

TABLE 15. Recent QPM Releases in Some Countries.

Name	Type	Pedigree	Country
HQ INTA-993	Hybrid	(CML-144 × CML-159) CML-176	Nicaragua
NB-Nutrinta	Open pollinated	Poza Rica 8763	Nicaragua
HB-PROTICTA	Hybrid	(CML-144 × CML-159) CML-176	Guatemala
HQ-61	Hybrid	(CML-144 × CML-159) CML-176	El Salvador
HQ-31	Hybrid	(CML-144 × CML-159) CML-176	Honduras
Zhongdan 9409	Hybrid	Pool 33 × Temp QPM	China
Zhongdan 3850	Hybrid		China
QUIAN2609	Hybrid	Tai 19/02 × CML-171	China
ICA-	Hybrid	(CML-144 × CML-159) CML-176	Colombia
Susuma*	Open pollinated	Across 8363SR	Mozambique
Obatampa*	Open pollinated	Across 8363SR	Mali
Obangaina*	Open pollinated	Across 8663SR	Uganda
Obatampa*	Open pollinated	Across 8363SR	Benin
BR-473	Open pollinated		Brazil
BR-451	Open pollinated		Brazil
Assum Preto	Open pollinated		Brazil
Obatampa*	Open pollinated	Across 8363SR	Burkina Faso
Obatampa*	Open pollinated	Across 8363SR	Guinea
QS-7705*	Hybrid		South Africa
GH-132-28*	Hybrid	P62, P63	Chana
INIA-	Hybrid	CML-161 × CML-165	Peru
FONAIAP	Hybrid	(CML-144 × CML-159) CML-176	Venezuela
HQ-2000	Hybrid	CML-161 × CML-165	Vietnam
SHAKTIMAN-1	Hybrid	(CML-142 × CML-150) CML-176	India
SHAKTIMAN-1	Hybrid	CML-176 × CML-186	India

In Mexico, 21 hybrids and 5 open pollinated varieties including . . .

44IC	Hybrid	CML-142 × CML-116	Mexico
H-551C	Hybrid	CML-142 × CML-150	Mexico
H-553C	Hybrid	(CML-142 × CML-150) CML-176	Mexico
H-519C	Hybrid	(CML-144 × CML-159) CML-170	Mexico
H-368EC	Hybrid	CML-186 × CML-149	Mexico
H-369EC	Hybrid	CML-176 × CML-186	Mexico
VS-537 C	Open pollinated	POZA RICA 8763	Mexico
VS-538 C	Open pollinated	ACROSS 8762	Mexico

* Sasakawa-Global 2000, a non-governmental organization dedicated to ending malnutrition and poverty in Africa and a leading promoter of QPM in the region, cooperated with national programs and CIMMYT for the release of these varieties.

CONCLUSION AND FUTURE OUTLOOK

The renewed interest in QPM is quite exciting. Several countries have re-initiated QPM breeding efforts and are anxious to release new QPM hybrids for commercial production. The private sector has also become involved in QPM research activities and indigenous companies in some countries are already producing QPM hybrid seeds. Based on the projections provided by the national program partners, the Sasakawa-Global 2000, and the CIMMYT maize program, more than 1.6 million hectares worldwide, may be sown to QPM by year 2003. There is tremendous optimism in countries like China, Mexico, India and others, for the promotion and dissemination of QPM. During the past 4-5 years, the CIMMYT maize program has expanded its research activities in QPM, boosted by additional funding from donors. Use of new molecular techniques in QPM research has already begun at CIMMYT and in other institutions. It is expected that these new tools will help in the understanding of various aspects of QPM and will accelerate the QPM conversion and germplasm development efforts. CIMMYT breeders also hope that the mechanism(s) controlling kernel modification and the role of gamma zein will be elucidated and better understood. Basic studies and strategies are needed to prevent contamination of QPM by normal pollen and simple techniques and procedures have to be developed to distinguish QPM from the normal kernels. As more QPM is grown, it will help alleviate malnutrition in many countries especially for the more vulnerable groups of children and pregnant women. Feed use of QPM will also be exploited for the purposes of feed efficiency ratio and for alleviating poverty and for increasing farmers' income. Therefore, QPM will certainly become an integral part of food and nutritional security of many nations in the future.

REFERENCES

Alexander, D.E. 1966. Problems associated with breeding opaque-2 corn and some proposed solutions. In *Proc. High Lysine Corn Conf.*, Mertz, E.T. and Nelson, O.E., Eds., Corn Refiners association Inc., Washington, DC, pp. 156-160.

Bjarnason, M. and S.K. Vasal. 1992. Breeding of quality protein maize (QPM), in *Plant Breeding Rev.*, Janick, J., Ed., pp. 181-216.

Bauman, L.F. 1975. Germ and endosperm variability, mineral elements, oil content and modifier genes in opaque-2. In *High-Quality Protein Maize*. Hutchinson Ross Publishing, Stroudsburg, PA, pp. 217-227.

Cordova, H.C. 2000. *2000 progress report on the improvement and promotion of Quality Protein Maize in selected countries*. Submitted to Nippon Foundation by CIMMYT, Dec. 2000.

Dudley, J.W., E.E. Alexander, and R.J. Lambert. 1975. Genetic improvement of modified protein maize. In *High-Quality Protein Maize*, Hutchinson Ross Publishing, Stroudsburg, PA, pp. 120-135.

Gevers, H.O. 1972. Breeding for improved protein quality in maize. *Trans. R. Soc. S. Afr.*, 40 (part 2): 81-92.

Gevers, H.O. and J.K. Lake. 1992. Development of modified opaque-2 maize. In *Quality Protein Maize*, E.T. Mertz, ed., American Association of Cereal Chemists, St. Paul, MN, pp. 49-78.

Glover, D.V. 1988. Corn protein and starch-genetics, breeding and value in foods and feeds. In *Proc. 43rd Annual Corn and Sorghum Industry Research Conference* American Seed Trade Assoc., Chicago, IL, pp. 106-130.

Glover, D.V. and E.T. Mertz. 1987. Corn. In *Nutritional Quality of Cereal Grains: Genetic and Agronomic Improvement*, R.A. Olson and K.J. Frey, eds., ASA Monograph 28, Am. Soc. Agronomy, Madison, WI, pp. 183-336.

Glover, D.V., P.L. Crane, P.S. Misra, and E.T. Mertz. 1975. Genetics of endosperm mutants in maize as related to protein quality and quantity. In *High-Quality Protein Maize*, Hutchinson Ross Publishing, Stroudsburg, PA, pp. 228.

Gupta, S.C., V.L. Asnani, and B.P. Khare. 1970. Effect of the opaque-2 gene in maize (*Zea mays* L.) on the extent of infestation by *Sitophilus orizae* L. *J. Stored Prod. Res.*, 6: 191-194.

Harpsted, D.D. 1969. High lysine maize in its proper perspective. In *Proc. 24th Annual Corn and Sorghum Research Conference*, American Seed Trade Assoc., Chicago, IL, pp. 74-80.

Ito, S. 1998. *General Overview on Exploding Maize Demand in Asia*. International maize Conference in Tottori, June 1-4, 1998.

Lambert, R.J., D.E. Alexander, and J.W. Dudley. 1969. Relative performance of normal and modified protein (opaque-2) maize hybrids. *Crop Sci.*, 9: 242-243.

Loesch, P.J. Jr., R.L. Grindeland, E.G. Hammond, and A.V. Paez. 1977. Evaluation of kernel hardness in normal and high lysine maize (*Zea mays* L.). *Maydica* 22: 197-212.

Lonnquist, J.H. 1964. Modification of the ear-to-row procedure for the improvement of maize populations. *Crop Sci.* 4:227-228.

Ma, Y. and O.E. Nelson. 1975. Amino acid composition and storage proteins in two new high-lysine mutants in maize. *Cereal Chem.* 52: 412-418.

McWhirter, K.S. 1971. A floury endosperm, high lysine locus on chromosome 10. *Maize Genet, Coop. News Lett.* 45: 184.

Mertz, E.T., L.S. Bates, and O.E. Nelson. 1964. Mutant gene that changes protein composition and increases lysine content of maize endosperm. *Science*, 145: 279-280.

Motto, M., C. Lorenzoni, E. Gentinetta, T. Maggiore, and F. Salamini. 1978. Expected genetic gain for protein related traits and allocation of resources in a modified opaque-2 synthetic. *Maydica*, 23: 35-43.

Nelson, O.E., E.T. Mertz, and L.S. Bates. 1965. Second mutant gene affecting the amino acid pattern of maize endosperm proteins. *Science*, 150 1469.

Nelson, O.E. 1969. Genetic modification of protein quality in plants. *Adv. In Agron.* 171.

Nelson, O.E. 1981. The mutants opaque-9 through opaque-13. *Maize Genet, Coop. News Lett.* 55: 68.

Ortega, A., C. De Leon, G. Granados, and S.K. Vasal. 1975. Disease-insect interactions in quality protein maize. In *High Quality Protein Maize*, Hutchinson Ross Publishing, Stroudsburg, PA, pp. 178-192.

Osborne, T.B. and L.B. Mendel. 1914a. Amino acids in nutrition and growth. *J. Biol. Chem.*, 17: 325.

Osborne, T.B. and L.B. Mendel. 1914b. Nutritive properties of protein of the maize kernel. *J. Biol. Chem.*, 18: 1-16.

Osborne, T.B. 1897. The amount and properties of the proteins of the maize kernel. *J. Am Chem. Soc.* 19: 525-532.

Paez, A.V., J.L. Helm, and M.S. Zuber. 1969. Lysine content of opaque-2 maize kernels having different phenotypes. *Crop Sci.* 251-252.

Paez, A.V. 1973. Protein quality and kernel properties of modified opaque-2 endosperm corn involving a recessive allele at the sugary-2 locus. *Crop Sci.* 13: 633-636.

Salamini, F., N. Di Fonzo, E. Fornasari, E. Gentinetta, R. Reggiani, and C. Soave. 1983. Mucronate, Mc. A dominant gene of maize which interacts with opaque-2 to suppress zein synthesis. *Theor. Appl. Genet.* 65:123-128.

Salamini, F., N. Di Fonzo, E. Gentinetta, and C. Soave. 1979. A dominant mutation interfering with protein accumulation in maize seeds. In *Seed Protein Improvement in Cereals and Grain Legumes*, IAEA, Vienna, pp. 97-106.

Sceeramulu, C. and L.F. Bauman. 1970. Yield components and protein quality of opaque-2 and normal dialles of maize. *Crop Sci.* 10: 262-265.

Schnieder, B.H. 1955. The nutritive value of corn. In *Corn and Corn Improvement*, Spraque, G.F., Ed., American Society of Agronomy, Madison, WI, pp. 637-678.

Singh, J. and V.L. Asnani. 1975. Present status and future prospects of breeding for better protein quality in maize through opaque-2. In *High-Quality Protean Maize*, Hutchinson Ross Publishing, Stroudsburg, PA, pp. 86-99.

Singh, S.V., J. Singh, D. Singh, and D.K. Bahl. 1977. Genetic environmental interactions in a diallel cross of opaque-2 maize. *Maydica* 22: 89-95.

Sriwatanapongse, S., E.C. Johnson, S.K. Vasal, and E. Villegas. 1974. Inheritance of kernel vitreosity in opaque-2 maize. *SABRAO, J.* 6: 1-7.

St. Martin, S.K., P.J. Loesch Jr., J.T. Demopulos-Rodriquez, and W.J. Wiser. 1982. Selection indices for the improvement of opaque-2 maize. *Crop Sci.* 22: 478-485.

Tsai, C.Y. 1979. Tissue-specific zein synthesis in maize kernel. *Biochem. Genet.* 17:1109-1119.

Vasal, S.K. 1986. Approaches and methodology in the development of QPM hybrids. In *Anais do XV Congresso National de Milho e Sorgo*, Maceio, Embrapa, CNPMS, p. 419-430.

Vasal, S.K., A. Ortega, and S. Pandey. 1982. *CIMMYT's Maize Germplasm Management, Improvement and Utilization Program.* CIMMYT, El Batan, Mexico.

Vasal, S.K., G. Srinivasan, C.G. Gonzales, D.L. Beck, and J. Crossa. 1993a. Heterosis and combining ability of CIMMYT's QPM maize germplasm. II. Subtropical. *Crop Sci.* 33: 51-55.

Vasal, S.K., G. Srinivasan, S. Pandey, C.F. Gonzalez, D.L. Beck, and J. Crossa. 1993b. Heterosis and combining ability of CIMMYT's QPM maize germplasm. I. Lowland Tropical. *Crop Sci.* 33: 46-50.

Vasal, S.K. 1975. Use of genetic modifiers to obtain normal-type kernels with the opaque-2 gene. In *High-Quality Protein Maize*, Hutchinson Ross Publishing, Stroudsburg, PA, pp. 197-215.

Vasal, S.K., E. Villegas, and C.Y. Tang. 1984. Recent advances in the development of quality protein maize at the Centro Internacional de Mejoramiento de Maiz y Trigo. In *Cereal Grain Protein Improvement*, IAE, Vienna, pp. 167-189.

Vasal, S.K., E. Villegas, M. Bjarnason, B. Gelaw, and P. Goertz. 1980. Genetic modifiers and breeding strategies in developing hard endosperm opaque-2 materials. In

Improvement of Quality Traits of Maize for Grain and Silage Use, Pollmer, W.G. and Phipps, R.H., Eds., Nighoff, The Hague, pp. 37-71.

Vasal, S.K., E. Villegas, C.Y. Tang, J. Werder, and M. Read. 1984. Combined use of two genetic systems in the development and improvement of quality protein maize. *Kulturpflanze*, 32: 171-185.

Vasal, S.K. 1987. *Development of Quality Protein Maize Hybrids*. A keynote paper presented at the First Symposium on Crop Improvement, Ludhiana, India 23-27 Feb, 1987. Eds. K.S. Gill et al., pp. 57-75.

Vasal, S.K. 1994. High Quality protein corn. In *Speciality Corns* (first edition), Ed. A.R. Hallauer. CRC Press. pp. 79-121.

Vasal, S.K., B.S. Dhillon, and S. Pandey. 1997. Recurrent selection methods based on evaluation-cum-recombination block. *Plant Breeding Reviews* 14: 139-163.

Vasal, S.K. 2001. High quality protein corn. In *Speciality Corns* (second edition), Ed. A.R. Hallauer. CRC Press. pp. 85-129.

Villegas, E., S.K. Vasal, and M. Bjarnason. 1992. Quality protein maize–What is it and how was it developed. In *Quality Protein Maize*, Mertz, E.T., Ed., American Association Cereal Chemists, St. Paul, MN, pp. 27-48.

Wall, J.S. and J.W. Paulis. 1978. Corn and sorghum grain protein. *Advanced Cereal Science Technology*, 2: 135-219.

Wessel-Beaver, L., R.H. Beck, and R.J. Lambert. 1984. Rapid method for measuring kernel density. *Agron. J.* 76: 307-309.

Zorilla, H.L. and P.L. Crane. 1982. Evaluation of three cycles of full-sib family selection for yield in the Colus o_2 variety of maize. *Crop Sci.* 22: 10-12.

Improving Rice to Meet Food and Nutritional Needs: Biotechnological Approaches

S. K. Datta
G. S. Khush

SUMMARY. The livelihood and calorie needs of large populations based in developing countries is dependent on rice cultivation. More than three billion people consume rice as a staple food. To meet the future demands of the human population, innovative tools such as genomics are being used to improve rice yield increase, for the incorporation of stress resistance/tolerance in rice varieties, and for the improvement of the nutritional quality of rice. These new tools include: sequencing, large-scale analysis of expressed sequence tags, high throughout microarray analysis and genetic transformation. Rice now serves as a model for a science based crop design for the agronomic, nutritional, and economic benefit of farmers. This article discusses the use of biotechnology as a tool to improve the rice plant for the benefit of mankind. *[Article copies available for a fee from The Haworth Document Delivery Service: 1-800-HAWORTH. E-mail address: <getinfo@haworthpressinc.com> Website: <http://www. HaworthPress.com> © 2002 by The Haworth Press, Inc. All rights reserved.]*

S. K. Datta is Plant Biotechnologist, and G. S. Khush is Principal Plant Breeder (and recipient of World Food Prize, 1996), Department of Plant Breeding, Genetics, and Biochemistry Division, DAPO Box 7777, Metro Manila, Philippines (E-mail: s.datta@cgiar.org or g.khush@cgiar.org).

Financial support from the USAID, USA, BMZ/GTZ, Germany and DANIDA, Denmark is gratefully acknowledged. The authors would like to thank Bill Hardy and Palit Kataki for editorial assistance.

[Haworth co-indexing entry note]: "Improving Rice to Meet Food and Nutritional Needs: Biotechnological Approaches." Datta, S. K., and G. S. Khush. Co-published simultaneously in *Journal of Crop Production* (Food Products Press, an imprint of The Haworth Press, Inc.) Vol. 6, No. 1/2 (#11/12), 2002, pp. 229-247; and: *Food Systems for Improved Human Nutrition: Linking Agriculture, Nutrition, and Productivity* (ed: Palit K. Kataki, and Suresh Chandra Babu) Food Products Press, an imprint of The Haworth Press, Inc., 2002, pp. 229-247. Single or multiple copies of this article are available for a fee from The Haworth Document Delivery Service [1-800-HAWORTH, 9:00 a.m. - 5:00 p.m. (EST). E-mail address: getinfo@haworthpressinc.com].

229

KEYWORDS. Biotechnology, genetic transformation, iron, microarray analysis, nutrition, rice, sequencing, vitamin A

INTRODUCTION

Rice provides 40-70% of the total calorie needs in Asia, making it the number one food staple crop in the region. The development of improved rice varieties during the Green Revolution era prompted enormous changes in the agricultural practices in the rice growing regions of the world (Khush, 1995; 1999), significantly contributing to yield increases and calorie supplies (Hossain et al. 2000). Despite the progress made, an estimated 800 million people of the world still suffer from malnutrition, particularly micronutrient deficiency related malnutrition. Staple crops, including rice, are therefore being targeted as an alternative, long-term sustainable delivery mechanism of dietary micronutrients for humans. However, efforts to increase the micronutrient content of staple grains will have to be coupled with the satisfactory agronomic performances of yield increases, pest resistance, and tolerance to other environmental stresses.

In this context, genetic engineering is being used in innovate ways as an effective tool to facilitate and accelerate the progress towards achieving these multi-faceted goals of nutritional and economic benefits of rice to farmers (Datta, 2000; 2001). Nutritional improvement of the rice plant includes loading and harvesting rice grains with higher than normal levels of micronutrients such as iron, zinc, provitamin A, and lysine. Such improved "Nutritious Rice" by conventional and molecular (genetic engineering) breeding techniques, provides an excellent opportunity to reduce malnutrition, particularly micronutrient deficiency related malnutrition in humans (Ye et al. 2000; Datta and Bouis, 2000). In recent years, collaboration with the private sector in the field of biotechnology has also increased, as is evident with the donation of the technology-driven "Golden Rice" containing genes for β-carotene biosynthesis for social welfare (IRRI Website). Such public-private institutional collaboration will further accelerate the pace of the development of improved rice varieties in the future.

GLOBAL RICE PRODUCTION AND THE PROGRESS TOWARDS INCREASING THE YIELD POTENTIAL

During the last four decades, the use of conventional plant breeding methods has significantly contributed towards increasing the global rice production. The cultivation of modern rice varieties in irrigated ecosystems coupled with better management practices has increased the total cereal production at a rate greater than the population growth rate. The increase in rice production has resulted in the lowering of its price, which has benefited a majority of consumers and small and marginal producers (Hossain et al. 2000). In 1966, IRRI released IR8, the first high yielding modern rice cultivar for the irrigated tropical lowlands (Figure 1). Since then, 44 indica-inbred cultivars from IRRI have been released in the Philippines. These cultivars and their derivatives have been widely grown in South and Southeast Asia and account for 80% of the total rice cultivated and produced in this region.

Since the release of IR8, efforts to improve the rice plant for higher yield coupled with other desirable characteristics continues, since the population continues to grow, especially in developing countries. To break the yield barrier of rice, the development of New Plant Type (NPT) and hybrid rice using the tools of biotechnology has been explored (Figure 1). Under tropical conditions, hybrid rice between the indicas has increased the yield potential by 9%. Incorporation of the grain filling gene *glgC* in NPT (unpublished data) and the further improvement of hybrid rice by incorporating *Bt* and *Xa21* genes for plant protection has also yielded excellent results (Alam et al. 1999; Tu et al. 1998a,b; 2000a,b; Datta, 1999). There has been a 28% yield advantage for hybrid Bt rice over the hybrid non-Bt rice in China (Tu et al. 2000b). IR64 is at present the most widely cultivated rice variety in the world, grown in an esti-

FIGURE 1. Progress in the yield potential of rice

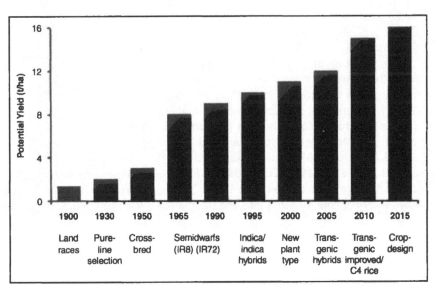

mated 13 million ha of rice land in Asia that includes Indonesia, Philippines, Vietnam, and the Indian states of Andhra Pradesh and Orissa (Hossain et al. 2000). Therefore, transgenic IR64 with *Bt*, *Xa21*, and *PR* genes are being developed and evaluated for enhancing yield and environmental protection. The goal is to grow transgenic IR64 rice without the application of pesticides and to obtain good yields.

GENOMICS AND RICE

Genomics now implies DNA sequencing, the routine use of DNA microarray technology to analyze gene expression profiles at the mRNA level and the use of improved information tools to organize and analyze such data. Cereal crops and other grasses have much homology in their genome sequence though they differ in many agronomic characteristics, which can be used to an advantage for learning and creating new crop varieties for tomorrows needs. Genomics-based strategies for gene discovery coupled with high-throughout gene technology can accelerate the identification of candidate genes (Figure 2). There are several advantages of working with rice as a major staple crop: a small genome size, a diploid plant (2n = 24), a well characterized phenotype and chromosome structural genetics (Khush, 1999), and has an excellent genetic transformation system (Datta et al. 1990; Datta and Datta 2001; Christou, Ford, and Kofron, 1991; Hiei et al. 1994) supported by a worldwide research network on rice improvement and biotechnology. The major genes of rice have been identified and their locations in the rice chromosomes have been characterized. It is envisaged that several of these genes will help researchers design rice varieties with a better phenotype for higher yield.

Domestication of rice over many centuries has resulted in a limited diversity of the cultivated rice varieties of today. Many wild species can potentially provide genes that could substantially increase the yield of rice (Xiao et al. 1996). It is important to characterize the wild species and use the genes of interest rather than placing them in the gene bank. Insertional mutagenesis is now an attractive method for functional analysis. This method screens the T-DNA insertion in a known gene and recovers the sequences flanking the insertions (Jeon et al. 2000). This activity is in addition to transposon tagging using the Ac/Ds system (Enoki et al. 1999). The recent breakthrough on the rice genome sequencing by Monsanto, the International Rice Genome Sequencing Project (IRGSP, rgp.dna.affrc.go.jp), and Syngenta (syngenta.com/en/media/article) (asp.article-id=126) will further accelerate the gene discovery and crop improvement endeavors (Figure 2). However, the following questions need to be addressed.

• How do we reorganize rice-breeding efforts in the genomic era?

- How does the rice genome discovery work of the IRGSP, Monsanto, and Syngenta help us in such an endeavor?
- How do we present such a knowledge-based intensive technology and obtain public acceptance?
- How do we convince policy makers of national governments to combine the advantages of "green and gene revolution" to reach more rice farmers whose livelihood can be improved by such knowledge-based intensive technology?

Invariably, such a task poses many challenges and rewards for human welfare.

MICRONUTRIENTS AND RICE

The bioavailability of micronutrients and its absorption by humans depends upon a number of factors and includes: genetic variation amongst the people, presence of dietary antinutrients, and dietary promoters. Green vegetables and fruits are a good source of essential micronutrients provided that the recom-

FIGURE 2. Application of genomics in rice improvement

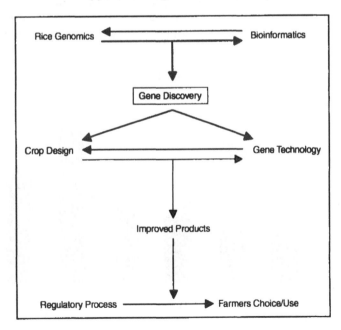

mended 73 kg/capita/year is consumed. Unfortunately, the production of and intake of vegetables and fruits in most Asian countries are well below the recommended intake levels.

The development of improved crop cultivars (staples) at the CGIAR centers for higher crop yield has significantly reduced malnutrition by increasing the calorie supplies during the last few decades (Figure 3, FAO 2000). However, micronutrient deficiency related malnutrition in humans is still alarming in many regions of the world. Since rice provides 40-70% of the total calorie intake for several Asian countries, it is envisaged that by increasing the micronutrient content in the grains rice and other staple crops will aid in the reduction of micronutrient deficiency related malnutrition amongst humans, without changing the dietary pattern of different population groups.

During the course of the CGIAR micronutrient project, it has been demonstrated that rice genotypes differ significantly in their ability to accumulate iron and zinc in its seeds (Table 1; and also Senadhira, Gregorio, and Graham, 1999; Graham et al. 1999). Screening and breeding for micronutrient dense seeds has helped in the development and selection of a few rice breeding lines that contain a higher than normal levels of iron and zinc in its seeds (Gregorio et al. 2000). Most aromatic rice cultivars contain higher levels of iron and zinc compared to non-aromatic rice cultivars (Graham et al. 1999). However, the potentials of this screening and cultivar selection process has not been fully exploited for human nutritional benefits, because nearly all of the iron and zinc are localized in the peripheral parts of the cereal grain. Paddy rice is composed

FIGURE 3. Benefits of international agricultural research (Adapted from Evenson, 2000)

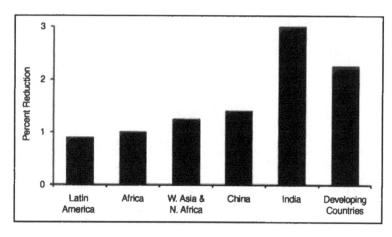

TABLE 1. Iron and Zinc Content of Varieties of Brown Rice Grown Under Similar Conditions in Eight Different Sets

Variety set	No. of samples	Iron	Zinc
		Mean ± SE mg/kg (range)	
Traditional and improved varieties	140	13.2 ± 2.9 (7.8-24.4)	24.2 ± 4.6 (13.5-41.6)
IR breeding lines	350	10.7 ± 1.6 (7.5-16.8)	25.0 ± 7.6 (15.9-58.4)
Tropical japonicas	250	12.9 ± 1.5 (8.7-23.9)	26.3 ± 3.8 (15.0-40.1)
Popular varieties and donors	199	13.0 ± 2.5 (7.7-19.2)	25.7 ± 4.6 (15.3-37.3)
Promising lines (NCT)	83	8.8 ± 1.3 (6.3-14.5)	25.4 ± 4.2 (17.0-38.0)
New plant types	44	16.7 ± 2.1 (11.5-24.0)	29.6 ± 3.2 (23.0-36.0)
Wild rice and derivatives	21	15.3 ± 2.3 (11.8-21.0)	37.9 ± 8.6 (23.0-52.0)
Aromatic rices	51	14.6 ± 3.2 (10.8-23.2)	31.9 ± 6.0 (23.0-50.0)

(Adapted from Gregorio et al. 2000)

of several essential micronutrients such as iron, iodine, and zinc, most of it being lost during the rice milling process (Welch and Graham 1999).

Experiments with different milling regimes on high iron rice cultivars have shown that 50% of the minerals are lost during the milling process (Gregorio et al. 2000). In general, iron is stored in a vesicle of ferritin consisting of 24 polypeptide sub-units that can sequester some 4,000-iron atoms in a safe form as hydrous ferric oxide-phosphate. Ferritin serves the dual purpose of providing iron for the synthesis of chlorophyll and iron proteins (ferredoxin and cytochromes) that prevents damage from free radicals produced by iron/dioxygen interactions. Ferritin genes have been isolated from a large number of plant species, including soybean, cowpea, *Arabidopsis*, maize, and *Medicago* sp. Iron in particular is partially mobilized from the leaves during its senescence. A 25-50 fold higher iron content is found in the leaves than in the seeds of rice. Therefore, it is still an open question whether plant ferritin can be mobilized from the source to the sink. Goto et al. (1999) reported a 3-fold increase in the iron content of japonica rice by genetically engineering the *ferritin* gene driven by the endosperm specific promoter.

The transgenic research laboratory at IRRI is also working on both the *ferritin* gene driven by endosperm specific promoter and 35SP of CaMV and *FRO2* gene that gets activated in iron deficient soils. The objective is to transport adequate amounts of iron into the indica rice seeds, irrespective of the iron status of the soil.

Polished or milled rice does not contain any provitamin A, although the β-carotene pathway operates in the rice plants, particularly in the leaves. Though the lysine content in rice is low, it may be possible to enhance lysine content in the rice grain by incorporating the *dapA* gene cloned from *Corynoebacterium*, as has been done in maize and canola by Falco et al. 1995.

GENETIC ENGINEERING AND TRANSGENIC RICE

The incorporation of novel traits/genes for crop improvement programs is possible by genetic engineering (Schell 1987). Major crops such as rice, maize, wheat, barley, cotton, potato, soybean, sunflower, and canola have been transformed using various gene transfer technologies such as micro-injection, laser beam techniques, pollen tube pathways, dry seed inhibition, and cell/tissue electroporation (Potrykus 1991). However, reproducible and unambiguous results have been obtained for rice by the protoplast, biolistic, and *Agrobacterium* methods (Figure 4). Detailed description of the methodologies for gene transfer technologies is available elsewhere (Datta et al. 1997; Datta and Datta 2001). Chloroplast engineering as an alternative to nuclear genetic engineering which has also been reported to be a successful strategy (Danielle 1999; Bogorad 2000). Studies on transgenic rice are continuing to explore the possibilities of conferring such traits as resistance to bacterial blight (Tu et al. 1998b), stem borer (Datta et al. 1998; Alam et al. 1998; 1999), sheath blight (Lin et al. 1995; Nishizawa et al. 1999; Baisakh et al. 2000; Datta et al. 1999a; Datta 2000; 2001), submergence tolerance (Quimio et al. 2000), towards N_2 fixation (Reddy et al. 1998), provitamin A, and rice with enhanced iron content (Ye et al. 2000, Goto et al. 1999, Table 2). Field evaluation of transgenic rice, resistant to bacterial blight and stem borer, has performed well in China (Tu et al. 2000a,b; Ye et al. 2001). Such field-testing of transgenic rice is now in progress in India (ICAR, DRR-IRRI collaborative work).

Potential for C_4 Rice

Most plants, including rice, fix atmospheric carbon dioxide by the C_3 photosynthetic pathway. Oxygen is released because of the oxygenase reaction of Rubisco, and this activity inhibits the carbon fixation and leads to a loss of CO_2 through photorespiration. Environmental stresses such as high temperature and water stress could further decrease photosynthetic efficiency.

Modifying C_3 plants to C_4 will enable plants to overcome O_2 inhibition and photorespiration of C_3 photosynthesis and increase the net carbon gain in rice. Transgenic japonica rice has already been developed with the intact gene of maize phosphoenolpyruvate carboxylase (PEPC) with a high level of expression in rice (Ku et al. 1999). The amount of the PEPC mRNA transcribed from one copy of the transgene in the haploid rice genome is comparable to that of the C_4 maize genome. The next step is to understand how this strategy can be extended to the tropical indica rice for improving its photosynthetic efficiency

FIGURE 4. A schematic protocol for the production of transgenic rice plants using biolostic, protoplast, and *Agrobacterium* system

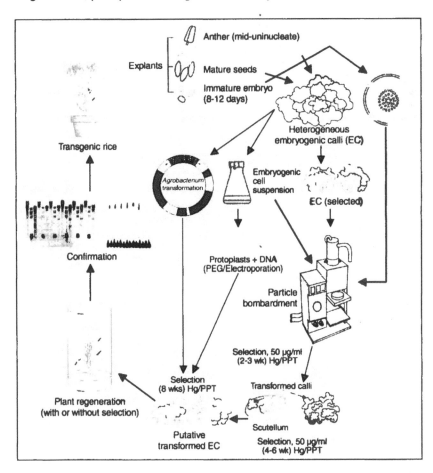

based on our work with transgenic indica rice developed with the maize PEPC gene (unpublished work).

Transgenic Hybrid Bt Rice

Crossing homozygous (restorer) Ming Hui 63 Bt rice with (CMS) ZS97 line that has been field evaluated in China has resulted in the commercial hybrid Bt rice "Shan You 63." This commercial hybrid has a 28.8% yield advantage over the non-Bt hybrid rice (Tu et al. 2000b).

TABLE 2. Development and Use of Transgenic Rice with Agronomically Important Genes

Rice	Method used	Genes transferred	Traits	Reference
Indica (IR72)	Protoplast (PEG)	*bar*	Resistant to herbicide	Datta et al. 1992
Japonica	Protoplast (electroporation)	cp-stripe	Resistant to stripe virus	Hayakawa et al. 1992
Japonica	Protoplast (electroporation)	*Bt*	Resistant to insects	Fujimoto et al. 1993
Japonica	*Agrobacterium*	*Bt*	YSB & SSB	Cheng et al. 1998
Indica	Protoplast (PEG)	*chi11*	Resistant to sheath blight	Lin et al. 1995
Japonica	Protoplast	cc	Resistant to insects	Irie et al 1996
Japonica	Biolistic	*Xa-21*	Resistant to bacterial blight	Wang et al. 1996
Indica	Protoplast and biolistic	*Bt*(DWR)	Resistant to stem borer	Alam et al. 1998
Japonica	Biolistic and protoplast	pin*II*	Resistant to insects	Duan et al. 1996
Indica	Biolistic	*Bt*	Resistant to stem borer	Nayak et al. 1997
Indica/ Japonica	Biolistic and protoplast	early nodulin	Biological N_2 fixation	Reddy et al. 1998
Indica/ Japonica	Biolistic and protoplast	early nodulin	Biological N_2 fixation	Dey et al. 1999
Indica	Biolistic	*Bt*	Resistant to stem borer	Tu et al. 1998a
Indica/ Japonica	Biolistic and protoplast	*Bt* (tissue-specific)	Resistant to stem borer	Datta et al. 1998
Indica (IR72)	Biolistic	*Xa-21*	Resistant to bacterial blight	Tu et al. 1998b
Indica	Biolistic	*Bt* ML for hybrid rice	Resistant to stem borer	Alam et al. 1999
Indica	Biolistic	*Bt* restorer for hybrid rice	Resistant to stem borer field evaluated	Tu et al. 2000b
Japonica	*Agrobacterium*	Ferritin	High iron storage	Goto et al. 1999
Japonica	*Agrobacterium*	pepc	Higher photosynthesis	Ku et al. 1999
Indica	Biolistic	viral replicase CP1, CP2, CP3	Resistance to RTSV and RTBV	Ang et al. 1999
Indica	Biolistic	PR genes	Resistant to sheath blight	Datta et al. 1999b Baisakh et al. 2000
Indica	*Agrobacterium*	PR-genes	Resistance to sheath blight	Datta et al. 2000, 2001
Japonica	*Agrobacterium*	psy, lyc, crt1	β-carotene synthesis	Ye et al. 2000
Japonica	Biolistic	adh, pdc	Submergence tolerance	Quimio et al. 2000
Japonica	Biolistic	waxy gene	Amylose content	Terada et al. 2000
Japonica	Biolistic	Bt	Resistance to insects	Ye et al. 2001

DWR = deep water rice; ML = maintainer line

High-Yielding Rice

Ja-Ock et al. (2000) and Venture Company Scigen Hamert introduced the *protox* gene (cloned from the soil microbe *Bacillus subtillis*) into rice and demonstrated a 20% increase in yield. This "super rice," a japonica type, is also called Makdong rice and is usually used in Korea and Japan. There is scope for increasing the yield of indica rice, with the successful expression of the *protox* gene in it.

Biotechnology as a tool has been used creatively for improving the performance of the rice plant. Figure 5 shows the progress made in improving the performance of the rice plant using biotechnology as a tool.

GOLDEN RICE: CONCEPT AND PRODUCT DEVELOPMENT

"Golden Rice" is genetically engineered rice that has β-carotene in its seeds, the term being given by a Thai businessman who has been an active par-

FIGURE 5. Progress in biotechnology toward rice improvement

Year	Event	Reference
1968	Anther culture in rice	Niizeki & Oono
1986	Protoplast regeneration to plants	Abdullah et al.
1987	Single microspore embryogenesis in wheat	Datta & Wenzel
1988	DNA finger printing in rice	Dallas
1988	First molecular map of rice based on RFLPs	McCouch et al.
1988	First transgenic japonica rice plantlets regenerated from protoplast	Toriyama et al.
1989	Artificial encapsulated seeds in cereals	Datta & Potrykus
1990	First transgenic homozygous indica rice regenerated from protoplast	Datta et al.
1990	Dicot-intron splicing in monocot-rice	Peterhans et al.
1991	Gene tagging for the first time in rice for blast resistance gene	Yu et al.
1991	Biolistic transformaion in rice	Christou et al.
1992	Use of RFLP to study gene introgression	Jena et al.
1993	First microsatellite mapped	Zhao & Kochert
1993	Marker assisted selection carried out for bacterial blight resistance gene, *Xa21*	Abenes et al.
1993	First observation of synteny between cereal genomes	Ahn & Tanksley
1994	*Agrobacterium* transformation in rice	Hiei et al.
1994	A new technique called restriction landmark genome scanning (RLGs) developed	Kawase
1995	Map based cloning of the first gene from cereals	Song et al.
1995	Gene pyramiding in a single cultivar conferring resistance to bacterial blight	Yoshimura et al.
1996	Advanced backcross QTL analysis	Tanksley & Nelson
2000	First successful field evaluation of hybrid *Bt* rice	Tu et al. (2000b)
2000	First genetically engineered rice with β-carotene	Ye et al.
2000	Rice genome sequenced	Monsanto
2001	Rice genome sequenced	Syngenta

FIGURE 6. Biosynthetic pathway of β-carotene

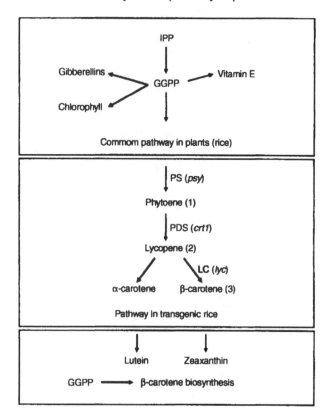

ticipant of family planning programs, that ensure food security. This term became very popular, particularly with the media, and "as the popular media live by selling news, "catchy" names are especially useful in attracting the interest of media consumers" Potrykus (2001).

β-Carotene is a precursor to vitamin A and is generally deficient in the diets of people in the highly populated regions of Asia, Africa, and Latin America. Four genes are required for the completion of the β-carotene synthesis pathway (Figure 6). Misawa et al. 1993 showed that phytoene desaturase cloned from a bacterium *Erwinia*, driven by the endosperm specific promoter glutelin 1, and combined with *tpII* is useful in expressing the gene in the endosperm of rice. Xudong Ye, working at ETH-Zurich, used this construct in addition to two other genes, *phytoene synthase*, and *lycopene cyclase* (published before by Peter Beyer) in collaboration with Peter Beyer's group that transformed japonica rice T309 by *Agrobacterium* system with hygromycin phosphotransferase (*hph*) as a selectable marker gene. Molecular (Southern) and biochemical (HPLC) analysis confirmed the integration of the three genes and of the β-carotene biosynthesis. In one of the transgenic line, the β-carotene level was as high as 1-6 µg/g dry seed (Ye et al. 2000). These events led to the development of the Golden Rice, a scientific breakthrough in introducing a desirable value added trait into the rice seed using biotechnology as a tool. Ingo Potrykus led this work in collaboration with Peter Beyer (Ye et al. 2000). We are now working on transferring this trait into tropical indica rice.

Where Do We Go from Here?

With the development of the Golden Rice, several questions have emerged that need to be addressed:

- Is the β-carotene level in Golden Rice adequate for the daily requirement of people who consume rice? And, how does it work?
- Can this trait/gene be efficiently transferred to other cultivars, popularly grown and used by the people in developing countries of Asia and elsewhere?
- Issues of biosafety, food safety, and environmental trade-off due to the incorporation of β-carotene genes need to be resolved.
- How can the public perception and acceptability of Golden Rice be dealt with?
- Will this material be freely available to all farmers?
- Will it reduce poverty, hunger, and malnutrition?
- What else can complement Golden Rice?

β-Carotene, the precursor of vitamin A, is naturally present in green leafy vegetables, red palm oil, and yellow fruits. Vitamin A retinol is a fat-soluble substance found in the liver, egg yolk, and dairy products. Approximately, six times as much of β-carotene for the comparable effect of one unit of retinol. The availability of stored vitamin A also depends on a child's general nutritional status.

Once the transgenic material is produced in an indica background, it will be rigorously tested for food and nutritional safety followed by its field evaluation to monitor its agronomic performances and trade-offs if any should be found. Based on all the supporting data, a few cultivars/lines will be recommended for their further evaluation at the country level. The national programs will then release these improved materials to the subsistence farmers and consumers. Materials from IRRI will be freely available to the NARS, along with all the relevant scientific data and food and nutritional information as a package. The relevant national institutions will then have to accelerate the wide-spread distribution and adoption of these materials. Besides provitamin A, the IRRI research program is also working towards enhancing iron and protein (lysine) contents of elite indica rice by genetic engineering. There is a lot of hope and confidence that these elite rice varieties with value added traits will provide improved nutrition and a better life for many people in the near future.

FOOD, NUTRITIONAL SECURITY, AND RICE

Cereal crops, including rice, will continue to be the mainstay of food and nutritional security of nations. However, there is continuous need for increasing its yield and total production. The green revolution technologies successfully tackled hunger related malnutrition problems. However, macro- and micronutrient deficiency related human health and productivity problems are still a major constraint in many regions of the world. Conventional plant breeding will have to be supported by the newer tool of biotechnology to shorten the turn-around time and hence, accelerate the pace of incorporating desirable traits into cereal crops. The use of this strategy is particularly true for increasing micronutrient contents of the rice grain and such research programs will have to be coupled with widely acceptable agronomic performances of the rice varieties. Public and private sector collaboration can be highly beneficial to further accelerate the pace of such developmental efforts.

REFERENCES

Abdullah, R., E.C. Cocking, and J.A. Thompson. 1986. Efficient plant regeneration from rice protoplasts through somatic embryogenesis. *Bio/Technology* 4:1087-1090.

Abenes, M.L.P. E.R. Angeles, G.S. Khush, and N. Huang. 1993. Selection of bacterial blight resistant rice plants in the F_2 generation via their linkage to molecular markers. *Rice Genet. Newsl.* 10:120-123.

Ahn, S. and S.K. Tanksley. 1993. Comparative linkage maps of the rice and maize genomes. *Proc. Natl. Acad. Sci. USA.* 90(17):7980-7984.

Alam, M.F., K. Datta, E. Abrigo, A. Vasquez, D. Senadhira, and S.K. Datta. 1998. Production of transgenic deepwater indica rice plants expressing a synthetic *Bacillus thuringiensis cryIA(b)* gene with enhanced resistance to yellow stem borer. *Plant Sci.* 135:25-30.

Alam, M.F., K. Datta, A. Vasquez, J. Tu, S.S. Virmani, and S.K. Datta. 1999. Transgenic insect resistant maintainer line (IR68899B) for improvement of hybrid rice. *Plant Cell Report* 18:572-575.

Ang, C.O., H. Huet, E. Sivamani, L. Chen, M.D. Hassan, A. Kochko, R.N. de Beachy, and C. Fauquet. 1999. Pathogen-derived resistance to rice tungro spherical virus. In: Abstract of the Rockefeller Foundation General Meeting of Int. Prog. on Rice Biotechnology. September 20-24, Phuket, Thailand. pp. 48.

Baisakh, N., K. Datta, N. Oliva, I. Ona, G.J.N. Rao, T.W. Mew, and S.K. Datta. 2000. Rapid development of homozygous transgenic rice using anther culture harboring rice *chitinase* gene for enhanced sheath blight resistance. *Plant Biotechnol.* 18: 101-108.

Bogorad, L. 2000. Engineering chloroplasts: an alternative site for foreign genes, proteins, reactions and products. *Trends in Biotechnol.* 18:257-263.

Cheng, X.Y., R. Sardana, H. Kaplan, and I. Altosaar. 1998. *Agrobacterium*-transformed rice plants expressing synthetic *cryIA(b)* and *cryIA(c)* genes are highly toxic to striped stem borer and yellow stem borer. *Proc. Natl. Acad. Sci.* USA 95(6): 2767-2772.

Christou, P., T.F. Ford, and M. Kofron. 1991. Production of transgenic rice (*Oryza sativa*) plants from agronomically important Indica and Japonica varieties via electric discharge particle acceleration of exogenous DNA into immature zygotic embryos. *BioTechnology* 9:957-962.

Dallas, J.F. 1988. Detecting of DNA fingerprinting of cultivated rice by hybridization with a human minisatellite DNA probe. *Proc. Natl. Acad. Sci.* USA. 85(18): 6831-6835.

Danielle, H. 1999. New tools for chloroplast genetic engineering. *Nature Biotechnology* 17:855-856.

Datta, K., and S.K. Datta. 2001. Plant transformation. In: *Molecular Plant Biology*, Gilmartin P. and Bowler C. (eds.). Vol. 1. A Practical Approach, Oxford University Press, UK (in press).

Datta, K., Z. Koukolíková-Nicola, N. Baisakh, N. Oliva, and S.K. Datta. 2000. *Agrobacterium*-mediated engineering for sheath blight resistance of indica rice cultivars from different ecosystems. *Theor. Appl. Genet.* 100:832-839.

Datta, K., S. Muthukrishnan, and S.K. Datta. 1999a. Expression and function of PR-protein genes in transgenic plants. In: *Pathogenesis-related proteins in plants*. S.K. Datta and S. Muthukrishnan, eds. CRC Press, USA. pp. 261-277.

Datta, K., J. Tu, N. Oliva, I. Ona, R. Velazhahan, T.W. Mew, S. Muthukrishnan, and S.K. Datta. 2001. Enhanced resistance to sheath blight by constitutive expression of infection-related rice chitinase in transgenic elite indica rice cultivars. *Plant Science* 160:405-414.

Datta, K., A. Vasquez, J. Tu, L. Torrizo, M.F. Alam, N. Oliva, E. Abrigo, G.S. Khush, and S.K. Datta. 1998. Constitutive and tissue-specific differential expression of *cryIA(b)* gene in transgenic rice plants conferring resistance to rice insect pest. *Theor. Appl. Genet.* 97:20-30.

Datta, K., R. Velazhahan, N. Oliva, T. Mew, G.S. Khush, S. Muthukrishnan, and S.K. Datta. 1999b. Over-expression of cloned rice thaumatin-like protein (PR-5) gene in transgenic rice plants enhances environment-friendly resistance to *Rhizoctonia solani* causing sheath blight disease. *Theor. Appl. Genet.* 98:1138-1145.

Datta, S.K. 1999. Transgenic cereals: *Oryza sativa* (rice). In: I.K. Vasil (ed.) *Molecular improvement of cereal crops*. Kluwer Acad. Pub. UK. pp. 149-187.

Datta, S.K. 2000. Transgenic rice: development and products for environmentally friendly sustainable agriculture. In: *Challenge of plant and agricultural sciences to the crisis of biosphere on the earth in the 21st century* (Eds. K. Watanabe and A. Komamine), Landes Bioscience, Texas, USA, pp. 237-246.

Datta, S.K. 2001. *The need for genetically engineered food when enough is produced and unused.* Scope Genetically Modified Food Controversy Forum, April 16. pp. 1-7.

Datta, S.K., and H.E. Bouis. 2000. The potential of biotechnology in developing nutrient-dense rice varieties. *Food and Nutrition Bulletin* 21:451-456.

Datta, S.K., K. Datta, N. Soltanifar, G. Donn, and I. Potrykus. 1992. Herbicide-resistant indica rice plants from IRRI breeding line IR72 after PEG-mediated transformation of protoplasts. *Plant Mol. Biol.* 20:619-629.

Datta, S.K., A. Peterhans, K. Datta, and I. Potrykus. 1990. Genetically engineered fertile Indica-rice recovered from protoplasts. *Bio/Technology* 8:736-740.

Datta, S.K., L. Torrizo, J. Tu, N. Oliva, and K. Datta. 1997. *Production and molecular evaluation of transgenic rice plants.* IRRI Discussion Paper Series No. 21. International Rice Research Institute. Manila, Philippines.

Datta, S.K. and I. Potrykus. 1989. Artificial seed in barley: encapsulation of microspore derived embryos. *Theor Appl. Genet.* 77:820-824.

Datta, S.K. and G. Wenzel. 1987. Isolated microspore derived plant formation via embryogenesis in *Triticum aestivum. Plant Science* 48:49-54.

Dey, M., L.B. Torrizo, R.K. Chaudhuri, P.M. Reddy, J.K. Ladha, K. Datta, and S.K. Datta. 1999. Transgenic rice harboring legume ENOD40 gene. *Rice Genet. Newsl.* 16:147-149.

Duan, X., X. Li, Q. Xue, M. Abo-El-Saad, D. Xu, and R. Wu. 1996. Transgenic rice plants harboring an introduced potato proteinase inhibitor II gene are insect resistant. *Nature Biotechnol.* 14:494-498.

Enoki, H., T. Izawa, M. Kawahara, M. Komatsu, S. Koh, J. Kyozuka, and K. Shimamoto. 1999. Ac as a tool for the functional genomics of rice. *Plant Journal* 19(5):605-613.

Evenson, R. 2000. *Crop genetic improvement and agricultural development,* TAC Secretariat, CGIAR, May 2000.

Falco, S.C., T. Guida, M. Locke, J. Mauvais, C. Sanders, R.T. Ward, and P. Webber. 1995. Transgenic canola and soybean seeds with increased lysine. *Bio/Technology* 13:577-582.

FAO. 2000. Dynamics of change. The dividends of food security. In: *The state of food insecurity in the world.* pp. 19-20.

Fujimoto, H., K. Itoh, M. Yamamoto, J. Kyozuka, and K. Shimamoto. 1993. Insect resistant rice generated by introduction of a modified δ-endotoxin gene of *Bacillus thuringiensis. Bio/Technology* 11:1151-1155.

Graham, R., D. Senadhira, S. Beebe, C. Iglesias, I. Monasterio, and R.M. Welch. 1999. Breeding for micronutrient density in edible portions of staple food crops: conventional approaches. *Field Crops Res.* 60(1-2): 57-80.

Goto, F., T. Yoshihara, N. Shigemoto, S. Toki, and F. Takaiwa. 1999. Iron fortification of rice seed by the soybean ferritin gene. *Nature Biotechnol.* 17(3):282-286.

Gregorio, G.B., D. Senadhira, T. Htut, and R.D. Graham. 2000. Improving the micronutrient value of rice for human nutrition. In: *Impact of Agriculture on human health and nutrition.* Encyclopedia of Life Support Systems UNESCO (ed. I. Cakmak), in press.

Hayakawa, T., Y. Zhu, K. Itoh, Y. Kimura, T. Izawa, K. Shimamoto, and S. Toriyama. 1992. Genetically engineered rice resistant to rice stripe virus, an insect-transmitted virus. *Proc. Natl. Acad. Sci.* USA. 89:9865-9869.

Hiei, Y., S. Ohta, T. Komari, and T. Kumashiro. 1994. Efficient transformation of rice (*Oryza sativa* L.) mediated by *Agrobacterium* and sequence analysis of the boundaries of the T-DNA. *Plant J.* 6(2):271-282.

Hossain, M., J. Bennett, S.K. Datta, H. Leung, and G.S. Khush. 2000. Biotechnology research in rice for Asia: priorities, focus and directions. In: *Agricultural biotechnology in developing countries: towards optimizing the benefits for the poor* (eds. M. Qaim, A. Kratigger, and J. von Braun). Kluwer Academic Publishers.

Irie K., H. Hosoyama, T. Takeuchi, K. Iwabuchi, H. Watanabe, M. Abe, K. Abe, and S. Arai. 1996. Transgenic rice established to express corn cystatin exhibits strong inhibitor activity against insect gut proteinases. *Plant Mol. Biol.* 30:149-157.

Ja-Ock, G., et al. 2000. <http://www.chonnam.ac.kr/~cnutoday/200019-5/english/news/y-bians.htm#Prof.%20Guh%20Ja-ock>.

Jena, K.K., G.S. Khush, and G. Kochert. 1992. RFLP analysis of rice (*Oryza sativa* L.) introgression lines. *Theor. Appl. Genet.* 84:608-616.

Jeon, J.S., S. Lee, K.H. Jung, S.H. Jun, D.H. Jeong, J. Lee, C. Kim, S. Jang, S. Lee, K. Yang, J. Nam, K. An, M.J. Han, R.J. Sung, H.S. Choi, J.H. Yu, J.H. Choi, S.Y. Cho, S.S. Cha, S.I. Kim, and G. An. 2000. T-DNA insertional mutagenesis for functional genomics in rice. *Plant J.* 22(6):561-570.

Kawase M. 1994. Application of restriction landmark genomic scanning (RLGs) method to rice cultivars as a new fingerprinting technique. *Theor. Appl. Genet.* 89(7/8):861-864.

Khush, G.S. 1995. Breaking the yield frontier of rice. *Geojournal.* 35(3): 329-332.

Khush, G.S. 1999. Green Revolution: preparing for the 21st century. *Genome.* 42:646-655.

Ku, M.S.B., S. Agarie, M. Nomura, H. Fukayama, H. Tsuchida, K. Ono, S. Hirose, S. Toki, M. Miyao, and M. Matsuoka. 1999. High-level expression of maize phosphoenol carboxylase in transgenic rice plants. *Nature Biotechnol.* 17:76-80.

Lin, W., C.S. Anuratha, K. Datta, I. Potrykus, S. Muthukrishnan, and S.K. Datta. 1995. Genetic engineering of rice for resistance to sheath blight. *Bio/Technology* 13:686-691.

Misawa, N., S. Yamono, H. Linden, M.R. de Felipe, M. Lucas, H. Ikenga, and G. Sandmann. 1993. Functional expression of the *Erwinia uredovora* carotenoid biosynthesis gene *crtI* in transgenic plants showing an increase of β-carotene biosynthesis activity and resistance to the bleaching herbicide Norflurazon. *Plant J.* 4:833-840.

McCouch, S.R., G. Kochert, Z.H. Yu, Z.Y. Wang, G.S. Khush, and S.D. Tanksley. 1988. Molecular mapping of rice chromosomes. *Theor. Appl. Genet.* 76(6):815-829.

Monsanto. 2000. <http://www.monsanto.com/monsanto/media/00/00apr4_rice.html>.

Nayak, P., D. Basu, S. Das, A. Basu, D. Ghosh, N.A. Ramakrishna, M. Ghosh, and S.K. Sen. 1997. Transgenic elite indica rice plants expressing *CrylAc* δ-endotoxin of *Bacillus thuringiensis* are resistant against yellow stem borer (*Scirpophaga incertulas*). *Proc. Natl. Acad. Sci. USA.* 94:2111-2116.

Nishizawa, Y., Z. Nishio, K. Nakazono, M. Soma, E. Nakajima, M. Ugaki, and T. Hibi. 1999. Enhanced resistance to blast (*Magnaporthe grisea*) in transgenic japonica rice by constitutive expression of rice chitinase. *Theor. Appl. Genet.* 99:383-390.

Niizeki, H. and K. Oono. 1968. Induction of haploid rice plan from anther culture. *Proc. Jpn. Acad.* 44:554-557.

Peterhans, A., S.K. Datta, K. Datta, G.J. Goodall, I. Potrykus, and J. Paszkowski. 1990. Recognition efficiency of *Dicotyledoneae*-specific promoter and RNA processing signals in rice. *Mol. Gen. Genet.* 22:361-368.

Potrykus, I. 1991. Gene transfer to plants: assessment and perspective. *Physiol. Plant.* 79:125-134.

Potrykus, I. 2001 Golden Rice and beyond. *Plant Physiol.* 125:1157-1161.

Quimio, C.A., L.B. Torrizo, T.L. Setter, M. Ellis, A. Grover, E.M. Abrigo, N.P. Oliva, E.S. Ella, A.L. Carpena, O. Ito, W.J. Peacock, E. Dennis, and S.K. Datta. 2000. Enhancement of submergence tolerance in transgenic rice overproducing pyruvate decarboxylase. *J. Plant Physiol.* 156:516-521.

Reddy P.M., J.K. Ladha, M.C. Ramos, F. Maillet, R.J. Hernandez, L.B. Torrizo, N.P. Oliva, S.K. Datta, and K. Datta. 1998. Rhizobial lipochitooligosaccharide nodulation factors activate expression of the legume early nodulin gene *ENOD12* in rice. *Plant J.* 14:693-702.

Schell, J. 1987. Transgenic plants as tools to study the molecular organization of plant genes. *Science* 237:1176-1183.

Senadhira, D., G.B. Gregorio, and R.D. Graham. 1999. Breeding iron and zinc-dense rice. In Proceedings *"International workshop on micronutrient enhancement of rice for developing countries"* September 3, Rice, Research and Extension Centre, Stuttgart, Arkansas, USA. pp. 1-23.

Song, W.Y., G.L. Wang, L.L. Chen, H.S. Kim, L. Pi, T. Holsten, J. Gardner, B. Weng, W.X. Xhai, L.H. Chu, C. Fauquet, and P. Ronald. 1995. A receptor kinase-like protein encoded by the rice disease resistance gene, *Xa21*. *Science* 270:1804-1806.

Syngenta. 2001. <http://www.Syngenta.com/en/media/article.asp?article_id=126>.

Tanksley, S.D. and C.J. Nelson. 1996. Advanced backcross QTL analysis, a method for the simultaneous discovery and transfer of valuable QTLs from unadapted germplasm into elite breeding lines. *Theor. Appl. Genet.* 92:191-203.

Terada, R., M. Nakajima, M. Isshiki, R.J. Okagaki, S.R. Wessler, and K. Shimamoto. 2000. Antisense *waxy* genes with highly active promoter effectively suppress *waxy* gene expression in transgenic rice. *Plant Cell Physiol.* 41(7):881-888.

Toriyama, K., Y. Arimoto, H. Uchimiya, and K. Hinata. 1988. Transgenic rice plants after direct gene transfer into protoplasts. *Bio/Technology* 6:1072-1074.

Tu, J., K. Datta, M.F. Alam, G.S. Khush, and S.K. Datta. 1998a. Expression and function of a hybrid *Bt* toxin gene in transgenic rice conferring resistance to insect pests. *Plant Biotechnol.* 15:183-191.

Tu, J., I. Ona, Q. Zhang, T.W. Mew, G.S. Khush, and S.K. Datta. 1998b. Transgenic rice variety IR72 with *Xa21* is resistant to bacterial blight. *Theor. Appl. Genet.* 97:31-36.

Tu, J., K. Datta, G.S. Khush, Q. Zhang, and S.K. Datta. 2000a. Field performance of *Xa21* transgenic indica rice (*Oryza sativa* L.), IR72. *Theor. Appl. Genet.* 101:15-20.

Tu, J., G. Zhang, K. Datta, C. Xu, Y. He, Q. Zhang, G.S. Khush, and S.K. Datta. 2000b. Field performance of transgenic elite commercial hybrid rice expressing *Bacillus thuringiensis* δ-endotoxin. *Nature Biotechnol.* 18:1101-1104.

Wang, G.L., W.Y. Song, D.L. Ruan, S. Sideris, and P.C. Ronald. 1996. The cloned gene *Xa21* confers resistance to multiple *Xanthomonas oryzae* pv. *oryzae* isolates in transgenic plants. *Mol. Plant-Microbe Interact.* 9(9):850-855.

Welch, R.M., and R.D. Graham. 1999. A new paradigm for world agriculture: meeting human needs productive, sustainable nutrition. *Field Crops Res.* 60(1-2):1-10.

Xiao, J.H., S. Grandillo, S.N. Ahn, S.R. McCouch, S.D. Tanksley, J.M. Li, and L.P. Yuan. 1996. Genes from wild rice improve yield. *Nature* 386(6606):223-224.

Ye, X., S. Al-Babili, A. Klöti, J. Zhang, P. Lucca, P. Beyer, and I. Potrykus. 2000. Engineering the provitamin A (β-carotene) biosynthetic pathway into (carotenoid free) rice endosperm. *Science* 287:303-305.

Ye, G., J. Tu, C. Hu, K. Datta, and S.K. Datta. 2001. Transgenic IR72 with fused *Bt* gene cry1AB/cry1Ac from *Bacillus thuringiensis* is resistant against four lepidopteran species under field conditions. *Plant Biotech.* 18(2):125-133.

Yoshimura, A., A. Yoshimura, N. Iwata, S.R. McCouch, M. Lleva Abens, M.R. Baraoidan, T.W. Mew, and R.J. Nelson. 1995. Tagging and combining bacterial blight resistance genes in rice using RAPD and RFLP markers. *Mol. Breed.* 1(4):375-387.

Yu, Z.H., D.J. Mackill, J.M. Bonmann, and S.D. Tanksley. 1991. Tagging genes for blast resistance in rice via linkage to RFLP makers. *Theor. Appl. Genet.* 81:471-476.

Zhao, X.P. and G. Kochert. 1993. Clusters of interspersed repeated DNA sequences in the rice genome (*Oryza*). *Genome* 36(5):944-953.

Changing Significance of Inland Fisheries for Livelihoods and Nutrition in Bangladesh

P. Thompson
N. Roos
P. Sultana
S. H. Thilsted

SUMMARY. Fish is an essential and irreplaceable food in the rural Bangladesh diet. Inland capture fisheries are still the main source of fish in the diet. Although wetlands and fish habitat have been lost to drainage and flood control, the contribution of aquaculture to total fish production has been increasing in the last two decades.

The contribution of different species to fish intake as well as micronutrient intakes has been investigated based on food consumption studies. The main distinction is between small indigenous fish species (SIS), which typically are caught in open waters and floodplains, and larger species including carps (which are now largely cultured in ponds) and other fishes. The contribution of nutrient–minerals and especially vitamin A–from SIS is particularly important. Some SIS have very high vitamin A contents, whereas other fish, including carps have low vitamin A content. SIS that are eaten whole are also an important source of calcium. In addition, fish as part of a meal can enhance the intake of minerals present in other foods. Lastly, SIS are well-liked by the rural poor and are considered tasty and nutritious.

P. Thompson and P. Sultana are affiliated with the International Center for Living Aquatic Resources Management, Bangladesh (E-mail: p.thompson@cgiar.og).

N. Roos and S. H. Thilsted are affiliated with the Research Department of Human Nutrition, The Royal Veterinary and Agricultural University, Denmark (E-mail: Shakuntala.H.Thilsted@fhe.kvl.dk).

This is an ICLARM Contribution No. 1629.

[Haworth co-indexing entry note]: "Changing Significance of Inland Fisheries for Livelihoods and Nutrition in Bangladesh." Thompson, P. et al. Co-published simultaneously in *Journal of Crop Production* (Food Products Press, an imprint of The Haworth Press, Inc.) Vol. 6, No. 1/2 (#11/12), 2002, pp. 249-317; and: *Food Systems for Improved Human Nutrition: Linking Agriculture, Nutrition, and Productivity* (ed: Palit K. Kataki, and Suresh Chandra Babu) Food Products Press, an imprint of The Haworth Press, Inc., 2002, pp. 249-317. Single or multiple copies of this article are available for a fee from The Haworth Document Delivery Service [1-800-HAWORTH, 9:00 a.m. - 5:00 p.m. (EST). E-mail address: getinfo@haworthpressinc.com].

Case studies of fisheries and aquaculture interventions in Bangladesh indicate that SIS still contribute more to fish consumption than do cultured species for both poor and rich households. Fish consumption levels and the proportion of SIS in the diet are seasonal, peaking in and immediately after the wet season. Examples of community initiatives to protect over-wintering fish in local sanctuaries and to restore fish habitat and migration routes appear to have increased fish catches and consumption. Where beel (lake) fisheries were enhanced by stocking carps, the user communities benefited from higher catches and incomes. However, it seemed that fish consumption for non-participants increase where fishing was not limited, but fell where they were excluded from fishing by participants.

Extension efforts have encouraged rapid growth in aquaculture production in the last two decades. A case study indicated that increases in production were sustained and that practices had spread from extension participants. Declining capture fisheries and increasing carp production mean that carps have become relatively cheaper, and it has been seen that the proportion of carps to other fish sold doubled in less than a decade in some local markets. However, poor rural consumers without ponds are now more dependent on purchased fish, and increased production of carp from ponds does not compensate for substantial declines in their SIS catches from open waters. Aquaculture in flooded rice fields would normally exclude the poor, but there have been attempts where NGOs have organized landless people to benefit from stocking carps.

SIS can be included in pond aquaculture systems, and on-farm experiments show this can complement carp production by increasing production and cash returns. A focus on incorporating vitamin A rich SIS in aquaculture combined with widespread and concerted efforts to restore and sustainably manage the floodplain fisheries (which are dominated by SIS) can result in an important food-based strategy to improve micronutrient deficiencies in poor people in Bangladesh and similar floodplains. *[Article copies available for a fee from The Haworth Document Delivery Service: 1-800-HAWORTH. E-mail address: <getinfo@haworthpressinc.com> Website: <http://www.HaworthPress.com> © 2002 by The Haworth Press, Inc. All rights reserved.]*

KEYWORDS. Fish consumption, fish production, inland fisheries, nutrition, small indigenous fish species, vitamin A

THE BANGLADESH CONTEXT

Fish and rice play an important and intertwining role in the livelihoods and nutrition of the Bangladeshi population, especially in the rural areas. They dominate the diet of Bangladeshis to such an extent that the old proverb—"machee bhatee Bangali" which can be translated as fish and rice make a Bangali, continues to hold true.

Fish is an essential and irreplaceable food in the rural Bangladeshi diet. Together with boiled rice, which is eaten twice per day, small amounts of vegetables, pulses, and spices are also eaten. In the last national nutrition survey conducted in rural Bangladesh in 1981-82, the total food intake was 763 g of raw food/capita/day, of which 60% was rice, 30% vegetables, and 6% animal food. Fish intake was 23 g/capita/day and made up 53% of the animal food intake (Ahmad and Hassan, 1983).

Since the advent of the Green Revolution, Bangladesh has made tremendous strides in increasing rice production. This success has occurred through many changes in the overall agricultural production the management of land and water. More areas have been brought under rice production, irrigation has expanded greatly, and areas have been drained and protected by flood control embankments. These changes have been at the expense of fish: the area of inland waterbodies and the duration of inundation in some areas have fallen, and thereby, there has been a reduction in the habitat for fish.

THE ROLE OF FISH AND FISHERIES IN THE LIVELIHOOD SYSTEMS OF RURAL BANGLADESH

Fish provide the main source of income to perhaps 2 million households that either fish for a profession or are involved in related trades (World Bank, 1991). Many more households catch fish for part-time income and food. In communities around 19 waterbodies studied by the International Center for Living Aquatic Resources Management (ICLARM), an estimated 87% of all households caught fish for some time each year (Thompson and Hossain, 1998). Similarly, studies conducted by the Flood Action Plan (FAP) showed that 85% of households surveyed fished at some time, and of these, 63% fished for own consumption and 22% fished full- or part-time for income (FAP 16, 1995).

Although capture fisheries dominate total production, aquaculture has grown rapidly in the past two decades, producing freshwater fishes for domestic consumption and shrimp for export, while marine fish production has remained static. From July 1998 to June 1999, the Department of Fisheries (DOF) estimated fish production at 1.55 million metric tonnes (t) (DOF, 2000), amounting to about 10.5 t of fish per km^2 of land or 12 kg/person, some of the highest production levels in the world. Nevertheless, there are concerns that fish availability both in aggregate and especially for the rural poor is declining and with it a vital component of food security and nutrition.

Floodplain fisheries are a vital but declining component of the traditional floodplain livelihood systems. Over half of the country comprises floodplains, and in the past some 6.3 million ha of agricultural land were regularly inundated (Master Plan Organization [MPO], 1987; Ali, 1997). In these open floodplains, agriculture and natural fisheries complemented one another. As is typical of floodplain fisheries (Welcomme, 1985; Payne, 1997), in the dry season (approximately December-May) most land was cultivated and fish were restricted to *beels* (floodplain depressions and lakes) and rivers, which are government property. Fish on government property were caught by professional fishers working for leaseholders. In the monsoon to post-monsoon (June-November), the private land of the floodplain was inundated, but much was still cultivated with deepwater rice. This practice provided for an ideal habitat for the wide diversity of fishes, some 260 species (Rahman, 1989), that inhabit this riverine floodplain system, and during this period, anyone from the rural areas could catch fish. Dependence on rice and fish helped to even out annual variations. In drier years, rice yields might be higher although there was less habitat for fish. In flood years, crops might be damaged, but fish catches would be higher. Seasonal access patterns benefited poor people, who were able to catch fish and other aquatic resources for food as well as obtain an additional income in the monsoon and post-monsoon period.

Although these livelihood systems still exist, the fishery sector has been modified and became more complex since the 1960s. Inland capture fisheries have been modified and encroached, and there is increasing competition for access. Freshwater aquaculture has grown and now most people with a pond try to stock fish (mostly a mixture of carps) in their ponds. A few commercial fish farmers have emerged, but most people use existing ponds to produce fish for a mixture of sale and own consumption. Shrimp farming has developed as an extensive business on private lands in large areas near the coast, fuelled by collection of wild shrimp larvae by the coastal poor, and most recently by fry from hatcheries. Marine and coastal catches have grown with the use of mechanized trawlers and new gears (Rahman, Chowdury, and Saha, 2000).

TRENDS IN FISH PRODUCTION AND CONSUMPTION

The basis for fish production and consumption is the interaction of people with wetland habitats and the fish that inhabit them. Considering inland fisheries first, the floodplains are a key component of the system as shown in Figure 1. Although official figures show these catches have risen in the 1990s after falling in the 1980s, it is widely held that floodplain catches have been falling. The apparent discrepancy may be due to more intensive monitoring of floodplain stocking in the early-mid 1990s and problems over the validity of areas used in

FIGURE 1. Fish production in Bangladesh, 1983-84 to 1998-99.

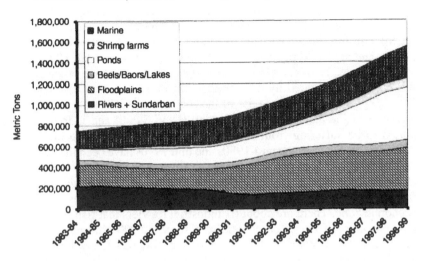

the estimates (Ali, 1999). Out of 6.3 million ha of floodplain agricultural land, about 0.8 million ha were reported to be inside flood control projects by 1985. This area had probably risen to 3.3 million ha by 1990 (Ali, 1997), while the Department of Fisheries estimated that 1.7 million ha of wetlands would be lost as fisheries between 1990 and 2010 (Ahmed, 1999). This estimation implies that most floodplain land is or will be affected by flood control and drainage. There is now a national policy not to further drain wetlands (National Water Policy 1998, see Habib, 1999), but past policies and water management projects have reduced the average depth and duration of monsoon flooding in much of the more shallow flooded parts of the floodplain. These shallow flooded areas have been shown by Environment and Geographic Information Systems (GIS) Support Project (1997) to be a vital habitat, supporting high densities of fish in the monsoon. Thus loss of wetlands and reduced access to waterbodies can have a negative effect on fish consumption in rural Bangladesh.

Not only has the area of fish habitat fallen, but embankments and water control structures have blocked the connections between rivers and the beels and floodplain land within embanked areas. This obviously affects the seasonal migrations of some fish species and the composition and diversity of fish stocks. Fish catches relative to area are reported to have fallen by 81% where there is full flood protection, but did not differ consistently within the remaining water area between partial flood control and unprotected floodplains—catches of about 120 kg/ha/year (FAP 17, 1994; Overseas Development Administration [ODA], 1997). Major carps have fallen from about 47% of floodplain catches to only 3% due to several factors including loss of habitat, loss of river-floodplain connections and over fishing (Payne and Temple, 1996). Thus a loss of 95% of migratory species and a 33% reduction in fish diversity were reported for full flood protection by ODA (1997). Use of agro-chemicals, pesticides, and industrial pollution also affect the fish habitat (Ali, 1997).

Meanwhile, the river and estuarine catch is reported to have fallen. Much of this catch is dominated by one species, hilsha, (*Tenualosa ilisha*) which in 1998-1999 comprised up to 65% of the river catch, 45% of the marine catch, and 14% of the national fish production (DOF, 2000) and is frequently reported to be suffering from over fishing. Notable changes to the Jamuna-Padma rivers between the mid-1980s and mid 1990s have been the decimation of the major carp spawn and fry fishery and increased fishing for shrimp larvae along the estuarine and coastal channels. This fishery connects with the marine fishery, the latter covering some 166,000 km^2 within Bangladesh's exclusive economic zone. There are about 67 industrial trawlers that fish in deeper waters, but most of the catch comes from some 50,000 artisanal boats (46% mechanized) and only a small part is exported (Rahman, Chowdury and Saha, 2000). Over the past two decades, this fishery grew up as a result of mechanization and by-catch of non-target shrimp larvae and other species is thought to be excessive.

One of the main contributors to the 7% per year growth in fish production from 1989-1990 to 1998-1999 (DOF, 2000) was pond aquaculture. Fish production from ponds tripled in this period. This growth has arisen due to increasing number of ponds, increasing proportion under culture, and improving technologies and culture practices (mostly carp polyculture, but also some tilapia [*Oreochromis mossambicus*]). This trend has been supported by a number of aquaculture extension projects of the Department of Fisheries (DOF) and extension messages in the mass media (Thompson et al., 2000). In Bangladesh, there are many freshwater ponds throughout the country. Official figures have been revised to 215,000 ha (DOF, 2000), but this is likely still to be an underestimate as updating has been partial. Islam and Collis (1998) estimated the area of perennial ponds to be 219,580 ha and seasonal ponds 73,194 ha. Perhaps because of the profitability of aquaculture, the number of ponds appears to have increased over the last decade faster than population growth: 8% per year in some areas of the south (Patuakhali Barguna Aquaculture Extension Project (PBAEP), 1998) and 5-8% per year in Gazipur, north of Dhaka (Thompson et al., 2000).

According to DOF (1996), the proportion of derelict (unused) ponds fell from 43% to 17% and the number cultured increased from 27% to 52% between 1984 and 1996. But locally, much higher values for cultured ponds have been reported; 85% (PBAEP, 1998) and 90% (Thompson et al., 2000). DOF (2000) estimated fish production of 3,080 kg/ha/year in cultured ponds and

2,610 kg/ha/year in all ponds in 1998-1999, but these figures may be higher than those normally achieved. Thompson et al. (2000) surveyed past participants of several extension projects and found production of 1,900-3,700 kg/ha/year compared with control farmers averaging 1,300-1,600 kg/ha/year. Non-cultured ponds may yield about 500 kg/ha/year (Ahmed, 1992). In addition, there are increasing areas of private farmland where fish are being stocked and grown together with or after a rice crop. There are no precise figures, but as part of integrated farming and pest management, fish are being grown in increasing areas of private farmland with average yields of about 210-230 kg/ha/year (Gupta et al., 1998).

About 85% of fish produced in ponds are carps (DOF, 2000): indigenous major carps or introduced species such as silver carp (*Hypophthalmichthys molitrix*) and common carp (*Cyprinus carpio*). As will be seen later, this form of carp introduction has important implications for the availability of fish to poor people and the nutritional value of the fish being consumed. Rotenone was used widely to kill undesired species (small fishes and predators) in ponds, but is not so widely recommended now, although most aquaculture extension projects still recommend that farmers catch wild fish before stocking. In the Second Aquaculture Development Project of Department of Fisheries in the early 1990s, rotenone was used to kill wild fish in beels so they could be used as nurseries to stock major carp fry that was later dispersed into the floodplain, through the monsoon but this was ended due to concern over environmental impacts (Payne and Cowan, 1998).

With a total fish production estimated at 1.55 million t from June 1998 to July 1999 and a population of about 128 million people, this would imply an average fish consumption of around 30 g/person/day, even allowing for almost all brackish water shrimps and some fish (marine and freshwater) being exported.

CATEGORIZATION OF FISH IN BANGLADESH

For the purposes of this article, "fish" in Bangladesh have been divided into six broad categories, defined as:

- Small indigenous fish species (SIS) (under 25 cm at maximum size).
- Shrimps and prawns (almost entirely small freshwater prawns).
- Cultured and carp species (all major carps and all other species cultured, i.e., introduced species), all these may be termed medium to large, growing to over 25 cm at maximum size.
- Hilsha—an important river and estuarine species that forms the single largest part of the official capture fishery catches.

- Medium and large catfish and carnivorous species, are high value freshwater species that are above 25 cm at maximum size.
- Other medium to large fishes, a miscellaneous group of variable values that include some brackish water fishes (above 25 cm at maximum size).

These categories are broadly consistent but simplify those that were used in past studies in Bangladesh. The key distinction is that of small indigenous species (SIS), which Felts, Rajts, and Akhteruzzaman (1996) defined as those growing at maximum length to not more than 25 cm. These SIS have been neglected in past statistics but are important as food for the poor and micronutrient sources. Appendix A gives the names of all species recorded in the various surveys reported in this paper, according to these six categories. The fish names used in the text are the common (Bangla) names which are widely used in Bangladesh. For all species mentioned in this article, scientific names following the taxonomy used in FishBase 2000 (Froese and Pauly, 2000) are given in Appendix A.

THE IMPORTANCE OF FISH FOR HUMAN NUTRITION

Several surveys and studies that have measured food intake have shown the importance of fish in the Bangladeshi diet. In terms of amount of food consumed, fish ranks third after rice and vegetables (Ahmad and Hassan, 1983). Fish intake is affected by several factors, such as year, season, location, water level, and income level. Table 1 shows a range of fish intakes from selected studies. The distributions of fish intake recorded at individual or household level are skewed, with higher mean than median values. Small fish contribute considerably to total fish intake. The values for Mymensingh suggest that the intake of large fish increases with income level (Bouis et al., 1998).

The Content of Nutrients in Fish

The importance of fish as a rich source of animal protein is well established and is frequently used to justify fish as a valuable food. However, very little focus has been given to the role of fish in supplying vitamin A and minerals in the diet.

Fish is a rich source of animal protein, providing essential amino acids such as lysine which are in low concentrations in rice. Protein content in fish ranges from 14 to 18 g/100 g raw edible parts (Darnton-Hill et al., 1988). From the last national survey in rural Bangladesh, the total protein intake was 48 g/person/day, of which fish contributed 3 g of total protein, but 84% of the animal protein intake (Ahmad and Hassan, 1983). However, the policy issues regarding fish in human nutrition are not centred on protein since the normal

Bangladeshi diet if it meets accepted standards of energy intake is sufficient to meet total protein requirements (Roos, 2001). The key issue is the composition of fish intake and additional nutrients–minerals, especially vitamin A–provided by different types of fish.

In 1981, two SIS, mola (*Amblypharyngodon mola*) and dhela (*Osteobrama cotio*) were reported as having high vitamin A content (Zafri and Ahmed, 1981). This resut was confirmed in minor studies, in which, high-performance liquid chromatography (HPLC) was used to analyze vitamin A components (Thilsted and Roos, 1999; Varming, 1996; Villif and Joergensen, 1993).

The categories in Table 2 are based on the vitamin A content of the most commonly consumed fish species in Bangladesh (Roos, 2001). Mola and chanda (*Parambassis baculis*) were categorized as having a very high content of vitamin A (over 1,500 RE/100 g raw edible parts). Dhela and darkina (*Esomus danricus*) were categorized as having a high content of vitamin A (500-1,500 RE/100 g raw edible parts). The values for vitamin A content in the different fish species suggest the vitamin A content is species specific. Species with very high, high, and medium vitamin A contents are all SIS. The cultured carp species, silver carp, rui (*Labeo rohita*), and mrigel (*Cirrhinus mrigela*) have low vitamin A contents.

Vitamin A content in mola is extremely high. However, 53% of the vitamin A is concentrated in the eyes (62,180 RE/100 g), and 39% in the viscera (3,622 RE/100 g), of the total amount contained in the whole fish. This distribution makes the cleaning of the fish before cooking extremely important. The cleaning practice depends on the fish species, size of fish, and the woman cleaning the fish. Waste included the gill cover, jaw, head, tail and/or viscera (partially or fully). It was found that the heads and eyes of mola were always regarded as edible parts (Roos, 2001).

Vitamin A in fish is found in the forms of retinol and dehydroretinol isomers, the relative contribution of which varies with species. In mola and chanda, 80-90% of the total vitamin A is present as dehydroretinol, while in darkina, 70% is present as all-*trans* retinol. The dehydroretinol isomers are calculated as having 40% of the biological activity of that of all-*trans* retinol (Shantz and Brinkman, 1950). Retinol and dehydroretinol, which are preformed vitamin A are more efficiently absorbed than carotenoids and are thus more effective in improving vitamin A status than vegetables and fruits (National Research Council, 1989).

The contents of iron, zinc, calcium, and selenium in commonly consumed Bangladeshi fish are shown in Table 3. As all small fish are eaten with bones (some bones may be discarded during cleaning and as plate waste), small fish are an excellent source of calcium. In large fish, most bones are discarded as plate waste. The contribution of small fish to calcium intake is especially important in countries such as Bangladesh where intake of milk and milk prod-

TABLE 1. Fish Intake in Bangladesh from Selected Studies.

Location	Year/Season	Small fish[1] Mean, g/capita/day ± SD (median)	Large fish[2] Mean, g/capita/day ± SD (median)	Total fish Mean, g/capita/day ± SD (median)	Method	Reference
Rural Bangladesh	1962-64			28[3]	700 hh, 14 locations, 24 h food weighing	US Department of Health, Education and Welfare, 1966
Rural Bangladesh	1975-76			23[3]	750 hh, 12 locations, 24 h food weighing	Institute of Nutrition and Food Science, 1997
Rural Bangladesh	1981-82			23[3]	600 hh, 12 locations, 24 h food weighing	Ahmad and Hassan, 1983
Tangail Surma–Kushiya Floodplains Singra Matlab	1992[4] 1992 1992 1992			12[5] 18[5] 22[5] 34[5]	520 hh, interview	Minkin et al., 1997
Manikganj	1991-92 Dec.-Jan.	13 ± 19 (5)[3]	5 ± 14 (0)[3]	18 ± 22 (12)[3]	119 hh, 24 h food weighing	Hels, 1995
Manikganj	1995 Oct.-Nov. 1996 Jan.-Mar.	28 ± 45 (8)[3] 25 ± 47 (0)[3]	29 ± 51 (0)[3] 12 ± 36 (0)[3]	57 ± 62 (42)[3] 37 ± 56 (19)[3]	152 hh, 769 individuals, 24 h food weighing 145 hh, 717 individuals, 24 h food weighing	Tetens et al., (2001)
Kishoreganj	1997 Jul. 1997 Oct. 1998 Feb.	28 ± 26 (21)[5] 65 ± 55 (45)[5] 38 ± 40 (25)[5]	10 ± 17 (5)[5] 18 ± 25 (7)[5] 16 ± 18 (12)[5]	37 ± 33 (27)[5] 82 ± 65 (64)[5] 55 ± 48 (42)[5]	84 hh, 5 d recall interview	Roos, 2001
Kapasia Small farm Medium farm Large farm	1998-99 Aug.-Jul. 1998-99 Aug.-Jul. 1998-99 Aug.-Jul.			83[6] 85[6] 96[6]	20 hh, 84 days 24 h fish weighing 36 hh, 84 days 24 h fish weighing 12 hh, 84 days 24 h fish weighing	Thompson et al., 2000

Mymensingh	1995	Oct.-Nov.	14±33 (0)[3]	24±38 (6)[3]	38±47 (25)[3]	152 hh, 765 individuals, 24 h food weighing	Tetens et al., (2001)
	1996	Jan.-Mar.	12±22 (0)[3]	20±34 (0)[3]	32±37 (24)[3]	146 hh, 729 individuals, 24 h food weighing	
Mymensingh							
Low income	1996	Jun.-Sep.	17±21 (8)[6]	9±18 (0)[6]	26±26 (21)[6]	104 hh, 24 h recall	Bouis et al., 1998
Medium income			22±26 (13)[6]	14±22 (2)[6]	35±31 (30)[6]	104 hh, 24 h recall	
High income			25±34 (11)[6]	17±27 (3)[6]	42±40 (31)[6]	105 hh, 24 h recall	
Low income	1996	Oct.-Dec.	26±41 (18)[6]	6±12 (0)[6]	32±42 (25)[6]	104 hh, 24 h recall	
Medium income			23±2 (19)[6]	19±49 (2)[6]	42±54 (34)[6]	104 hh, 24 h recall	
High income			25±24 (19)[6]	18±25 (4)[6]	43±32 (38)[6]	105 hh, 24 h recall	
Low income	1997	Feb.-May	12±17 (4)[6]	8±13 (2)[6]	20±21 (14)[6]	104 hh, 24 h recall	
Medium income			13±19 (4)[6]	12±18 (3)[6]	25±25 (19)[6]	104 hh, 24 h recall	
High income			14±19 (6)[6]	15±21 (3)[6]	29±26 (24)[6]	105 hh, 24 h recall	
Low income	1997	Jun.-Sep.	21±24 (13)[6]	9±16 (0)[6]	30±27 (23)[6]	104 hh, 24 h recall	
Medium income			30±38 (18)[6]	11±17 (3)[6]	41±38 (30)[6]	104 hh, 24 h recall	
High income			28±31 (21)[6]	13±25 (0)[6]	41±37 (32)[6]	105 hh, 24 h recall	
Tangail (Hamil Beel)	1999	Feb.-May	9±7 (6)[6]	6±6 (5)[6]	15±9 (12)[6]	90 hh, 24 h food weighing, 7 days per month	ICLARM (2001)
		Jun.-Sep.	11±9 (9)[6]	6±6 (5)[6]	17±12 (14)[6]		
		Oct.-Dec.	15±12 (13)[6]	7±8 (6)[6]	23±14 (20)[6]		
Dinajpur (Ashurar Beel)	1999	Feb.-May	8±7 (6)[6]	5±8 (3)[6]	13±11 (11)[6]	90 hh, 24 h food weighing, 7 days per month	
		Jun.-Sep.	24±19 (20)[6]	2±4 (0)[6]	26±19 (23)[6]		
		Oct.-Dec.	29±17 (25)[6]	5±7 (3)[6]	34±19 (31)[6]		
Kishoreganj (Kali Nadi)	1999	Jan.-May	18±9 (16)[6]	8±7 (6)[6]	26±14 (23)[6]	90 hh, 24 h food weighing, 7 days per month	
		Jun.-Sep.	20±10 (19)[6]	9±8 (7)[6]	28±13 (26)[6]		
		Oct.-Dec.	28±15 (25)[6]	12±12 (8)[6]	40±21 (36)[6]		

[1] Small fish include small indigenous fish species (SIS), shrimp (except in Hamil Beel, Ashurar Beel and Kali Nadi) and the following medium sized fish: magur, rita, baila, bara baim, bhangon and kakila as shown in Appendix A.
[2] Large fish include all other fish species as shown in Appendix A.
[3] Raw edible parts.
[4] Drought year.
[5] Raw edible parts. Cleaning waste; mean 13% for SIS; mean 22% for large fish (including 8% plate waste).
[6] Raw whole fish.
hh = households

TABLE 2. Categories of Bangladeshi Fish Species Based on Vitamin A Content in Edible Parts.

Category of Fish Species	Vitamin A Content (RE/100 g raw edible parts)	Common Name[1]	Scientific Name
Very high content	> 1,500	Mola	*Amblypharyngodon mola*
		Chanda	*Parambassis baculis*
High content	500-1,500	Dhela	*Osteobrama cotio*
		Darkina	*Esomus danricus*
Medium content	100-500	Ranga chanda	*Parambassis ranga*
		Koi	*Anabas testudineus*
		Golsha tengra	*Mystus bleekeri*
		Gol chanda	*Chanda nama*
		Taki	*Channa punctata*
		Chela	*Chela cachius*
Low content	< 100	Tara baim	*Macrognathus aculeatus*
		Guchi baim	*Macrognathus pancalus*
		Kachki	*Corica soborna*
		Gutum	*Lepidocephalus guntea*
		Chapila	*Gudusia chapra*
		Chala puti	*Puntius chola*
		Jat puti	*Puntius sophore*
		Khalisha	*Colisha fasciatus*
		Shing	*Heteropneustes fossilis*
		Magur	*Clarias batrachus*
		Bara baim	*Mastacembelus armatus*
		Tit puti	*Puntius ticto*
		Chata	*Trichogaster lalius*
		Tilapia	*Oreochromis niloticus*
		Mrigel	*Cirrhinus mrigala*
		Rui	*Labeo rohita*
		Silver carp	*Hypophthalmichthys molitrix*
		Hilsha	*Tenualosa ilisha*

Adapted from Roos, 2001.
[1]Fish species listed in descending order of vitamin A content in each category.

ucts, rich calcium sources, are very low. In studies with both humans and rats, it has been shown that the bioavailability of calcium from whole small fish (mola) is as high as that from milk (Hansen et al., 1998; Larsen et al., 2000). In humans, the fractional calcium absorption was 24 ± 6% from small fish and 22 ± 6% from milk.

The iron content of the fish species analyzed ranged from 1.8 to 12.0 mg iron/100 g raw edible parts. Within the same species, the range was also high, indicating that environmental factors, including contamination affects the iron content. In fish, iron is present as both haem and non-haem iron in variable proportions. In five batches of mola, the percentage of haem iron with respect to total iron ranged from 5.0% to 29.2% (Soerensen, 1998). The bioavailability of haem iron in the diet is 20%-30%, and it is constant with little influenced by diet composition in contrast to non haem iron which has a bioavailability of

TABLE 3. Mineral Content in Raw Edible Parts of Commonly Consumed Bangladeshi Fishes.

Common name	Scientific name	n[1]	Mineral content per 100 g raw edible parts					Dry matter % (SD)
			Fe mg (SD)	Zn mg (SD)	Ca mg (SD)	Ca[2] mg (SD)	Se µg (SD)	
Baim/ Chikra	*Macrognathus aculeatus, Macrognathus pancalus, Mastocembelus armatus*	5	2.4 (0.4)	1.2 (0.1)	462 (56)	203 (25)	20 (15)	25 (1)
Chanda	*Parambassis ranga, Parambassis baculis, Chanda nama*	5	1.8 (0.7)	2.3 (0.6)	955 (342)	878 (314)	19 (11)	24.3 (1.6)
Chapila	*Gudusia chapra*	3	7.6 (5.3)	2.1 (0.1)	1063 (51)	786 (38)	13 (3)	27 (3)
Darkina	*Esomus danricus*	3	12.0 (9.1)	4.0 (1.0)	891 (357)	775 (321)	12 (2)	23 (3)
Kachki	*Corica soborna*	2	2.8 (1.2)	3.1 (0.5)	476 (37)	347 (34)	8 (2)	16 (1)
Mola	*Amblypharyngodon mola*	3	5.7 (3.7)	3.2 (0.4)	853 (86)	776 (78)	5 (2)	20 (1)
Puti	*Puntius sophore, P. chola, P. ticto*	4	3.0 (0.9)	3.1 (0.5)	1171 (216)	784 (145)	12 (4)	25 (1)
Taki	*Channa punctuatus*	3	1.8 (0.4)	1.5 (0.2)	766 (183)	337 (81)	15 (3)	22 (1)
Tengra	*Mystus vittatus*	2	4.0 (0.4)	3.1 (0.8)	1093 (334)	480 (147)	24 (13)	26 (4)
Shrimp (Chingri)	*Macrobracium sp.*	3	3.1 (2.2)	1.5 (0.3)	687 (23)	687 (23)	9 (3)	21 (2)
Mrigel	*Cirrhinus mrigala*	3	2.5 (1.3)	1.5 (0.1)	960 (104)	0 (0)	19 (2)	24 (3)
Silver carp	*Hypophthamichthys molitrix*	3	4.4 (1.8)	1.4 (0.5)	903 (361)	37 (14)	12 (1)	23 (2)

Adapted from Roos, 2001.
[1]n = number of samples. A sample contained 10-300 fish for SIS and 1-2 fish for larger fish.
[2]Calcium content corrected for plate waste.

less than 10% (Carpenter and Mahoney, 1992). Selenium content ranged from 7 to 45 µg/100 g raw edible parts.

Many Bangladeshi fish analyzed have low fat contents, less than 5 g/100 g raw edible parts, except for hilsha with a fat content of 19 g fat/100 g raw edible parts (Darnton-Hill et al., 1988). Fat from fish is generally low in saturated fatty acids and high in mono- and polyunsaturated fatty acids. Hilsha, a popular fish for consumption contributes to fat intake, and especially, to the intakes of omega 3 essential fatty acids, eicosapentanoic and docosahexanoic acids. Omega 3 fatty acids are essential for eicosanoid metabolism, gene expression, and intracellular and cell-to-cell communication, thereby, influencing numerous biochemical and pathophysiological processes in the body (Simopoulos, 1996). They are also linked to the prevention of cardiovascular diseases and other chronic diseases.

Enhancing Effects of Fish on Mineral Bioavailability

The Bangladeshi rice based diet is considered to have a low bioavailability of iron and zinc due to the contents of bioavailability inhibitors such as phytic acid in rice (Tuntawiroon et al., 1990). Fish protein is acknowledged to be a potent enhancer of iron and zinc bioavailability (Sandström et al., 1985). In addition to providing easily absorbable haem iron, fish protein enhances the absorption of non haem iron in other foods in the meal. Non-haem iron absorption was increased by a factor of 4.4 with an addition of fish corresponding to 20 g protein to a maize porridge meal, while fish corresponding to 10 g protein enhanced the absorption by a factor of 1.5 (Björn-Rasmussen and Hallberg, 1979). Forty grams of catfish added to a Burmese rice based meal containing 7.6 mg non-haem iron increased iron absorption from 2.0% to 13.2% (Aung-Than-Batu, Thein-Than, and Thane-Tae, 1976).

Studies have demonstrated that there is an interaction between vitamin A deficiency and anaemia, and that vitamin A intake improves iron status as well as vitamin A status (Bloem, 1995; Bloem et al., 1989; Mejia and Chew, 1988). Also, adding retinol to a radio-iron labelled rice meal with a retinol content of 150-800 RE/100 g cooked rice doubled iron absorption (García-Casal et al., 1998). It has been suggested that vitamin A reduces the inhibiting effect of phytic acid and phenol on non-haem iron absorption.

Contribution of Fish Intake to Recommended Dietary Intakes of Nutrients

An intake of 17 g mola/day (2,680 RE/100 g raw edible parts) meets the full daily vitamin A recommended dietary allowance of 4-6-year-old children (450 RE/day) (Food and Agriculture Organization of the United Nations [FAO]/ World Health Organization [WHO], 1998). In addition, this amount of mola contributes 22% of the recommended intake of calcium. The contributions to iron and zinc intakes are 8% and 5%, respectively, of the recommended intakes, assuming a diet with low bioavailability of these nutrients. The contribution to selenium intake is 4% of the recommended intake. Less than 5% of the recommended protein intake of 4-6-year-old children is met with an intake of 17 g of fish.

Perceptions of Rural People on the Nutritional Value of Fish in Bangladesh

Figure 2 shows the perceptions of the importance of various fish species for health and wellbeing as expressed by Bangladeshi women in a village survey (Thilsted and Roos, 1999). The 11 fish species with the highest ratings are shown. Two SIS, mola and dhela, were reported by many women as being good for protecting the eyes. These species have been found to have high vitamin A content (Table 2). It may be worthwhile to investigate whether the fish species, shing (*Heteropneustes fossilis*), magur (*Clarias batrachus*), and koi (*Anabas testudineus*) which were rated as increasing blood volume have a high iron content.

FIGURE 2. The 11 species with the highest rankings are shown. Perceptions of fish species by Bangladeshi rural women.

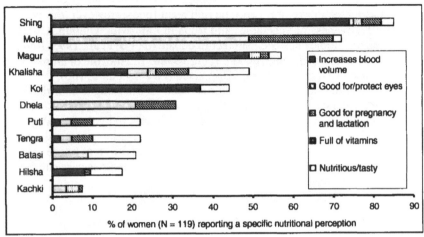

Adapted from Thilsted and Roos (1999).

In a household survey in Kishoreganj in 1997-1998, both male and female household members (n = 481) were asked to name the fish species which was most preferred for consumption. Rui, a large indigenous carp, was the most preferred fish species, mentioned by 24% of the persons. The second and third most preferred fishes were mola and hilsha, preferred by 13% and 11% of the respondents, respectively (Roos, 2001).

Overview of the Role of Fish in Human Nutrition

It can be concluded that fish are a vital part of the Bangladeshi diet, and an increase over current consumption levels will be generally nutritionally beneficial. Thus, all efforts to increase fish production and fish accessibility, especially to the poor are important. Fish contributes animal protein, which enhances the bioavailability of minerals. Moreover, certain SIS have very high vitamin A content and since small fish are eaten whole, or almost whole, they provide more calcium and other minerals than large fish, from which the bones are removed. This preference is of special importance in Bangladesh as vitamin A and iron deficiencies are recognized as public health problems, and there is evidence of low intakes of other minerals such as zinc and calcium (Ahmed, 1999; Ahmed, 2000; Seshadri, 1997). SIS can, therefore, play a very important role in food based strategies for improving vitamin A and mineral status in humans. At present, vitamin A deficiency in Bangladesh is sought to be prevented and controlled by high potency vitamin A capsule supplementation to preschool children, but food based strategies are needed to achieve long-term sustainability. Food based strategies to improve vitamin A status generally aim at increasing the intake of β-carotene rich plant foods. However, the evidence of the effectiveness of vegetables and fruits in improving vitamin A status in experimental studies has been subject to debate (de Pee et al., 1995; Reddy et al., 1996; Underwood, 1995; de Pee et al., 1998a) and the role of animal foods in food based strategies is being reappraised (de Pee et al. 1998b).

As fish is the most important animal food in the Bangladeshi diet, it is, therefore, necessary to understand the amounts of fish and types of fish actually produced, caught, bought, and eaten by different individuals and types of households, in different environments and seasons in order to assess the significance of fish for human nutrition and the potential of different future development paths in the fisheries sector. The next sections comprise case studies that provide this information.

INLAND FISHERIES IN BANGLADESH

In this chapter, we focus on the importance for fish consumption of inland fisheries and aquaculture because they produce 74% of fish in Bangladesh (Figure 3), which is almost all consumed within Bangladesh. Several key themes are explored through case study based evidence all of which focuses on implications for the consumption of fish by poor people. These include:

- The importance of fish species diversity in fish consumption. The "miscellaneous" small fish (SIS) caught from the floodplains by poor people have been termed "weed" or "trash" fish and have been neglected in official statistics, policies and recent development trends which have favoured expansion of carp production. SIS make up the everyday food of poor people, are well liked and are good sources of animal protein, vitamin A and minerals (Thilsted and Roos, 1999).
- Access to inland capture fisheries and the potential for user communities to establish common property or co-management regimes over local fisheries and then to take actions to restore fisheries and improve their food security. The fisheries of Bangladesh became state property under the jurisdiction of the Ministry of Land (MOL) with the break-up of large estates in 1950. The MOL has effectively continued colonial policy by dividing these fisheries into about 12,000 *jalmohals* or water estates and administering them to raise revenue by leasing out fishing rights to the highest bidder, usually for 1-3 years. Through successive attempts to improve on this system, the following now exist in different waterbodies: leasing to individuals or cooperatives, licensing of individual fishing units, group or community management, and open access (Farooque, 1997).

- The extent that pond aquaculture can expand to meet current and future demand for fish and nutrition, and whether, this expansion will compensate, complement or compete with capture fisheries. For example, the potential for higher production to replace declining capture fisheries and/or to match population growth, stocking of fish to enhance natural fisheries, the enclosure of floodplain fisheries for aquaculture, and the scope to include SIS, especially rich in vitamin A within aquaculture systems.

CASE STUDIES ON FISH PRODUCTION AND CONSUMPTION

Fish Catches and Consumption from Three Openwater Fisheries

This case study presents unpublished data from a detailed ongoing study of fishing and fish consumption in three representative inland fisheries in Bangladesh. It describes the trend in fish catches and consumption and relates these to access and management arrangements. It also investigates the composition of fish consumption and seasonal variations in consumption. In addition, it shows the consumption impacts of community based conservation measures in one beel, and of stocking-based management in another beel.

Background

From the early 1990s, there have been several projects in Bangladesh that introduced community or group management of fisheries (Middendorp, Thomp-

FIGURE 3. Sources of fish production in Bangladesh in 1998-1999.

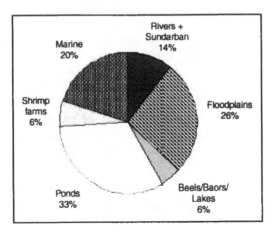

son, and Pomeroy, 1999). This case study is based on data from the Community Based Fisheries Management (CBFM) Project. This project was a partnership between the Department of Fisheries and five non-governmental organizations (NGOs): Banchte Sheka, Bangladesh Rural Advancement Committee (BRAC), Caritas, Center for Rural and Environment Development (CRED), and Proshika; and ICLARM-The World Fish Center (Hossain et al., 1999; Thompson et al., 1999). Out of 19 waterbodies under the CBFM project, the results from detailed monitoring of fishing and fish consumption during 1997-1999 from three waterbodies and their communities are presented. They represent three types of inland fishery found in Bangladesh. Table 4 summarizes the management institutions and actions taken in each waterbody by the communities and provides the context for the assessment of fishing patterns and fish consumption. Locations are shown on the map of Bangladesh (Appendix B).

- Hamil Beel is a small permanent closed lake of 16 ha with exclusive access for 136 Muslim households organized by the NGO Caritas into six groups from five villages; another 1,250 households live around the beel.
- Ashurar Beel is a large open lake extending to about 400 ha during the monsoon season with management by about 500 culturally diverse fishing households organized into groups by Caritas out of about 1,000 households in 17 villages around the beel.
- Kali Nadi is an open-access river branch of about 1,200 ha where the NGO, Proshika, supports with credit and training of 20 groups of about 330 traditional fisher households out of about 2,300 households living around the river.

For each of these sites, fish consumption and fishing in a random sample of 30 NGO participant households and 30 non-NGO participant households from the same villages were monitored daily for 7 days, each month by local girls who visited the households twice a day to weigh the fish being prepared for cooking. The NGO participants were expected to be fishing for an income and be involved in fishery management, while the non-participants represented the rest of the community that might be fishing for an income or only for food, but were not represented in management decisions. In 1999, fresh random samples for each site of 30 participants and 60 non-participants were drawn. The non-participants were split into equal samples of landless (LL), with under 0.2 ha of land (for direct comparison with the NGO participants who generally had under 0.2 ha of land) and landowners (LO), with over 0.2 ha of land.

Fishing Effort and Catches

Household survey data on fishing effort showed considerable differences between waterbodies according to the nature of the fishery and management

TABLE 4. Property Rights, Community Organizations and Institutions in Three Waterbodies Under the CBFM Project.

Attributes	Hamil Beel	Ashurar Beel	Kali Nadi
Property rights	Public jalmahal. NGO[2] participant fishers pay revenue for exclusive fishing rights.	Public jalmahal. Earlier fishers paid license fee for each gear for fishing rights. Now no revenue collected.	Public jalmahal. Open access, no revenue collection since 1996.
Management committee			
Year formed	1996	1997	1998
No. of members	18	25	30
Membership	NGO fishers	NGO fishers	Mixed
Executive members	Elected by all NGO group members	Elected by all NGO group members	Selected by DoF[3] and NGO, but non-functional
Composition	Secretary, President, Treasurer, and 3 leaders from each of 5 groups except leaders elected to executive posts	Secretary, Chairman, Vice Chairman, Assistant Secretary, and Cashier. All group leaders from whom executive elected	NGO group leaders, other fishers, brush-pile owners owners, DoF, NGO staff, and local council member
Financial responsibility	Yes since 1996	Yes since 2000	None
Institutions			
Decision-making process	Monthly BMC[4] meetings. Validation/acceptance of decisions from each group.	Monthly BMC meetings. Group leaders discuss and get members opinions. Decisions made based on consensus. Special emergency meeting if necessary	Initial RMC[5] meetings proposed conservation measures. No follow up and decisions not implemented
Resource management rules	All NGO members share costs and benefits equally. Exclude others. Stock carp, closed season, rotational harvest, and group guarding	Closed season, gear restrictions, permanent fish sanctuary, no FADs[6] (*katas*), and subsistence fishing by non-members permitted	Rotational and limited use of fine mesh seine net in "good fishing ground" by NGO group consensus
Compliance	Financial: high	Sanctuary: high	Not applicable/low
	Closed season: partial	Closed season: partial	

[1] CBFM–Community Based Fisheries Management.
[2] NGO–Non-Governmental Organization, here used to indicate the fishers organized for the project by NGOs.
[3] DoF–Department of Fisheries of the Government of Bangladesh.
[4] BMC–Beel Management Committee.
[5] RMC–River Management Committee.
[6] FADs–Fish aggregating devices, in this case brushpiles.

arrangements and actions, but there was less difference between years. Hamil Beel is typical of a small closed beel where the fishers annually stock carps, here the NGO participants fish in the waterbody half of their fishing time. They only fished in teams during the organized harvest time, at other times they fished individually for food either in the beel (averaging 3 days/household/month, despite a closed season) or elsewhere. Catches were low (2 kg/household/month), since most of the reported catches were from individual subsistence fishing, with little of the organized harvesting of stocked fish included. They successfully excluded other households from the same villages (non-NGO house-holds) from fishing in the waterbody, with, for example, significantly[1] lower non-participant catches in 1997.

Ashurar Beel is typical of larger beels that form capture fisheries. The participants spent 85% of their fishing effort in the waterbody, on average 8 days/household/month, but non-participants were not excluded from the beel although they fished only about half as often (the NGO participants included almost all households fishing for an income there). In mid-1997, the community initiated a permanent 8 ha fish sanctuary in the deepest part of the beel, and started a closed season in the early monsoon when fish were breeding. Within two years, this appeared to have been successful in helping to recover from overfishing since most of the SIS caught were at not more than one year old. Without a significant change in fishing effort, catches of NGO participants were significantly higher in 1998 and 1999 (13 kg/household/month in 1999 compared with 5 kg/household/month in 1997). The landless non-participants also caught significantly more in 1999 (7 kg/household/month) than in 1997 (2 kg/household/month).

In the river–Kali Nadi–open access and large traditional fishing communities represented in both NGO and non-NGO samples meant that effort was similar for both groups (6-8 days/household/month). Most fishers concentrated effort on the river, and in the high flood year of 1998 when more fish were available in the floodplains, the fishing effort by non-participant part-time fishers doubled and extended from the river into the floodplain. There was no specific management activity by the community and the catch increased to 32 kg/household/month in 1999, which appeared to be due to increasing effort in an open access situation.

In all cases, effort and catches were strongly seasonal, peaking in the monsoon and post-monsoon, but with a longer peak in sites with more permanent water (river and larger beel). In these two sites, there were more professional fishers and both NGO participants and other households sold over 60% of the fish they caught each year. In the small stocked beel, non-participants were subsistence fishers who hardly sold any fish (although they sold more in 1999), and even the participants usually sold less than 50% of their catch.

Fish Consumption

Compared with fish catches, consumption of fish was more uniform between years in each type of waterbody. Fish was still much more commonly consumed than other protein rich foods (pulses and meat), at least for households living near waterbodies (Table 5). However, there was a notable change in the frequency of fish consumption in Hamil Beel. In this cultured beel, production of carps was lower in 1998 and 1999 than in 1997, while more small fishes were available in the high floods of 1998, so overall fish availability was probably lowest in 1999. Although the households in the NGO sample were more involved in fishing for an income than their neighbours, they apparently did not eat fish more often than other neighboring households.

Fish consumption patterns are complex, with differences in species composition, seasonality of consumption, sources of fish, and quantities per household or per person. In the remainder of this section, these patterns are compared for the three sites monitored. Since each represents a different type of fishery, this consumption pattern provides an overview of the significance of fish in rural floodplain diets in Bangladesh.

The households living around the river had significantly higher fish consumption than those living around the two beels (Figure 4) reflecting higher fish availability (year-round water and fishing and a major fish market receiving fish from a wider area). On average, there was a lack of significant differences between NGO participant households (that tended to fish for an income) and those that were not organized by the NGOs (that tended to fish for food or part time income). However, the 1999 data revealed higher fish consumption by households with more land. The 3-year trend suggested a clear relation with fishery management. In the open access river, there was no change in fishing effort or management by the community and no change in fish consumption. In the capture fishery beel, where the community established a local fish sanctuary and closed season, fish catches increased and this increase was associated with significant increases in consumption for participants and non-participants. Consumption fell significantly for both participants and non-participants around the closed stocked beel (Hamil Beel) where there were conflicts among the organized fishing community; therefore catches of stocked fish fell. More-

TABLE 5. Frequency of Eating Protein Rich Foods in Three CBFM Project Waterbodies.

Food	Number of Days/Household/Month								
	Hamil Beel			Ashurar Beel			Kali Nadi		
	1997	1998	1999	1997	1998	1999	1997	1998	1999
NGO[2] participants (30 households per site per year)									
Fish	14.3	15.2	9.1	9.6	10.2	9.7	19.4	22.5	21.5
Pulses	5.8	4.2	5.2	1.9	2.0	2.4	8.6	6.7	7.8
Meat	1.5	1.1	0.9	2.2	1.0	1.0	0.4	0.2	0.3
Non-NGO (30 per site per year, except in 1999—60 per site)									
Fish	12.8	15.0	9.4	7.6	10.6	7.5	18.3	23.7	22.2
Pulses	7.9	6.3	5.9	2.0	3.0	2.5	7.1	6.2	8.0
Meat	2.0	1.4	1.2	2.3	2.0	1.4	1.6	1.2	1.4

[1] CBFM–Community Based Fisheries Management.
[2] NGO–Non-Governmental Organization, here used to indicate the fishers organized for the project by NGOs.

FIGURE 4. Changes[1] in fish consumption in CBFM[2] project sites.

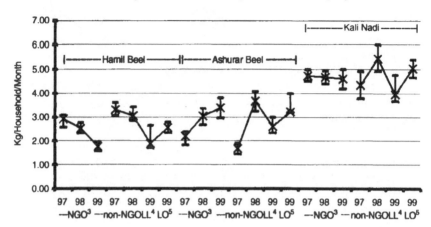

[1]Mean ±95% confidence intervals
[2]Community Based Fisheries Management
[3]Participants of Non-Government Organizations under the project
[4]Landless (> = 0.2 ha) Non-NGO households
[5]Landowning (> 0.2 ha Non-NGO households

over, in this last beel, there was no action to conserve indigenous fish. The data in Figure 4, converts to a consumption of 14-40 g/person/day.

Despite the recent trend of increasing aquaculture production, particularly of carps, wild-caught indigenous fishes especially SIS continue to be important to food systems. Larger cultured species may not be affordable to poor households compared with small fishes that can be bought in small quantities even if the price per kilogram are similar. The composition of fish consumption was recorded at species level.

Consumption was dominated by SIS in all of the sites for all three years, with higher levels of consumption of cultured species in the stocked beel (Figure 5). In 1999, households with over 0.2 ha of land ate relatively more cultured species by weight, but the differences were not large. At the species level, diversity of fish consumed was high. For example, samples of 30 households monitored for 84 days in a year (2,520 household-days) ate between 32 and 77 species of fish, but the diversity fell for the households around both the stocked and open beels over the three years. The main species eaten did not change between years, and over three years 70-71 species were recorded in the diets of households around both beels and 97 were recorded for the riverine households.

Fish consumption varies greatly between seasons. Figure 6 shows monthly fluctuations in consumption over three years. On average, the fluctuations

FIGURE 5. Composition of fish consumed by fish type and household category in 1999 in CBFM[1] project waterbodies.

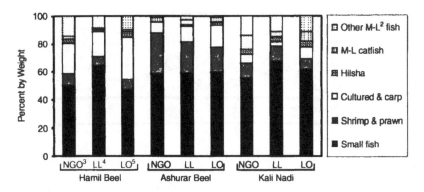

[1]Community Based Fisheries Management
[2]Medium to large
[3]Participants of Non-Government Organizations under the project
[4]Landless (< 0.2 ha) Non-NGO households
[5]Landowning (> 0.2 ha) Non-NGO households
Note: Fish categories are defined in Appendix A.

were greater for the open beel site (Ashurar Beel) which had the greatest annual fluctuation in water extent. The types of fish consumed varied by season around the beels. Figure 7 shows the variety of fish in the open beel (Ashurar Beel). There was little difference in composition of fish in diets in the river site, where fishing effort and catches were more uniform. Carps are cultured in Hamil Beel, and the consumption of carps and cultured species varied less over the year than in Ashurar Beel. There were very few indigenous medium-large fish in the Ashurar Beel diet, even though there was some increase in the catch of these fish after community conservation measures–these higher value fish were mainly sold. SIS were an important component of fish consumption in all months, but especially during July-December (monsoon and post-monsoon season).

Across the three sites, 55%-59% of fish consumed by weight were SIS. The ten highest ranking fish species consumed are shown in Table 6 which was based on three criteria for the three waterbodies. In the beels, these species contributed over 80% weight of total consumption, but contributed only 69% in the river site (where more species were eaten). In all three sites, weight, frequency of eating, and number of households ever eating a species, the SIS "jat puti" (which is likely to include more than one puti *Puntius* species) ranked number one. The one exception was the river where an even smaller fish, kachki (*Corica soborna*) ranked first by weight. Mola, a beel-resident fish

FIGURE 6. Monthly fluctuation in fish consumption in three CBFM[1] project waterbodies.

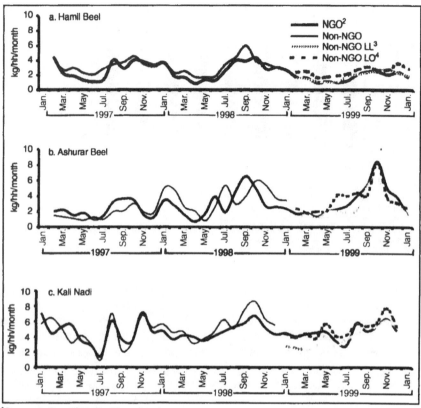

[1]Community Based Fisheries Management
[2]Participants of Non Government Organizations under the project
[3]Landless (< 0.2 ha) Non-NGO households
[4]Landowning (> 0.2 ha) Non-NGO households
hh = household

with its special importance for vitamin A, also ranked highy in diets, but comprised only 1-5% of fish consumed. Consistently across all three sites, major carps and cultured species ranked higher by weight consumed than by frequency of consumption (number of days and number of households). Small shrimps (gura icha) also ranked very high, again emphasizing the importance of floodplain catches of small aquatic organisms. The dominant carp species in the diets was the cheapest species–silver carp. In Hamil Beel, it was stocked and contributed to 10% of the fish eaten. In Ashurar Beel (9%) and Kali Nadi

FIGURE 7. Seasonal composition of fish consumption in Ashurar Beel.

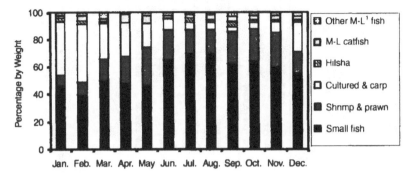

¹Medium to large
Note: Fish categories are defined in Appendix A.

(2%), these carp species must have come from ponds. By all measures, 10-14 out of the top 20 species eaten were SIS. These rankings show that SIS and small shrimp play an integral part in the everyday diet in rural Bangladesh, although the amounts consumed in each meal are small.

Implications

This study is ongoing, but the evidence so far indicates that simple community initiated management of a floodplain beel through sanctuary and closed season has increased catches, particularly of SIS. This strategy appeared to result in an increase in consumption of fish (mainly SIS) which is enjoyed both by households who implemented the management plan and by other households who catch fish for food. By comparison, only the households organized to manage a closed beel through stocking carp benefited substantially, and this benefit was through sale of fish for an income rather than higher fish consumption. There is no evidence from the river studied that open access has so far affected fish catches or consumption, although there are concerns among the fishing community that over-fishing is occurring.

Openwater Fishery Restoration

Local fish sanctuaries and closed seasons are not the only conservation measures possible for floodplain fisheries and may not be sufficient to restore fisheries that have been adversely affected by physical changes in the environment. This case study shows the potentially large gains for SIS production and consumption from small scale fishing where there is re-excavation of channels

TABLE 6. Ranking of Fish Species (by local names) Consumed in Three CBFM[1] Project Waterbodies During 1997-1999.

Rank	Hamil Beel (closed, stocked beel)			Ashurar Beel (open beel with sanctuary)			Kali Nadi (open access river)		
	Weight consumed (raw pre-cooked)	No. of days eaten	No. of households eating	Weight consumed (raw pre-cooked)	No. of days eaten	No. of households eating	Weight consumed (raw pre-cooked)	No. of days eaten	No. of households eating
1	Jat puti	Jat puti	Jat puti	Jat puti	Jat puti	Jat puti	Kachki	Jat puti	Jat puti
2	Silver carp	Gura icha	Baila	Gura icha	Gura icha	Gura icha	Jat puti	Kachki	Gura icha
3	Mrigel	Baila	Gura icha	Silver carp	Taki	Taki	Chapila	Gura icha	Baila
4	Baila	Taki	Taki	Taki	Bajari tengra	Gol chanda	Gura icha	Poa	Kachki
5	Gura icha	Kajuli	Fesha	Bajari tengra	Gol chanda	Bajari tengra	Baila	Fesha	Chapila
6	Taki	Mola	Mola	Gol chanda	Guchi baim	Silver carp	Guchi baim	Chapila	Fesha
7	Mola	Silver carp	Mrigel	Guchi baim	Silver carp	Guchi baim	Ilish	Baila	Gol chanda
8	Chapila	Gol chanda	Silver carp	Ilish	Mola	Mola	Rui	Guchi baim	Guchi baim
9	Guchi baim	Mrigel	Gol chanda	Boal	Ranga chanda	Darkina	Gol chanda	Gol chanda	Bajari tengra
10	Gol chanda	Fesha	Guchi baim	Cheng	Darkina	Poa	Taki	Bajari tengra	Ilish

[1] CBFM –Community Based Fisheries Management.
Note: Only the top 10 species are shown for each site and by each criterion.
Weight consumed: total weight eaten on survey days by all households.
No. of days eaten: total household days on which a species was eaten combining all households and survey days.
No. of households eating: number of households in the sample ever eating each species within the total survey days.
Bold = Small indigenous fish species (SIS) and shrimps, plain text = wild caught medium-large fishes, italic = cultured species including all major carps.

274

linking floodplains and rivers to restore inflow of water and fry during the monsoon.

Habitat restoration involves simple earthworks that are carried out by the poorest people under food-for-work programs, but it is uncertain how much maintenance work local communities are willing and capable to do themselves. A further benefit of such restoration is that movement of water and fish is not then dependent on operation of sluices and regulators. These are normally operated to benefit agriculture, and thus, often closed when fish and fry could enter into flood control project areas. Mechanisms to resolve conflicts between farming and fisheries are generally lacking, and the relative benefits and costs to farming and fish of opening or closing sluices are not considered.

Rahman et al. (1998) presented the results of community based habitat restoration undertaken by a NGO, Center for Natural Resources Studies, and the local community in Singharagi Beel in Tangail area. Fish catches and consumption were compared in the years before and after restoration of a link canal between the beel and main river. Before physical work began, general agreement was reached among fishers and farmers in the area that re-excavation would be beneficial to all. The catch from the beel and floodplain increased by about five times in the year after restoration but fell to about three times the earlier level in the next year which was drier, while the catch from fish aggregating devices (ditches or *pagars*) also increased (Table 7). Subsistence fishers (both landless and land owners) in aggregate gained since they caught almost twice as much. Landless households thereby reduced their dependence on purchased fish from 75% to about 50% of total consumption, but nevertheless ate only marginally more fish. The maximum gains from increased production went to full-time fishers, who moved into the beel and whose catches were marketed (Rahman et al., 1999) and to small farmers who recorded a substantial increase in fish consumption in the year after restoration.

In addition to increased fish catches and consumption, monitoring of catches in the beel for 7 months a year revealed that carps increased from 2% to over 20%. The share of SIS in total catch did not increase, and these species comprised over 30% of total consumption (Rahman et al., 1998). In this case, restoration of the link between river and beel appears to have benefited all households involved in fishing. Higher value carps and catfish were able to return to the beel, and these were mainly caught by people who sell fish, thereby, increasing incomes of those landowners who own ditches and of professional fishers (a poor section of the community). The landless subsistence fishers also benefited since they caught more fish and reduced their dependence on buying fish for food.

TABLE 7. Changes in Distribution of Fish Catch and Consumption in Singharagi Wetland with Habitat Restoration.

Category	Pre-intervention (1995)	Post-intervention (1996)	Post-intervention (1997)	Increase (1996 vs. 1995)	Increase (1997 vs. 1995)
Total catch (t)					
Pagar[1]	1.45	5.18	2.44	3.6	1.7
Beel/floodplain	2.48	12.22	8.69	4.9	3.5
Fishing effort (person days)					
Landless	434	624	402	1.4	0.9
Small farm	118	450	300	3.8	2.5
Medium-large farm	138	228	156	1.7	1.1
Fish consumption (g/person/day)					
Landless	18	22	19	1.2	1.1
Small farm	26	42	26	1.6	1.0
Medium-large farm	40	43	36	1.1	0.9
Percentage of consumed fish which were caught by household					
Landless	25	52	44	2.1	1.8
Small farm	22	46	56	2.1	2.5
Medium-large farm	34	38	51	1.1	1.5

[1] Privately owned ditches in the floodplain, most of the catch goes to the owners (medium and large farmers), with a share to professional fishers and some access for poor from gleaning.
Note that the production figures are the total during the monitoring period (December to June each year), the area represented is not reported.
The last two columns give the factor of increase over the respective pre-intervention figure (e.g., pagar catch increased 3.8 times in 1997 compared with 1995, but by only 1.7 times in 1997 compared with 1995).
Adapted from Rahman et al. (1998)

Culture-Based Fisheries and Openwater Stock Enhancement

The first case study included an example of a culture based beel fishery. This approach and stock enhancement of larger floodplains were major components of fisheries policies in Bangladesh in the 1990s. This case study examines some of the reported impacts on poorer people's catches, access to fish, consumption, and impacts on SIS from stocking carps.

During the early to mid-1990s, there was considerable effort from the Department of Fisheries to promote stocking of carps (native and exotic) in two types of waterbody: oxbow lakes (*baors*) and open floodplains. It aimed to increase total fish production from waterbodies that had lost major carp fisheries and to promote hatchery production. Technical and social aspects of these projects have been reported in Middendorp, Thompson, and Pomeroy (1999).

During 1991-1997 under the Oxbow Lakes Project II (OLPII), well-defined sets of fishers were organized and themselves invested in stocking carps in closed lakes each year with NGO assistance and Department of Fisheries ensuring access for the fishers on payment of the lease fee (Apu et al., 1999). Hamil Beel in the first case study represented a similar institutional arrangement. In the open floodplains, the Department of Fisheries through the Third

Fisheries Project during 1991-1996 (Islam, 1999) and the Second Aquaculture Development Project during 1989-1996 (Ahmed, 1999) released subsidized or free fingerlings of carps in large floodplain beels with low involvement of communities in decisions and management. These projects were not sustained after the projects ended, but a Fourth Fisheries Project that started in 2000 is attempting a similar approach with greater community mobilization and involvement (World Bank, 1999).

These enhanced fisheries may be more likely to be taken on lease by rich people, since productive fisheries tend to be controlled by richer and more powerful lessees. This trend seems most likely in open waters where fingerlings are provided by national projects and seen as almost a free good and in culture based systems where high profits are demonstrated (Thompson and Hossain, 1998). For example, in OLPII baors there was concern among the organized fishers managing these baors that at the end of the project richer people (who controlled the previous fishing cooperatives) would once again take control of access (Khan and Apu, 1998).

Stocking of baors by organized fishers under OLPII resulted in carp yields of about 490 kg/ha/year (Middendorp and Balarin, 1999), more than achieved in DOF managed baors. However, there were some negative impacts on fishers' access. BRAC (1995) found that 26% of the households around the OLPII baors had previously fished in their respective baor. Of these, 16% were displaced by the project and of those displaced 70% were poor. The same study found that participants' fish consumption increased by 38% over two years compared with a 14% increase among comparable non-participants, but the project participants already ate twice as much fish as the control group in the initial year. Carp consumption increased from 9% to 30% of fish consumption among participant households.

Nabi (1999) reported on the opinions of fishers regarding the distribution of benefits from floodplain stocking under the Third Fisheries Project. The fishers believed that owners of *kuas* (ditches) and larger gear (seine nets and lift nets) gained most, although catch monitoring apparently did not confirm this opinion. Few professional fishers reported any increase in their fish consumption, but 40-70% of households fishing mainly for consumption reported an increase in their fish consumption, indicating a widespread gain from the project including for some of the poor (Table 8). However, 21%-38% of professional fishers reported losses because landowners prevented them from fishing or they could not fish during an imposed closed season. Moreover, project-control comparisons failed to indicate any clear difference in the incomes of professional fishers.

The additional fish produced by stocking were carps, and the majority were harvested by leaseholders, owners of ditches, and professional fishers who sold the fish. The impacts of stocking on SIS harvests are not well understood.

TABLE 8. Reported Impacts of Stocking Beels by Third Fisheries Project.

Fisher type	Sample size	Percentage of households reporting			
		Income gain	Consumption gain	No impact	Loss
Stocked normal beels					
Professional, traditional	78	68	9	22	21
Professional, non-traditional	71	79	10	16	16
Casual, marginal	143	42	48	16	10
Casual, non-marginal		15	61	14	6
Stocked waterlogged beels					
Professional, traditional	42	45	2	28	38
Professional, non-traditional	80	83	6	15	13
Casual, marginal	126	48	40	15	0
Casual, non-marginal		39	70	6	8

Note: All respondents were asked directly if they experienced an income gain. The last three columns are percentages of respondents giving an answer to an open question, to which more than one response was possible, therefore the rows do not add up to 100%. Each figure is the percentage out of all respondents.
The sample size of casual fishers by sub-headings is not given, marginal indicates a landholding of up to 0.2 ha.
Adapted from Nabi (1999)

The argument behind stocking was that the decline in natural major carp populations had resulted in a gap that could be filled by re-stocking. However, these fish must be stocked each year as they either cannot reproduce in the wild in Bangladesh or do not reproduce due to unfavourable conditions for example blockage of potential migration routes. Islam (1999) reported that catches of non-stocked fishes increased in the Third Fisheries Project floodplains due to strict observance of a closed season, but this also prevented subsistence fishing by the poor. Hossain, Ehsan, and Mazid (1999) found no clear trend in fish diversity indices for some of these floodplains. In OLPII baors, there was evidence that catches of indigenous non-stocked fish in densely stocked baors were about half of those in lightly stocked baors, but the latter did not differ from non-stocked baors (Haque et al., 1999).

Stocking of larger waterbodies is a means of increasing overall fish production, but involves financial costs. Inability to contribute to these costs may exclude the poor from access to not just stocked fish, but also SIS. Usually organized fishing communities allow the poor to catch SIS if they are using small gears such as push nets that do not target stocked fish. However, catches and consumption of fish in a similar stocked beel in the CBFM case study fell for non-participants and the impacts on the overall catch of indigenous fish are uncertain.

Changes in Pond Aquaculture and Fish Consumption in Kapasia

Inland capture fisheries in Bangladesh appear to be declining due to conversion of floodplain wetlands to agriculture and very high levels of fishing effort.

In response, there is a focus on aquaculture extension that aims to improve use of private ponds and increase production so that per capita availability of fish will rise despite population growth. It is expected that some of this production will reach poorer consumers. This case study which took place in an area with seasonally flooded land where pond aquaculture was extended, summarizes some of the practices and production changes from pond culture, the levels and composition of fish consumption by pond owners, loss of fishing and fish consumption by non-pond owners, and overall market impacts.

Background

During 1990-1994, ICLARM and the Department of Fisheries undertook action research on aquaculture extension and its impact on farming systems in six unions (the smallest administrative unit comprising on average about ten villages) in Kapasia Upazila, Gazipur District. The study included a control area in the adjacent Upazila of Sreepur, which has not received any specific aquaculture extension effort up to the year 2000. A baseline survey (Ahmed, 1992) found 1,045 ponds in the project area with the average pond fish production in both project and control areas being 0.55 t/ha/year. Local fish markets were surveyed in 1991 before aquaculture extension (Ahmed, Rab, and Bimbao, 1993).

The main emphasis of the project was on pond aquaculture. The operators of 418 ponds were trained in basic aquaculture. They were expected to adapt either monoculture of tilapia or silver barb (*Barbodes gonionotus*), locally known as Thai sharputi, or polyculture of a mix of native and exotic carp species (typical of most pond aquaculture in Bangladesh) to their ponds using largely on-farm resources as feed and fertilizer. Detailed monitoring of participants in the first year revealed that carp polyculture and tilapia monoculture achieved production of just over 2 t/ha/year. Monoculture of silver barb was intended for seasonal ponds and was adopted by many farmers, but this species was particularly affected by disease (epizootic ulcerative syndrome) and its average production was only 1.1 t/ha/year (Ahmed, Rab, and Bimbao, 1995).

Method

In 1998-1999, a post-project impact assessment investigated changes in fish production and consumption. All 418-pond-operating households trained by the earlier project were identified and a fresh census was made of all pond-owning-households in the same six unions revealing an additional 1,641 households with ponds which were not extension recipients. There was faster growth in pond number (8% per year) in the project area than in the control upazila (5% per year), which may reflect the profitability of aquaculture and impact of extension. In Kapasia a random sample of 100 past-participants and

60 neighboring non-participants was made from the six unions, stratified by reported pond size. A control (without-project) sample of 60 households was also taken in the earlier control area (Sreepur) based on an updated list of pond owning households drawn up by the Department of Fisheries. Pond operation, farming system and socioeconomic data covering 1997-1998 were collected from each household by interview. In this case study, the three samples are termed "past-participants," "neighbors," and "control group," "non-partici-pants" is used to denote the combination of neighbors and control group.

Sixty-nine out of 100 past-participants were found to be stocking their ponds in 1998. For these households aquaculture practices, inputs and output were monitored each week, and children or students from the households were trained to record household fish consumption on each day for one week in each month for a year. However, severe flooding in July-September 1998 affected a number of the monitored ponds and consequently average production in 1998-1999 was lower than that reported in 1997-1998 from recall interviews.

On average, pond operators have substantial land holdings, very few were landless (under 0.02 ha), about 30% were marginal and small farmers (0.2-1.0 ha), about 40% were medium farm owners (1.0-3.03 ha), and over 20% owned large farms (3.03 ha and above). Pond size and landholding size were posi-tively correlated ($r = 0.34$, $p < 0.001$).

Production

The past-participants continued to follow improved aquaculture practices in respect to fingerling stocking, species composition and input use compared with control farmers. However, 10% of the past-participants no longer culti-vated fish (for example due to loss of access to ponds), while 6-7% of non-par-ticipant pond owners in Kapasia and Sreepur did not cultivate fish.

Past-participants and non-participants stocked large numbers of carp fry and fingerlings each year in their ponds. Past-participants stocked 5-times more fingerlings per ha than recommended, but the others reported stocking even more: 7-times more for neighboring non-participants and 10-times more for the control group. The preferred larger fingerlings were difficult to obtain after the project terminated so farmers mainly bought smaller fry and finger-lings. Carp polyculture comprising 7-8 species has continued as the single technology type with most pond operators adding silver barb and a few adding tilapia in their ponds.

Average annual fish production of 2.27 t/ha/year was achieved by past-par-ticipants who cultured fish in 1997-1998. This was about 10% more than pro-duction achieved during the previous extension project (Figure 8). In the flood affected year, 1998-1999, average production was only 1.7 t/ha for a 12 months' period for 69 out of the same 100 households. By comparison in

1997-1998, neighboring non-participants in Kapasia achieved only 1.6 t/ha/year. The past-participants' production was 77% above the fish production level of the control group.

The use of on-farm inputs (household bio-resources such as cow dung, rice bran and green grass) increased significantly irrespective of extension. Chemical inputs were reduced from the levels recommended, although past participants use substantially more than the control farmers, but high levels of organic fertilizer compensated for this. Nevertheless, fish production levels were low compared to the fingerlings stocked: too many small fingerlings were used for the sizes of ponds. On average, there was little difference in the proportion of production reported to be consumed by the household between production levels associated with past extension (past participants in 1998-1999 consumed 50%).

The gross return on investment (ratio of gross income to total costs) for carp polyculture was estimated to be about 200% for past-participants compared with 150% for the non-participants, but the return could have been much more if the stocking densities were lower. Diffusion of technology to neighbors in Kapasia appeared to have taken place, since they had intermediary pond management practices and yields.

Production function analysis of 1997-1998 data (when ponds were not affected by floods) indicated that smaller ponds were more intensively used and had higher production. It confirmed a positive influence of extension that was not reflected only in the quantities or value of inputs used but presumably also related to better management practices. Most of the ponds had high feed rates (bran and oilcake), and neither feed nor nitrogen inputs were significant fac-

FIGURE 8. Changes in carp polyculture production in Kapasia and Sreepur.

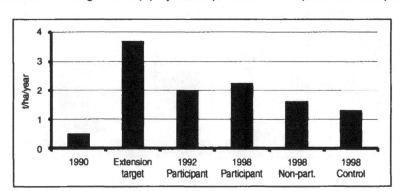

Note: 1990 production was the same in Kapasia and Sreepur. 1992 and 1998 data are all for Kapasia, except the 1998 control data which is for Sreepur.

tors in the function. The only significant fertilizer input in the relationship was phosphate.

Had the trend for aquaculture development in the control area (Sreepur) occurred in the project area of Kapasia (the "without project" scenario), then the production of fish from ponds would have been about 40% lower than it was in 1998, reflecting both lower production and less growth in pond numbers (Figure 9). This implied that in 1998, 44% of the higher aquaculture production in Kapasia could be attributed to the earlier extension project's influence over and above general extension activities within Bangladesh. Roughly, 42% of the incremental growth in Kapasia pond fish production could be attributed to direct benefit to participants, 58% was attributed to demonstration effects on other people: pond operators with ponds in 1991, and induced growth in pond numbers.

Household Incomes

Income increases during 1990-1998 for the households came mainly from non-farm sources associated with improved communications and household members moving elsewhere for work and remitting incomes, and not from ponds. Average household income increased 2.8 times between 1990 and 1997-1998 for the past-participants (compared with 1.9 times for non-participants in Kapasia and 2.3 times for Sreepur). Pond owners in Kapasia were rich

FIGURE 9. Total estimated fish production from aquaculture by source in six unions of Kapasia.

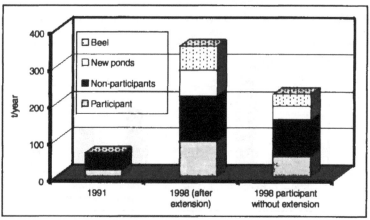

[1]Based on trends in the control area, Sreepur, estimated to have applied in Kapasia without a project. New ponds are ponds excavated after 1991.

compared with rural households as a whole (average annual income per household from all sources of the medium farmers was Tk. 141,800 and that of the large farmers was Tk. 251,500 in 1997-1998). Even marginal and small farmers' average annual income of about Tk. 85,500 was much higher than the annual average income of a Bangladeshi household of Tk. 11,300 (Bangladesh Bureau of Statistics [BBS], 1997).

Fish Consumption

On average, all pond operating households monitored ate fish almost every day in a month. Fish consumption was highest in October when fish from the floodplains were caught in maximum numbers (in 1998, there were more wild fish available in the area due to high floods). Consumption was lowest in June when the water level was rising and there were few fish to catch in the rivers or other waterbodies (Figure 10). Fish consumption had a positive correlation to wild fish catch and a negative or lagged correlation to water level.

On average, fish consumption of the 69 surveyed households was about 17.6 kg/household/month or 211 kg/household/year. There was no significant difference in consumption according to pond size (16.8 kg/household/month for small pond owners and 18.4 kg/household/month for medium-large pond owners). Small farm households consumed 14.8 kg/household/month or 83 g/person/day, medium farm households consumed 17.7 kg/household/month or 85 g/person/day, and large farm households consumed 22.2 kg/household/month or 96 g/person/day. Thus large farm households consumed 49% more than small farmers on a household basis but only 15% more per person

FIGURE 10. Fish consumption in Kapasia 1998-1999.

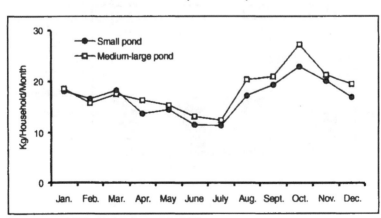

Note: Small pond < = 0.06 ha, Medium-large pond > 0.06 ha

per day. Large landowners on average have more people eating each day due to a larger household size, permanent laborers, servants, and guests.

Eighty-two species of fishes were consumed by all the 69 pond owning households during 25% of the days in the 12 months' period, of which 41% by weight were cultured species (carps) and 35% were SIS, the remainder were medium-large native species and shrimps. A small fish, jat puti (*Puntius sophore*) and the most prized cultured species, rui jointly topped the list of species eaten, by weight consumed (each about 10%). However, 52 species combined contributed less than one third of the total amount consumed. The breakdown of fish consumption by type of fish did not differ much between landholding sizes (Figure 11), except that the landless household ate more of the cheaper silver carp and less medium-large catfish. Non-cultured fishes were important throughout the year as were cultured fishes, but only one-third of fish consumption was cultured species in the monsoon peak which coincided with hilsha being in season.

All the landed participant pond owners bought more than half of the total fish they consumed (Figure 12). The one "landless" household having under 0.2 ha of land did little fishing in flooded fields and open waters. About 25% of the fish consumed by large farmers was caught from other places. Large farmers by definition own more land and they excavate ditches to reserve water for irrigation during the dry season and also for house building. During the monsoon when fields flood, fish from beels, canals, and rivers enter into these

FIGURE 11. Composition of fish consumed by pond owners in Kapasia in 1998-1999.

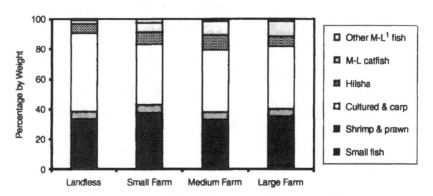

[1]Medium-large
Landholdings were defined as: landless < = 0.2 ha, small farm 0.2-1.01 ha, medium farm 1.01-3.03 ha, large farm > 3.03 ha.
Note: Fish categories are defined in Appendix A.

FIGURE 12. Source of fish consumed by pond owners in Kapasia in 1998-1999.

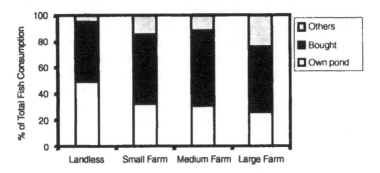

Landholdings were defined as: landless < = 0.2 ha, small farm 0.2-1.01 ha, medium farm 1.01-3.03 ha, large farm > 3.03 ha.
Note: Others almost all came from the households' own catch in flooded fields and openwaters, while bought fish were purchased in local markets.

fields and when water recedes after the monsoon fish become trapped in the ditches. During the monsoon, the owners fish in their fields and after the monsoon they catch fish from the ditches. Landless and small farm owners can fish in these areas when water levels are high but have very little access to these areas during the post-monsoon peak fishing season.

Medium and large landowners consumed more cultivated species by quantity (7.8 kg/household/month and 9.5 kg/household/month, respectively) than small land owners (6.1 kg/household/month), and a slightly higher proportion of cultured species, but a smaller percentage came from their own ponds. They reported that they sold a large part of the fish from their ponds in a lot and bought other (preferred and mainly higher value) fish throughout the year to eat. Discussion with the participant farmers in a workshop revealed that some do not like to eat fish from ponds heavily fertilized with manure, and that silver carp is not preferred compared for example with rui.

Consumer Impacts

In the six unions studied, there were about 41,000 households in 1999 (1991 census adjusted for population growth) and only 2,059 pond operating households (5%). Even allowing for some underestimation of small ponds and ditches, most households cannot grow fish and, therefore, eat fish from other sources. Focus group discussions were held in each union with separate groups of landless and landed households without ponds to investigate changes in fishing pattern and fish consumption.

In 1990, the small beels in the area were the main source of fish consumed by both categories of households and during the fishing season (monsoon and post-monsoon) about 75% of all households caught fish on roughly 50% of days. By 1999, at least 25% had stopped fishing and the rest fished less frequently than before. Among the landless group, 40% were marginal farmers in 1990 and consequently had some time and land on which to fish. Similar types of fish were still caught except that large catfish had disappeared from their catches. All groups reported a fall in daily catches, despite using the same gear types (traps, cast and push nets and rod-and-line), from 0.8-1.0 kg/person/day in 1990 to 0.2-0.3 kg/person/day in 1999. In 1990, these catches were reported to have contributed 50% of landless and 25% of landed household fish consumption. By 1999, however, own catch contributed only about 10% of consumption for both categories.

Hence, non-pond owners were more dependent on the markets for fish, but they also reported reduced fish consumption–by about 50% for landed and by almost two-thirds for landless households. The focus groups implied that both landless and landed non-pond operating households had reduced the amount of fish they bought to about 60-63% of the earlier level. The composition of their consumption had also changed in favour of low priced and smaller cultivated fish-silver carp and Thai sharputi. In the same period, the landed households increased meat consumption by 40% while the landless households reported a more than 50% reduction in meat consumption (Table 9).

Although the estimates of changes in fishing effort and catch obtained from the focus groups were not precise, they indicated a massive fall in capture fish catch in the area-from about 90 kg/household/year in 1990 to about 8 kg/household/year in 1999. This implied a loss of some 3,000 t/year of fish catch from floodplains and small beels over nine years which was much more than that replaced by aquaculture. An increasing landless population means that a large number of people who can no longer catch as much fish as before and who have no pond, now buy different types of fish (mainly cheap cultured species) but cannot afford to buy as much fish as they once ate.

Fish Markets and Fish Prices

A baseline market survey carried out in November 1991 covering the upazila market and 14 other markets (Ahmed, Rab, and Bimbao, 1993) was repeated in February 1999. From this, changes in fish availability and market characteristics were assessed comparing the time just before first aquaculture harvests with the situation some 5 years after extension work ended. Local markets in general have grown in size to accommodate increasing numbers of buyers, this reflected population growth (about a 15% increase between the

TABLE 9. Changes in Fishing and Fish Consumption of Non-Pond Owners in Kapasia.

Characteristic	Landless		Landed	
	1990	1999	1990	1999
Proportion of households who never fish (%)	2	29	3	25
Proportion of households who go fishing 2+ times per week (%)	75	38	82	56
Catch in main fishing season (kg/household/day)	0.8	0.2	1.0	0.3
Average consumption (kg/household/day)	0.43	0.16	0.60	0.30
Proportion of fish bought (%)	50	89	74	91
Meat consumption (kg/household/day)	0.10	0.04	0.10	0.14

Note: typical figures based on averages of six focus group discussions with 32 landed male household heads and five focus group discussions with 24 landless male household heads. The consensus or average views from each focus group have been averaged for this table.

two surveys) and growing market dependence. The number of fish sellers per market increased by a much greater factor (5.8 times), reducing the number of potential customers per trader (Table 10). The massive increase in volume of fish in the markets reflected the increase in traders and that each one traded about 50% more than before. However, there was a fall in the number of people selling fish that they themselves caught in openwaters in these markets: in 1991, 48% of traders were selling their own openwater catch but in 1999 this had fallen to 29%.

Cultured species were found on sale in virtually all markets in 1999, while before they were present in less than a quarter (types of fish are those used in the 1991 study) (Table 11). In the 1991 survey, 39% of the volume of fish traded were carps (some of which were caught wild), in 1999, 80% were cultured species (including all carps). The increase in total volume in the markets suggested a major impact of aquaculture.

Associated with these changes have been changes in the relative prices of fish and in trader's margins. The consumer price of major carp had hardly changed in the area from 1991 to 1999, although the price of common carp increased by about 60%, similarly the price of SIS increased by about 68%, and prices of some types increased by even higher proportions (Table 12). By comparison, the official national inflation between the two surveys was about 31%. So while the real prices of wild fish caught had increased substantially, those of "chinese carp" (virtually all silver carp) and major carp had fallen, resulting in a major change in relative prices-silver carp being 23% cheaper than small fishes in the local markets of Kapasia in 1999. Traders reported local sources for much of the cultured fish they sold, reflecting the four-fold increase in pond aquaculture production.

TABLE 10. Characteristics of 15 Sample Markets in Kapasia.

Characteristic	1991	1999	% change
Average number of fish buyers/day	1,700	2,567	+51
Average number of fish sellers/day	9	52	+478
Buyer/seller ratio	189	49	-76
Average volume of fish/market/operating day (kg)	91	801	+780
Average amount of fish per trader (kg/seller/day)	10.1	15.4	+52
Availability of fish in the market (g/buyer/day)	54	312	+478

TABLE 11. Types of Fish Marketed in Kapasia in November 1991 and February 1999.

Type of fish	% markets where recorded		% of volume of fish sampled	
	1991	1999	1991	1999
SIS[1]	100	53	32	14
Airbreathers[2]	80	87	10	2
Shrimps and prawns	8	33	6	1
Indian major carps	27	93	29	50
Chinese carps	20	93	4	22
Common carp	13	87	6	4
Thai sharputi	0	87	0	3
Tilapia	7	27	0	1
Hilsha	13	20	7	1
Marine fish	7	7	0	0
Other medium-large fish	40	67	6	2
Total (kg)	Na[3]	Na	1,367	3,346

[1] SIS–Small indigenous fish species.
[2] Certain SIS which have an auxiliary air breathing capability and so can be sold live, for example, koi and shing.
[3] Na–Not applicable

Conclusions

This case study shows that aquaculture is generating little additional income and food for most pond owning households. Also pond owners are more dependent on capture fisheries for consumption than their own cultured carps. Aquaculture in Kapasia has only partly compensated for the loss of local capture fisheries in seasonal beels, poor people now catch fewer fish themselves for food, and depend more on buying fish, including the cheaper cultured species. Despite the increased availability of carps, the poor eat substantially less fish in total and eat less of the nutritionally more valuable SIS. Households with land and diversified livelihoods have been better able to maintain their fish consumption through increased purchasing power and buy both cultured

TABLE 12. Changes in Consumer Prices for Main Types of Fish in Kapasia Between 1991 and 1999.

Fish type	Price (Tk/kg) in 1991	Price (Tk/kg) in 1999	Inflation (% change 1991-1999)	Traders' 1999 margin as % of 1991 margin
SIS[1]	26.9	45.3	69	15
Airbreathers[2]	53.0	65.2	23	13
Small/large prawn	27.6	80.0	190	6
Indian major carps	59.4	58.9	−1	88
Chinese carps	30.0	35.2	17	72
Common carps	38.0	61.5	62	66
Hilsa	51.3	140.0	173	27
Other wild fish	49.6	78.8	59	53

[1] SIS–Small indigenous fish species.
[2] Certain SIS which have an auxiliary air breathing capability and so can be sold live, for example koi and shing.

fish and wild-caught SIS in the market, despite increasing real prices for wild caught fishes.

Production and Consumption Impacts of Rice-Fish Culture in Floodplains

Rice-fish culture is now spreading in Bangladesh since it gives good returns where individual farmers can protect their fields from external flooding with bunds (Gupta et al., 1998), but group-based fish culture in larger deeper flooded rice field areas is a new concept.

In 2000-2001, trials on group-based fish culture in rice fields were implemented in eight sites comprising four pairs of sites located in: Narail and Muktagacha in shallow flooded ecosystems, and Brahmanbaria and Kuliarchar in deeply flooded ecosystems. The project was undertaken by an NGO, Proshika, Bangladesh Fisheries Research Institute (BFRI), Bangladesh Rice Research Institute (BRRI), and ICLARM. Areas of 2-14 ha in size bounded partly by high land were selected. Groups of landless households who had earlier caught wild fish in these fields were organized and assisted to negotiate with the landowners the right to stock fish in these fields in return for giving the landowners a share of the catch. Fences were constructed to prevent stocked fish from escaping from the project sites. In the deeply flooded sites, the groups stocked a range of carps during July-January in the fallow fields after winter rice was harvested. In the shallow flooded sites, carps were cultured concurrently with transplanted deepwater rice varieties, again during July-January.

Cultured fish yields varied considerably but averaged 990 kg/ha/year for deeply flooded sites and 450 kg/ha/year for shallow flooded sites. Catches of wild fish averaged 120 kg/ha/year in the project sites and 50 kg/ha/year in similar nearby control sites, although species diversity was higher in the control sites. The annual catches reported were those recorded during July 2000-January 2001, as these areas are dry and no fish are caught for the remainder of the year.

Data on fish consumption were collected from random samples of eight landless and eight landowning households participating in each trial, and from similar sized samples of households from adjacent areas of the same ecosystem (designated as "control"), a total of 256 households. Fish that were ready to be cooked by the households were weighed each day for one week, each month for 8 months, starting from August 2000 (after stocking fish in the rice fields). During this period, data on total fish catch for those households were also collected.

The first five months were designated the "peak period" when fish were grown and caught in the rice fields. The next three months after harvest were designated as the "lean period." Average fish consumption per month was highest during the peak (fish culture) period in all project sites. Per capita fish consumption was higher in the project sites (39 g/capita/day) than in the control sites (29 g/capita/day) during the peak harvesting months. There were no differences in fish consumption during the lean period between project and control sites (Table 13).

Access to catch wild fish was restricted for the project area households as the groups did not allow non-participants to fish in the project fields, but for control area households there was no such restriction in their areas. Over-fishing may have occurred in the control areas as some project households also fished in the control areas since fishing was restricted in the project areas.

The control area households bought about 70% of the fish they ate, with a lower proportion of wild caught fish in their diet than the project area households. The latter households from the shallow flooded areas ate more own caught fish than bought fish. This was partly because the enclosed habitat for stocking also protected wild fish which were eaten by the project area households. The project area beneficiaries did not harvest wild fish right after stocking. To allow stocked fish to grow, they only started catching wild fish in the area two months after stocking, and this also allowed SIS to grow. Consequently in the project areas, the dominant fishes consumed were SIS and small

TABLE 13. Fish Consumption (kg/household/month) in Eight Rice-Fish Sites in 2000-2001.

Type of site	Project			Control		
	Peak period	Lean period	All	Peak period	Lean period	All
Deeply flooded	7.7	4.0	6.3	6.1	4.0	5.0
Shallower flooded	7.3	4.0	6.0	6.2	4.3	5.3

prawns. In the control areas, households consumed more (purchased) cultured carps, even though they did not stock fish in their fields.

Despite being stratified and matched by landholding size, the monthly income of the control area households was on average 14% higher than that of the project area households, and this may have influenced their fish purchases. The sub-samples of land owners in both project and control areas ate more fish than the landless reflecting their higher incomes and ownership of ponds–the landless mostly have no ponds. Over 75% of fish consumed by landowners were purchased, irrespective of area, whereas the landless were more dependent on their own catches of wild fish.

Similar areas of ricefields are increasingly being stocked with fish by private landowner initiatives, but unless landless households who previously caught SIS in those fields are organized and helped to take a leading role in managing these small fisheries they may lose access to fish and as a consequence have lower SIS consumption. This case study shows that landless people can be organized by an NGO so that they gain access to moderate to deeply flooded rice field areas through sharing agreements with the landowners, where they then enhance fish production by stocking carps. This generated an additional income for the landless participants as well as landowners. In addition, fish consumption increased slightly. Because the landless participants had rights over the fish, they delayed all fishing which had a small positive impact on catches and consumption of SIS. Further piloting is needed to determine the sustainability of the institutional arrangements.

The Production and Nutritional Benefits of Integrating SIS in Carp Polyculture in Small Seasonal Ponds in Rural Bangladesh

This case study presents the results from a field study in Kishoreganj district in which the production and nutritional contribution from integrating SIS with carps in polyculture in small seasonal ponds was surveyed. By integrating the nutrient dense SIS, mola in polyculture with carps, the nutritional quality of the production was improved without hampering the carp production. SIS naturally inhabit seasonal ponds, and therefore are suitable to include in aquaculture systems in these waterbodies. Fish production systems in seasonal ponds need to be developed in order to benefit the rural poor. This study was motivated specifically by vitamin A and iron deficiencies being public health problems in Bangladesh (Ahmed, 1999; Ahmed, 2000; Seshadri, 1997), along with evidence of insufficient intakes of other minerals, such as zinc and calcium which are important for human nutrition.

Background

The on-going development of aquaculture in Bangladesh focuses mainly on production systems developed for perennial ponds with water quality suitable for carp production. Production of SIS has only been investigated in small-scale experimental studies (Kohinoor, 2000; Mazumder, 1998; Felts, Rajts and Akhteruzzaman, 1996). A quarter of all ponds in Bangladesh are believed to be seasonal ponds (Islam and Collis, 1998). A large number of these small seasonal waterbodies are unexploited or under-exploited, as they are not considered suitable for the existing production systems. Seasonal ponds typically belong to poor households (Gupta et al., 1992) and few research and extension programs have addressed fish production in these ponds. These production systems need to be improved and further developed through field trials in order to increase fish production. They must also be appropriate for the physical conditions of the ponds as well as to the needs and available resources of the pond owners.

As seasonal ponds are a natural habitat of SIS, it is technologically simple to stimulate the production of these fish. In contrast with commonly cultured carps, SIS breed in the pond, eliminating the need for developing hatching technology and establishing hatcheries. In a survey in Choromonkathi, southeast Bangladesh, the perception of culturing SIS was surveyed among 95 fish farmers (Mazumder, 1998). The farmers cultured carps in their ponds, and most of them harvested a small amount of wild SIS as well. Sixty percent of the farmers responded that they wished to culture SIS if the technology was available.

A major concern among farmers and aquaculture extensionists about having SIS in fish ponds is the potential of a negative impact on carp production. However, polyculture production systems with carps and SIS are merely an extension of the well-known principle of polyculture in which different fish species exploit different food resources in the fish pond. The integration of SIS in carp culture therefore should be based on combinations of fish species, which fit into the ecosystem of semi-intensive fish ponds.

Methods of Carp-SIS Polyculture

The production potential of culturing carps and SIS in polyculture in small seasonal ponds was surveyed in an intervention trial in four upazilas in Kishoreganj district in 1997-1998. This is an area where the Mymensingh Aquaculture Extension Project (MAEP) had been extending carp-polyculture technology to farmers.

The production system selected for the intervention trial was a polyculture of commonly cultured carps and SIS. The carps cultured in the intervention ponds were silver carp, grass carp (*Ctenopharyngodon idella*), mrigel (replaceable by common carp), and rui. The stocking densities were 4,000/ha for silver carp, 2,000/ha for grass carp and mrigel, and 500/ha for rui. The carps were stocked with a mean size of 35 g/fish.

Two models of carp-SIS polyculture were practiced:

- Carp-mola ponds: in 34 ponds, all native SIS were removed by treatment with the piscicide, rotanone. The carps were stocked together with the vitamin A rich SIS, mola at a density of 25,000/ha with a mean size of 1.6 g/fish.
- Carp-native SIS ponds: in 25 ponds, carps were stocked without removal of the native population of SIS present in the ponds. The species and numbers of SIS were unknown until harvest.

The details on stocking of mola are described in Roos et al. (1999). The ponds were managed by the farmers under close supervision of the MAEP extension staff. Urea and TSP were applied as fertilizers in rates corresponding to approximately 0.3 g N/m^2/week and 0.5 g P/m^2/week. Rice bran was applied as a low-grade feed at a daily rate of approximately 3% of the biomass of carps. Fertilization and feeding rates were flexible, and adjusted to pond conditions. Grass, duck weed, banana leaves, and cow manure were applied daily according to availability. At the final harvest, rotenone was used in all ponds to ensure all fish were harvested in order to record the complete production. Rotenone was used only for trial purposes, and is not in general recommended to be used in fish ponds.

Fish Consumption Survey Methods

The total fish consumption, including fish bought in local markets, captured from wild stocks and from the pond was surveyed in the 59 households participating in the carp-SIS production intervention trial. The fish consumption in a control group, consisting of 25 neighboring non-fish producers (households with or without ponds but who did not cultivate fish) was also surveyed. The nutritional contribution from fish was calculated and expressed relative to the WHO recommendations for intakes of vitamin A, iron, zinc, and calcium (FAO/WHO, 1998). The households were selected from MAEP's target group of poor farmers, defined as owning less than 0.8 ha of land, with an annual income less than 35,000 taka/year (approximately US$ 800/year, 41 taka approximately equalled US$ 1 in 1998) and a general impression of poor living standard.

Fish consumption was surveyed by recall interviews, covering 5 days. The head of the household and the housewife were jointly interviewed about the fish consumption in the household in the past 5 days. Fish species, origin, price, amount of raw fish cooked and which parts of the fish were consumed were recorded. The amount of fish was estimated by the use of food models, and expressed as raw edible parts by subtracting the cleaning waste (Roos, 2001). The average waste from cleaning SIS was 13% of the whole fish, and for large fish 22% of the whole fish, including 8% plate waste, which was mainly of bones. The total amount of fish harvested from the fish ponds and consumed in the fish producing households was also recorded.

The fish intake was converted to the intake of vitamin A and minerals based on chemical analyses of samples of the most commonly consumed fish species (Tables 2 and 3).

SIS Production in Seasonal Ponds

The mean total fish production in the trial fish ponds was 2.87 t/ha/season in carp-native SIS ponds (SD = 0.92) as well as in carp-mola ponds (SD = 0.84) (Figure 13). The season in which the ponds were cultivable ranged from 6 to 8 months, averaging 7 months, from June to December 1997. In the carp-native SIS ponds, SIS contributed on average 16% of the total fish production and in carp-mola ponds, mola contributed on average 11% and other SIS 2% of the total fish production. Within the range of total fish production of 0.6-4.1 t/ha/season recorded in the 59 trial ponds, there was no indication of a negative correlation between the production of SIS and the total carp production, using both parametric and non-parametric statistical methods (Roos, 2001).

The feeding biology of mola is similar to that of silver carp, as both species filter-feed exclusively on plankton. Since silver carp contributed 50% of the production in the ponds, the impact of mola on the pond ecology, in particular the possibility of food competition between mola and silver carp was analyzed (Roos, 2001). The results indicated that the co-production of these two fil-

FIGURE 13. Fish production in two version of carp-SIS polyculture in small seasonal ponds.

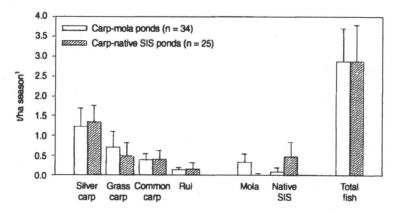

[1]The production season ranged from 6 to 8 months, depending on the water level in the ponds.

ter-feeding species resulted in a more efficient utilization of planktonic food resources in the ponds, compared to a polyculture in which silver carp is the only filter-feeding species.

The net profit from fish production was 136 taka/decimal/season (US$ 830/ha/season) in the carp-native SIS ponds and 112 taka/decimal/season (US$ 687/ha/season) in carp-mola ponds. The mean net income from fish production was 1,230 taka/household/season (US$ 30/household/season). The value of fish consumed in the households was included in the calculation of profit. The difference in the net profit between the two production systems was mainly due to the expenditure of buying and transporting mola for stocking in the carp-mola ponds. However, further development of the culture of mola can possibly reduce these expenses. The mean gross return on investment (ratio of gross income to total costs) was 195% for the carp-native SIS ponds, and 150% for the carp-mola ponds. If the expenditures on mola were excluded, the gross return was 180% for the carp-mola ponds. Mola harvested from carp-mola ponds was sold at a higher price (mean 24 taka/kg) than mixed batches of native SIS (mean price 17 taka/kg). Silver carp was sold at an average price of 19 taka/kg.

Fish Consumption

Fish was consumed frequently in all households, but in small amounts and with high seasonal variations. There was no difference in fish intake in the fish-producing households (n = 59) and the non-fish producing control households (n = 25), and there was no correlation between fish intake and land ownership or educational level in the households. The average amount of fish consumed in the 84-surveyed households was 37 g raw edible parts/person/day (median = 27) in July 1997, 82 g raw edible part/person/day (median = 64) in October 1997, and 55 g raw edible parts/person/day (median = 42) in February 1998. The average fish intake for the period, July 1997 to February 1998 was 60 g raw edible parts/person/d; 59 g raw edible parts/person/day in the fish producing households and 62 g raw edible parts/person/day in the non-fish producing households.

Fish was consumed daily in 48% of the households in October and in 25% of the households in July and February. The mean amount of fish eaten in a fish meal almost doubled from the season with low intake to the season with high intake; 24 g raw edible part/person/fish meal (median = 16) in July compared to 43 g raw edible parts/person/fish meal (median = 34) in October.

The fish species diversity in the diet was high. A total of 44 fish species by common names were recorded in the diet, covering up to 60 scientifically distinct species. However, five species contributed 57% of the intake, and puti (mainly *Puntius sophore*) alone contributed 26% of the intake. Puti was eaten both fresh and fermented. Fermented puti was recalculated to fresh wet weight by the conversion factor 2.64, based on measurements of dry matter content. The ranking of fish species in the diet is shown in Table 14, according to amount consumed frequency of consumption and number of households eating the species. By all measures, SIS dominated the fish intake. Of large fish species, silver carp ranked high, second in amount consumed and fourth in frequency of consumption. The majority of the silver carp in the diet, also in the fish producing households originated from the local fish markets, where it was available at a low price. The mean consumer price of silver carp in October 1997 was 21 taka/kg, compared to 47 taka/kg for rui.

Fish species defined as SIS or as medium sized catfish (Appendix A) contributed in total 84% of the fish intake, and were consumed in 98% of the households. SIS, often as fermented puti was consumed in all households in July, the season of low intake. Cultured and large fish species were consumed in small amounts by 60-70% of the households, depending on the season (Figure 14).

The mean intake of fish from the pond in the fish producing households in the period July 1997 to February 1998 is shown in Table 15. The consumption of SIS originating from the pond was highest in the carp-native SIS producing households, partly because the SIS production was higher, but also because a higher proportion of the harvested SIS was consumed. In the carp-native SIS producing households, 57% of the SIS harvested from the ponds was con-

TABLE 14. Ranking of Fish Species Consumed in Rural Households in Kishoreganj, 1997-1998.

Rank	Weight Consumed (% of total amount of fish recorded eaten by raw edible parts)		No. of Fish Meals Eaten (% of total surveyed fish meals in which the species was recorded)		No. of Households[1] Eating (% of household in which the species was consumed)	
1	26	Puti	49	Puti	98	Puti
2	11	*Silver carp*	15	Taki	72	Mola
3	9	Taki	15	Mola	68	Baim/chikra
4	6	Baim/chikra	12	*Silver carp*	66	*Silver carp*
5	5	Mola	11	Baim/chikra	66	Taki
6	4	Magur	9	Chanda	59	Chingri
7	4	*Rui*	9	Chingri	56	Chanda
8	3	Hilsha	9	Darkina	50	Darkina
9	2	Chingri	6	Shing	41	*Rui*
10	2	*Common carp*	6	Gutum	39	Gutum

[1]n = 84

Note: Only the top 10 species are shown for each site and by each criterion.

Bold = Small indigenous fish species (SIS) and shrimps, plain text = wild caught medium-large fishes, italic = cultured species including all major carps.

FIGURE 14. Intake of fish by categories of fish species.

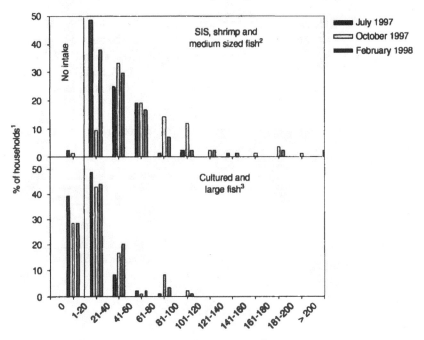

Fish intake intervals, g raw edible parts/person/day

[1]n = 84 households
[2]See Appendix A for grouping of fish species. Medium sized fish include: magur, rita, baila, bara baim, bhangon, and kakila.
[3]Include all other fish species as shown in Appendix A.

sumed in the households, while 47% of the harvested mola from the carp-mola ponds was consumed. The remaining fish were sold.

Of the total consumption of SIS, that harvested from own ponds was a minor source. More than 60% of the SIS in the diet originated from the local markets, and own-caught fish were the second most important source, contributing about 30% of the total amount of fish consumed. However, 32% of the households never consumed own-caught fish.

Nutritional Contribution from Fish and Pond Culture

The nutritional contribution from fish is calculated as a Nutrient Contribution Ratio (NCR), expressing the intake of a nutrient from fish as a percentage of the WHO recommendations for nutrient intakes (FAO/WHO, 1998). The fish consumption was recorded on household level, and the recommended intake was cumulated for the households based on gender and age specific recommendations.

Fish in the diet was an important source of dietary vitamin A and calcium (Figure 15), while the contribution to iron and zinc intakes was modest, depending on assumptions made for bioavailability. In October 1997, the mean NCR from fish was 40% (median = 23%) for vitamin A and 32% (median = 26%) for calcium. SIS contributed over 99% of vitamin A and calcium intakes

TABLE 15. Fish Harvested from Ponds and Consumed in the Households in a Production Season.[1]

Consumption	Carp-native SIS producing households (n = 25) Mean (median), g raw edible parts/person/day	Carp-mola producing households (n = 34) Mean (median), g raw edible parts/person/day
Mola	0	4 (3)
Native SIS	9 (7)	1 (0.5)
Carps	9 (7)	9 (5)
Total	18 (14)	13 (10)

[1]Production season: June 1997-January 1998

FIGURE 15. NCR[1] for the contribution of vitamin A and calcium from total fish intake in rural households[2] in Kishoreganj.

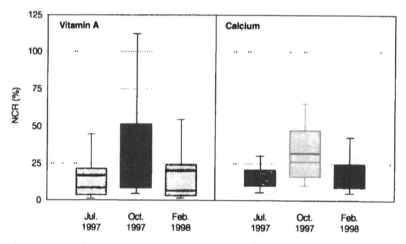

Box-and-whisker plot: 10th, 25th, 50th, 75th and 90th percentile. Dotted line: Mean
[1]Nutrient Contribution Ratio (NCR): The nutrient contributed from fish as a percentage of the recommended nutrient intake of the households (FAO/WHO, 1998).
[2]n = 84, of which 59 households were fish producing households. The mean fish intake was the same in the fish producing households as the non-fish producing households (n = 25).

of the total amounts derived from fish. The mean NCR for iron was 9% (median = 7%), assuming 5% bioavailability, and the mean NCR for zinc was 15% (median = 9%), assuming low bioavailability. Fish contributed less than 10% of the recommended protein intake.

The supply of vitamin A from mola was the most important nutritional contribution of culturing SIS in small seasonal ponds. The mola harvested from the 34 carp-mola ponds and consumed in the households, contributed an average of 4 g raw edible parts/person/day. This amount of mola in the diet is sufficient to cover 21% (median = 18%) of the recommended intake of vitamin A in the production season. The NCR for vitamin A from SIS other than mola harvested in the ponds was low, less than 5%. Also, NCRs for iron, zinc, and calcium from SIS harvested from the ponds were all low, less than 5%.

Conclusion and Perspectives

SIS are an important food in the rural Bangladeshi diet. These fish were consumed in nearly all households, and were an important source of vitamin A and calcium. Of large and cultured fish species, silver carp ranked high in the diet. Fish-producing as well as non-fish-producing households depended on buying fish in local fish markets. The fish intake was highly seasonal, with peak intake in October 1998

The most important nutritional contribution from culturing SIS in fish ponds is obtained through the culture of species with high to very high vitamin A contents. By integrating vitamin A dense SIS, such as mola, with carps in semi-intensive cultured ponds, the nutritional quality of the production is improved without any negative impact on the total fish production. Mola fits well in a carp polyculture which includes silver carp, and inclusion of mola in these systems offers a great potential as a valuable source of dietary vitamin A in rural Bangladesh. If only 10 kg of mola per year can be produced in each of the estimated 1.3 million ponds in Bangladesh, the annual recommended vitamin A intake of more than 2 million children will be met.

Forty-four of the 59 trial farmers continued to culture their ponds with carp-native SIS or carp-mola polyculture in the following season, demonstrating that they were interested in adopting the production technology. Their willingness to do so indicated that they perceived the technology to be attractive and the economical risk as being acceptable. Further efforts should be directed towards manipulating SIS to optimize their contribution to the polyculture production.

The potential for culturing other vitamin A rich species than mola, such as dhela, chanda and darkina should be investigated and tested. The simple practice of leaving native SIS in ponds used for carp polyculture should be implemented in all production strategies, and further developed to manipulate the native species composition in order to obtain the most favorable production as well as nutritional quality of the production.

CONCLUSIONS OF CASE STUDIES AND LESSONS LEARNED

In spite of the species composition of fish intake being highly dependent of location, season and access to water resources, there is a high species diversity in the rural Bangladeshi diet. A large proportion of the fish consumed can be termed "gura mach" (the Bangla term for mixed SIS). This is important nutritionally, since increased fish intake will lead to greater intakes of fish protein, iron, and other minerals, while increased intake of SIS in particular will improve vitamin A and calcium intakes.

The accessibility of SIS to poor households is affected by many factors. Drainage and enclosure of seasonal floodplains affect total production and squeeze the area of seasonal common fisheries that are usually open for anyone from the neighboring villages to fish in. Seasonally, SIS are still a major component of consumption–in the monsoon subsistence fishing in floodplains and other waterbodies is practiced by many households and the major proportion of the fish caught are SIS. In this season, many SIS are affordable for the poor and can be bought in small quantities in local markets.

For poorer households to have continued and sustainable access to SIS largely depends on the establishment of common property regimes based on institutional arrangements that protect the rights of poor people to catch fish for food but also limit fishing to ensure resource sustainability. This can be augmented by community actions to restore fish habitat or create local fish sanctuaries. These have been shown to bring benefits to communities in general–both landless and landowners. To maintain access for the poor to SIS, the critical issue is to help them to organize themselves so that they can hold access rights to these fisheries and to support them in taking appropriate management actions.

Pond aquaculture has expanded hugely and is dominated by production of carps (both native and exotic). In some areas people without ponds are now more dependent on purchase of cultured fish in local markets than on catching fish from seasonal common property floodplains due to the increased availability and lower relative prices of cultured species. Unfortunately the case studies suggest that the recent sustained increase in production from aquaculture may have failed to compensate for the loss to landless people of access to and catches from local capture fisheries due to drainage and enclosure. There are, however, some technical options that can help to mitigate loss of wild-caught SIS. It has been shown that micronutrient rich SIS can be grown as part of carp polyculture systems, and this results in both financial and nutritional gains.

RECOMMENDATIONS

Greater efforts are needed to maintain and even increase fish intake in general, as this is an irreplaceable food in the Bangladeshi diet. This should focus on maintaining and enhancing SIS in the diet since these fishes are a major source of essential nutrients. This has implications for floodplain land use planning, for fisheries management and for aquaculture development.

The floodplain fisheries still are the main source of fish eaten by rural people, and the main type of fish caught are SIS. Sustainable management and restoration of these fisheries are a higher priority than stocking them with carps since these measures are more easily managed by rural communities and can generate significant increases in catches of SIS in a short time thanks to the short generation spans of these fishes. These species are important in the diet of all rural people but have the advantages of being accessible for poor households to catch or to buy regularly in affordable small quantities.

However, past drainage of floodplains for agriculture and increasing population pressure limit the scope for this strategy to continually increase per capita fish supply. Moreover sustainable management implies restrictions on fishing at least in time and/or place. To expand the long-term availability of SIS, and meet the needs of a growing urban poor population, these fishes need to be incorporated in the continuing expansion of aquaculture as a means of adding nutritional and financial value to these systems. This should target species that are particularly rich in vitamin A, such as mola. SIS, including vitamin A rich species, can be incorporated in aquaculture systems that benefit poor households, for example group management of flooded fields and carp-SIS technologies for small seasonal ponds. Thus SIS can be used in sustainable food based strategies to improve micronutrient deficiencies in poor people.

In Bangladesh, emphasis in inland fisheries management is moving towards community based management approaches and restoration of fisheries through several governmental institutions, international organizations, bilateral agencies and NGOs. This should improve the access of poor people to fishery resources and help to restore and manage capture fisheries at higher yet sustainable levels. Carp polyculture in ponds is still a major emphasis of development efforts in the sector, but there is a growing interest in adapting carp polyculture to carp-SIS polyculture, especially carp-mola polyculture.

These recommendations are not just relevant to Bangladesh. The inhabitants of other floodplains in the humid tropics such as the Mekong basin also depend on similar water resources and fisheries. Population pressure and human interventions are creating similar pressures and SIS, being poor people's food that is often not marketed but eaten by the catcher, may well be neglected in development policies, as they have in the past in Bangladesh. Already a number of organizations, including ICLARM, are involved in initiatives to pilot community based fisheries management in several countries in the Mekong basin based on protection and restoration of fish habitat and SIS stocks. Danida (Danish International Development Assistance, Ministry of Foreign Affairs, Denmark) and the Mekong River Commission (MRC) aim–to identify commonly consumed fish species in the Mekong basin that are vitamin A and mineral rich, as a first step towards influencing capture fishery management to maintain and enhance production and consumption of these fishes.

AUTHORS NOTE

These case studies include data from four studies undertaken by the authors. The CBFM project was undertaken by a partnership of ICLARM, Department of Fisheries, Banchte Sheka, BRAC, Caritas, CRED, and Proshika and was funded by the Ford Foundation. The study of aquaculture extension impact in Kapasia was undertaken by ICLARM and the Department of Fisheries and was funded by the International Fund for Agricultural Development (IFAD), which also funded the earlier project in Kapasia. The study of rice-fish culture in moderately-deep flooded areas was undertaken by ICLARM, Bangladesh Fisheries Research Institute, Proshika and Bangladesh Rice Research Institute and was funded by the IFAD. The study on integrating SIS in carp polyculture in small seasonal ponds was undertaken by the Research Department of Human Nutrition, The Royal Veterinary and Agricultural University, Denmark, in close collaboration with the Mymensingh Aquaculture Extension Project (MAEP). MAEP is implemented by the Department of Fisheries with assistance from Danida.

The views expressed in this paper are the authors' and do not reflect the views of the agencies that funded the research reported. The authors thank the authors of the other studies summarized for additional insights into their projects, particularly the participants in a workshop in Bangladesh organized by ICLARM and Danida OLPII in 1997. The authors are grateful to Dr. Mahfuzuddin Ahmed, ICLARM, for advice. The authors aslo thank all their colleagues in the ICLARM Bangladesh office, in MAEP, the various teams of extension staff and interviewers, and particularly the many families who contributed to the studies.

NOTE

1. All notes of significant differences in this and subsequent sections of this chapter relate to $p < 0.05$ in two-tailed t-tests of differences in means.

REFERENCES

Ahmad K. and N. Hassan. 1983. Nutrition survey of rural Bangladesh 1981-1982. Institute of Nutrition and Food Science, University of Dhaka, Bangladesh.

Ahmed, F. 1999. Vitamin A deficiency in Bangladesh: a review and recommendations for improvement. *Public Health Nutrition*. 2:1-14.

Ahmed, F. 2000. Anaemia in Bangladesh: a review of prevalence and aetiology. *Public Health Nutrition* 3(4):385-393.

Ahmed, M. 1992. *Status and potential of aquaculture in small waterbodies (ponds and ditches) in Bangladesh*, ICLARM, Manila: ICLARM.

Ahmed, M., M.A. Rab, and M.A.P. Bimbao. 1993. *Household socioeconomics, resource use and fish marketing in two thanas of Bangladesh*, ICLARM Technical Report 40, Manila: ICLARM.

Ahmed, M., M.A. Rab, and M.A.P. Bimbao. 1995. *Aquaculture technology adoption in Kapasia Thana, Bangladesh: some preliminary results from farm record-keeping data*, ICLARM Technical Report 44, Manila: ICLARM.

Ahmed, M.N. 1999. Fingerling stocking in openwaters. pp. 201-208. *In* H.A.J. Middendorp, P.M. Thompson and R.S. Pomeroy (eds.) *Sustainable inland fisheries management in Bangladesh*. ICLARM Conf. Proc. 58, Manila.

Ali, M.Y. 1997. *Fish, water and people*. Dhaka: University Press Ltd.

Ali, M.Y. 1999. Openwater fisheries management issues and future strategies, paper presented at the National Workshop on Community Based Fisheries Management and Future Strategies for Inland Fisheries in Bangladesh, 24-25 October 1999, Dhaka.

Apu, N.A., M.A. Satar, D. Nathan, J.D. Balarin, and H.A.J. Middendorp. 1999. Fisheries co-management and sustainable common property regimes based on security of tenure in oxbow lakes in Bangladesh. pp. 19-30. *In* H.A.J. Middendorp, P.M. Thompson and R.S. Pomeroy (eds.) *Sustainable inland fisheries management in Bangladesh*. ICLARM Conf. Proc. 58, Manila.

Aung-Than-Batu, Thein-Than, and Thane-Toe. 1976. Iron absorption from Southeast Asian rice-based meals. *American Journal of Clinical Nutrition*, 29:19-225.

Bangladesh Bureau of Statistics. 1997. *Statistical yearbook of Bangladesh*. Bangladesh Bureau of Statistics, Dhaka.

Björn-Rasmussen, E. and L. Hallberg. 1979. Effect of animal protein on the absorption of food iron in man. *Nutrition and Metabolism*, 23:192-202.

Bloem, M.W. 1995. Interdependence of vitamin A and iron: an important association for programmes of anaemia control. *Proceedings of the Nutrition Society*, 54: 501-508.

Bloem, M.W., M. Wedel, R.J. Egger, A.J. Speek, J. Schrijver, S. Soawakontha, and W.H.P. Schreurs. 1989. Iron metabolism and vitamin A deficiency in children in Northeast Thailand. *American Journal of Clinical Nutrition*, 50:332-338.

Bouis, H., B. de la Briére, K. Hallman, N. Hassan, O. Hels, W. Quabili, A. Quisumbing, S.H. Thilsted, Z.H. Zihad, and S. Zohir. 1998. Commercial vegetable and polyculture fish production in Bangladesh: their impacts on income, household resource allocation, and nutrition. Final Project Report to DANIDA and USAID. Washington, DC: International Food Policy Research Institute.

BRAC. 1995. *Impact of the Oxbowlakes Project on participant households.* Research and Evaluation Division, Bangladesh Rural Advancement Committee, Dhaka.

Carpenter, C.E. and A.W. Mahoney. 1992. Contribution of heme and nonheme iron to human nutrition. *Critical Review of Food Science and Nutrition,* 31:333-367.

Darnton-Hill, I., N. Hassan, R. Karim, and M.R. Duthie. 1988. *Tables of nutrient composition of Bangladeshi foods,* English version with particular emphasis on vitamin A content. Dhaka: Helen Keller International.

de Pee, S., C.E. West, Muhilal, D. Karyadi, and J.G.A.J. Hautvast. 1995. Lack of improvement in vitamin A status with increased consumption of dark-green leafy vegetables. *Lancet,* 346:75-81.

de Pee, S., C.E. West, D. Permaesih, S. Martuti, Muhilal, and J.G.A.J. Hautvast. 1998a. Orange fruit is more effective than are dark-green, leafy vegetables in increasing serum concentrations of retinol and β-carotene in schoolchildren in Indonesia. *American Journal of Clinical Nutrition,* 68:1058-1067.

de Pee, S., M.W. Bloem, J. Gorstein, M. Sari, Satoto, R. Yip, R. Shrimpton, and Muhilal. 1998b. Reappraisal of the role of vegetables in the vitamin A status of mothers in Central Java, Indonesia. *American Journal of Clinical Nutrition,* 68: 1068-1074.

DOF. 1996. *Fish catch statistics of Bangladesh 1995-1996,* Dhaka: Department of Fisheries.

DOF. 2000. *Fish catch statistics of Bangladesh 1998-1999,* Dhaka: Department of Fisheries.

Environment and GIS Support Project. 1997. *Floodplain fish habitat study.* Water Resources Planning Organization, Ministry of Water Resources, Dhaka.

FAO/WHO. 1998. Preliminary report on recommended nutrient intake. Joint FAO (Food and Agriculture Organization of the United Nations)/WHO (World Health Organization) Expert Consultation on Human Vitamin and Mineral Requirements; 1998 Sep 21-30; Bangkok, Thailand. Available from: URL http://www.fao.org/waicent/faoinfo/economic/ESN/vitrni.pdf [cited June 1, 2001].

FAP 16. 1995. *Potential impacts of flood control on the biological diversity and nutritional vale of subsistence fisheries in Bangladesh.* Flood Action Plan 16 Environmental Study, Flood Plan Coordination Organization, Ministry of Water Resources, Dhaka. (Report prepared by Irrigation Support Project for Asia and the Near East).

FAP 17. 1994. *Fisheries study and pilot project final report* Main Volume. Government of Bangladesh, Dhaka (Report prepared for Overseas Development Agency).

Farooque, M. 1997. *Regulatory regime on inland fisheries in Bangladesh: Issues and remedies.* Bangladesh Environmental Lawyers Association, Dhaka.

Felts, R.A., F. Rajts, and M. Akhteruzzaman. 1996. *Small indigenous fish species culture in Bangladesh.* Project ALA/92/05/02. Integrated Food Assisted Development Project (IFADEP) Sub-Project 2 Development of Inland Fisheries, Dhaka.

Froese, R. and D. Pauly (Eds.). 2000. *FishBase 2000: concepts design and data sources.* ICLARM, Los Banos, Philippines.

García-Casal, M.N., M. Layrisse, L. Solano, M.A. Baron, F. Arguello, D. Llovera, J. Ramirez, I. Leets and E. Tropper. 1998. Vitamin A and β-carotene can improve nonheme iron absorption from rice, wheat and corn by humans. *Journal of Nutrition,* 128:646-650.

Gupta, M.V., M. Ahmed, M.A.P. Bimbao, and C. Lightfoot C. 1992. *Socioeconomic impact and farmers assessment of Nile tilapia (Oreochromis niloticus) culture in Bangladesh.* International Center for Living Aquatic Resources Management (ICLARM) Technical Report 35. ICLARM, Manila.

Gupta, M.V., J.D. Sollows, M.A. Mazid, A. Rahman, M.G. Hossain, and M.M. Dey. 1998. *Integrating aquaculture with rice farming in Bangladesh: feasibility and economic viability, its adoption and impact.* International Center for Living Aquatic Resources Management (ICLARM) Technical Report 55. ICLARM, Manila.

Habib, E. 1999. Legal and regulatory issues in inland fisheries in Bangladesh. pp. 77-84. *In* Papers presented at the national workshop on community based fisheries management and future strategies for inland fisheries in Bangladesh, Department of Fisheries, October 1999, Dhaka, Bangladesh.

Hansen, M., S.H. Thilsted, B. Sanstrom, K. Kongsbak, T. Larsen, M. Jensen, and S.S. Sorensen. 1998. Calcium absorption from small soft-boned fish. *J. Trace Elements in Medical Biology,* 12:148-154.

Haque, A.K.M.A., M.A. Islam, M.F.A. Mollah, and M.R. Hasan. 1999. Impact of carp stocking on non-stocked indigenous fish in the oxbow lakes of southwest Bangladesh. pp. 51-58. *In* Papers presented at the national workshop on community based fisheries management and future strategies for inland fisheries in Bangladesh, Department of Fisheries, October 1999, Dhaka, Bangladesh.

Hels, O. 1995. Dietary intake of nutrients from fish and rice in rural Bangladesh. M.Sc. thesis. Copenhagen: Research Department of Human Nutrition, The Royal Veterinary and Agricultural University.

Hossain, M.M., Kabir, S., Thompson, P.M., Islam, M.N., and M. Kadir. 1999. Overview of the Community Based Fisheries Management Project. pp. 9-18. *In* H.A.J. Middendorp, P.M. Thompson and R.S. Pomeroy (eds.) *Sustainable inland fisheries management in Bangladesh.* ICLARM Conf. Proc. 58, Manila.

Hossain, M.S., M.A. Ehsan, and M.A. Mazid. 1999. Fish biodiversity study of three floodplains in Bangladesh. pp. 229-234. *In* H.A.J. Middendorp, P.M. Thompson and R.S. Pomeroy (eds.) *Sustainable inland fisheries management in Bangladesh.* ICLARM Conf. Proc. 58, Manila.

ICLARM. 2001. Beel fisheries managed by communities: the contribution of stocked and wild fish. (Unpublished data)

Institute of Nutrition and Food Science. 1977. *Nutrition survey of rural Bangladesh, 1975-76.* Dhaka, Bangladesh: Institute of Nutrition and Food Science, University of Dhaka, Bangladesh.

Islam, M.A. and W.J. Collis. 1998. Fourth Fisheries Project preparatory phase. Final report, freshwater aquaculture, Vol. 4. Department of Fisheries, Dhaka, Bangladesh.

Islam, M.Z. 1999. Enhancement of floodplain fisheries: experience of the Third Fisheries Project. pp. 209-218. *In* H.A.J. Middendorp, P.M. Thompson and R.S. Pomeroy (eds.) *Sustainable inland fisheries management in Bangladesh.* ICLARM Conf. Proc. 58, Manila.

Khan, M.S. and N.A. Apu. 1998. *Fisheries co-management in the ox-bow lakes of Bangladesh.* ICLARM, Dhaka.

Kohinoor, A.H.M. 2000. Development of culture technology of three small indigenous fish–mola (*Amblypharyngodon mola*), puti (*Puntius sophore*) and chela (*Chela cachinus*) with notes on some aspects of their biology. Ph.D. Thesis. Department of Fisheries Management, Bangladesh Agricultural University, Mymensingh, Bangladesh.

Larsen, T., S.H. Thilsted. K. Kongsbak, and M. Hansen. 2000. Whole small fish as a rich calcium source. *British Journal of Nutrition*, 83:191-196.

Mazumder, D. 1998. The context of developing small native species (SNS) for aquaculture in Bangladesh: local environmental change, markets and farmers perception. M.Sc. Thesis. Imperial College of Science, Technology and Medicine, University of London, London.

Mejia, L.A. and F. Chew. 1988. Hematological effect of supplementing anemic children with vitamin A alone and in combination with iron. *American Journal of Clinical Nutrition*, 48:595-600.

Middendorp, H.A.J. and J.D. Balarin. 1999. Fisheries enhancement and participatory aquatic resource management: two types of management in the oxbow lakes projects in Bangladesh. pp. 31-34. *In* H.A.J. Middendorp, P.M. Thompson and R.S. Pomeroy (eds.) *Sustainable inland fisheries management in Bangladesh*. ICLARM Conf. Proc. 58, Manila.

Middendorp, A.J., Thompson, P.M., and R.S. Pomeroy (eds.). 1999. *Sustainable inland fisheries management in Bangladesh*. ICLARM Conf. Proc. 58, Manila.

Minkin, S.F., M.M. Rahman, and S. Halder. 1997. Fish biodiversity, human nutrition and environmental restoration in Bangladesh. pp. 183-198. *In* Tsai C. and M.Y. Ali (eds.) *Openwater fisheries of Bangladesh*. Dhaka: The University Press Limited.

Ministry of Water Resources. 1999. *National water policy*. Ministry of Water Resources, Dhaka.

MPO. 1987. *Fisheries and flood control, drainage and irrigation development*. Master Plan Organization Technical Report 17, Ministry of Irrigation Water Development and Flood Control, Dhaka (Report prepared by Harza Engineering Company Int., Chicago).

Nabi, R.U. 1999. Attitudes of fishing communities to floodplain stocking in Southwestern Bangladesh. pp. 219-224. *In* H.A.J. Middendorp, P.M. Thompson and R.S. Pomeroy (eds.) *Sustainable inland fisheries management in Bangladesh*. ICLARM Conf. Proc. 58, Manila.

National Research Council. 1989. *Recommended dietary allowances*. National Academy Press, USA.

ODA. 1997. Impacts of Flood Control and Drainage with or without Irrigation Projects (FCD/I) on fish resources and fishing communities in Bangladesh: executive summary of Food Action Pan (FAP)-17 Final Report. pp. 199-212. *In* Chu-fa Tsai and M. Youssouf Ali (Eds.) *Openwater fisheries of Bangladesh*. Dhaka: University Press Ltd.

PBAEP 1998. Result of the pond survey Amtoli Thana, Barguna District. Patuakhali Barguna Aquaculture Extension Project, Patuakhali.

Payne, I. 1997. Tropical floodplain fisheries. pp. 1-26. *In* Chu-fa Tsai and M. Youssouf Ali (Eds.) *Openwater fisheries of Bangladesh*. Dhaka: University Press Ltd.

Payne, A.I. and V. Cowan. 1998. Review of stock enhancement in the floodplains of Bangladesh. pp. 153-158. *In* T. Petr (ed.) *Inland fishery enhancements*: papers presented at the FAO/DFID expert consultation on inland fishery enhancements, Dhaka, Bangladesh, 7-11 April 1997. FAO Fisheries Technical Paper No. 374. Rome, FAO.

Payne, A.I. and S.A. Temple. 1996. *River and floodplain fisheries in the Ganges Basin: final report.* London: Overseas Development Administration Fisheries Science Management Programme.

Rahman, A.K.A. 1989. *Freshwater fisheries of Bangladesh*, Zoological Society Bangladesh, Dhaka.

Rahman, M.M., Z.A. Chowdury, and M.N.U. Saha. 2000. National fisheries situation, component coastal resources management policy/planning (Bangladesh). Paper presented at the National Consultative Workshop on Sustainable Management of Coastal Fish Stocks, Dhaka, 3-5 October 2000.

Rahman, M.M., A. Islam, S. Halder, and D. Capistrano. 1998. Benefits of community managed wetland habitat restoration: experience from Bangladesh. Paper presented at the seventh annual conference of the International Association for the Study of Common Property, 10-14 June, Vancouver, Canada.

Rahman, M., D.A. Capistrano, S.F. Minkin, A. Islam, and S. Halder. 1999. Experience of community managed wetland habitat restoration. pp. 111-121. *In* H.A.J. Middendorp, P.M. Thompson and R.S. Pomeroy (eds.) *Sustainable inland fisheries management in Bangladesh.* ICLARM Conf. Proc. 58, Manila.

Reddy, M.B., R.F. Hurrell, M.A. Juillerat, and J.D. Cook. 1996. The influence of different protein sources on phytate inhibition of nonheme-iron absorption in humans. *American J. of Clinical Nutrition*, 63:203-207.

Roos, N. 2001. Fish consumption and aquaculture in rural Bangladesh: nutritional contribution and production potential of culturing small indigenous fish species. Ph.D. Thesis. The Department of Human Nutrition, The Royal Veterinary and Agricultural University, Copenhagen, Denmark.

Roos, N., M.M. Islam, S.H. Thilsted, M. Ashrafuddin, M. Mursheduzzaman, D.M. Mohsin, and A.B.M. Shamsuddin. 1999. Culture of mola (*Amblypharyngodon mola*) in polyculture with carps-experience from a field trial in Bangladesh. *Naga, The ICLARM Quarterly* 22(2):16-19.

Sandström, B., L. Davidson, A. Cederblad, and B. Lönnerdal. 1985. Oral iron, dietary ligands and zinc absorption. *J. of Nutrition*, 115:411-414.

Seshadri, S. 1997. Nutritional anaemia in south Asia. pp. 75-124. *In* S. Gillespie (ed.) *Malnutrition in South Asia: a regional profile.* UNICEF Regional Office for South Asia (ROSA).

Shantz, E.M. and J.H. Brinkman. 1950. Biological activity of pure vitamin A_2. *Journal of Biological Chemistry*, 183:467-471.

Simopoulos, A. 1996. Omega-3 fatty acids. Part 1: Metabolic effects of omega-3 fatty acids and essentiality. *In* G.A. Spiller (ed.) *Handbook of lipids in human nutrition.* CRC Press, Boca Raton.

Soerensen, G. 1998. Impact of mola fish on iron absorption from rice. M.Sc. thesis. Copenhagen: Research Department of Human Nutrition, The Royal Veterinary and Agricultural University.

Tetens, I., N. Khan, O. Hels, S.H. Thilsted, and N. Hassan. 2001. Rice-based diets in rural Bangladesh: seasonal changes in energy balance and nutritional status in different age groups. (Unpublished data)

Thilsted, S.H. and N. Roos. 1999. Policy issues on fisheries in relation to food and nutrition security. pp. 61-69 *In* M. Ahmed, C. Delgado, S. Sverdrup-Jensen, and R.A.V. Santos (eds.) *Fisheries policy research in developing countries: issues, priority and needs.* Manila: International Center for Living Aquatic Resources Management (ICLARM). ICLARM Conf. Proc. 60, Manila.

Thompson, P.M. and M.M. Hossain. 1998. Social and distributional issues in open water fisheries management in Bangladesh. pp. 351-370. *In* T. Petr (ed.) *Inland fishery enhancements*: papers presented at the FAO/DFID expert consultation on inland fishery enhancements Dhaka Bangladesh 7-11 April 1997. FAO Fisheries Technical Paper No. 374. Rome, FAO.

Thompson, P.M., P. Sultana, M.N. Islam, M.M. Kabir, M.M. Hossain, and M.S. Kabir. 1999. An assessment of co-management arrangements developed by the Community Based Fisheries Management Project in Bangladesh. Paper presented at the international workshop on fisheries co-management, 23-28 August 1999, Penang, Malaysia.

Thompson, P.M., P. Sultana, M. Nuruzzaman, A.K.M.F. Khan, and S.M.N. Islam. 2000. Fisheries Extension Evaluation Project Final Report. ICLARM and Department of Fisheries, Dhaka.

Tuntawiroon, M., N. Sritongkul, M. Brune, L. Rossander-Hulten, R. Pleehachinda, R. Suwanik, L., and L. Hallberg. 1990. Dose-dependent inhibitory effect of phenolic compounds in foods on nonheme-iron absorption in men. *American Journal of Clinical Nutrition*, 53:554-557.

Underwood, B.A. 1995. Vitamin A status and dark green leafy vegetables. Letter to the editor. Lancet, 346, pp. 165.

US-DEHW. 1966. Nutrition survey of East Pakistan, 1962-1964. Bethesda: United States Department of Education, Health and Welfare. National Institutes of Health.

Varming C. 1996. Vitamin A in Bangladesh. B.Sc. thesis. Copenhagen: Research Department of Human Nutrition, The Royal Veterinary and Agricultural University.

Villif A. and Joergensen L.B. 1993. Analyse af næringsstoffer i dambrugsfisk og traditionelle fish i Bangladesh med henblik på at vurdere den ernæringsmæssige betydning. B.Sc. thesis. Research Department of Human Nutrition, The Royal Veterinary and Agricultural University, Denmark (in Danish, English title: Analysis of nutrient content in fish species in aquaculture and in indigenous fish species in Bangladesh).

Welcomme, R.L. 1985. *River fisheries*, FAO Fisheries Technical Paper 262, FAO, Rome.

World Bank. 1991. *Bangladesh fisheries sector review.* World Bank Report No. 8830-BD, World Bank, Washington, DC.

World Bank 1999. Project appraisal document on a proposed credit in the amount of SDR20.6 million (US$ 28.0 million equivalent) and a GEF grant in the amount SDR3.7 million (US$ 5.0 million equivalent) to the People's Republic of Bangladesh for a Fourth Fisheries Project. Report 19344-BD. World Bank South Asia Region, Dhaka.

Zafri A. and K. Ahmad. 1981. Studies on the vitamin A content of fresh water fishes: content and distribution of vitamin A in mola (*Amblypharyngodon mola*) and dhela (*Rohtee cotio*). *Bangladesh Journal of Biological Science*, 10:47-53.

APPENDIX A. Names and Categorization of Common Bangladeshi Fish Species Recorded in the Surveys.

Common Name	English Name (where available)	Scientific Name
Small indigenous fish species (SIS)		
Along	Bengal barb	*Rasbora elanga*
Anju		*Danio rerio*
Baim/Chikra	Eel sp	*Macrognathus* sp.
Bajari tengra	Long bled catfish	*Mystus tengara*
Balitora	Minnow	*Psilorhynchus balitora*
Banspata	River catfish	*Ailia punctata*
Batasi	River catfish	*Pseudeutropius atherinoides*
Batasi tengra	Catfish	*Batasio batasio*
Bhangra	Carp	*Labeo boga*
Bozri		*Chandramara chandramara*
Bud koi	Mottled loach	*Acanthocobitis botia*
Chaka	Talking catfish	*Chaca chaca*
Chala puti	Swamp barb	*Puntius chola*
Chanda	Perch, Glass fish	*Parambassis baculis*
Chapila	Herring, Indian river shad	*Gudusia chapra*
Chela/Chep chela		*Chela cachius*
Cheng	Snakehead	*Channa orientalis*
Chep chela		*Danio devario*
Chuna kholisha	Perch	*Trichogaster chuna*
Darkina	Minnow	*Esomus danricus*
Dhela		*Osteobrama cotio*
Ekthota	Wrestling halfbeak	*Dermogenys pusilla*
Foli	Bronze featherback	*Notopterus notopterus*
Gachua	Snakehead	*Channa orientalis*
Gang tengra	Catfish	*Gagata gagata*
Gol chanda	Perch (Glass fish)	*Chanda nama*
Golsha	Catfish	*Mystus cavasius*
Golsha tengra	Long bled catfish	*Mystus bleekeri*
Guchi baim	Spiny eel	*Macrognathus pancalus*
Gutum	Loach	*Lepidocephalichthys guntea*
Jat puti	Spotfin swamp barb, Pool barb	*Puntius sophore*
Jhili puti	Golden barb	*Puntius gelius*
Kachki	Minnow, Ganges river sprat	*Corica soborna*
Kajuli	River catfish	*Ailia coila*
Kanchan puti	Rosy barb	*Puntius conchonius*
Kash khaira		*Chela laubuca*
Katari	Minnow	*Salmostoma bacaila*
Kauwa	River catfish	*Gagata cenia*
Khalisha	Perch	*Colisa fasciatus*
Koi	Climbing perch	*Anabas testudineus*
Lal khalisha/Chata	Perch	*Trichogaster lalius*
Meni	Perch, Gangetic leaffish	*Nandus nandus*
Mola	Mola carplet	*Amblypharyngodon mola*

APPENDIX A (continued)

Mola puti	Glass barb	*Puntius guganio*
Napit koi	Mud perch	*Badis badis*
Narkeli chela	Minnow	*Salmostoma acinaces*
Neftani	Perch	*Ctenops nobilis*
Pabda	Butter catfish	*Ompok pabda*
Phutani puti	Dwarf barb, Spottedsail barb	*Puntius phutunio*
Piali	Aspidobara	*Aspidoparia morar*
Puti	Barb sp	*Puntius* sp.
Putul	Reticulate loach	*Botia lohachata*
Ranga chanda	Perch, Glass fish	*Parambassis ranga*
Rani	Necktie or Bengal loach	*Botia Dario*
Shing	Stinging catfish	*Heteropneustes fossilis*
Taki	Spotted snakehead	*Channa punctata*
Tara baim	Spiny eel	*Macrognathus aculeatus*
Tengra	Catfish	*Mystus vittatus*
Tepa	Puffer fish	*Tetraodon cutcutia*
Teri puti	One spot barb	*Puntius terio*
Tin chouka	Top minnow	*Aplocheilus panchax*
Tit puti	Ticto barb	*Puntius ticto*

Shrimps and Prawns (chingri)

Chingri	Shrimp	*Machrobrachium* sp.
Chatka icha	Shrimp	*Macrobrachium malcolmsoni*
Dimua icha	Shrimp	*Macrobrachium villosimanus*
Golda icha	Giant freshwater prawn	*Macrobrachium rosenbergii*
Gura icha	Shrimp	*Macrobrachium styliferus*
Thengua icha	Shrimp	*Macrobrachium birmanicus*

Cultured Fish and Carps

African magur	African catfish	*Clarias gariepinus*
Bighead carp	Bighead carp	*Aristichthys nobilis*
Catla	Carp	*Catla catla*
Common carp	Common carp	*Cyprinus carpio*
Grass carp	Grass carp	*Ctenopharyngodon idella*
Kalibaus	Carp	*Labeo calbasu*
Mrigel	Carp	*Cirrhinus mrigala*
Nilotica/Tilapia	Nile tilapia	*Oreochromis niloticus*
Rui	Carp	*Labeo rohita*
Silver carp	Silver carp	*Hypophthalmichthys molitrix*
Thai sarputi	Thai sarputi/Silver barb	*Barbodes gonionotus*
Tilapia	Mozambique tilapia	*Oreochromis mossambicus*

Hilsha

Ilish	Hilsa shad	*Tenualosa ilisha*

Medium-Large Catfish and Carnivorous Native Fish

Ayre	Long barb catfish	*Aorichthys aor*
Bacha	River catfish	*Eutropiichthys vacha*

Bagha ayre	River catfish	*Bagarius bagarius*
Bhetki	Giant perch	*Lates calcarifer*
Boal	Freshwater shark	*Wallago attu*
Chital	Featherback, Clown knife fish	*Chitala chitala*
Gajar	Snakehead	*Channa marulius*
Gang magur	River catfish	*Plotosus canius*
Ghaura	River catfish	*Clupisoma garua*
Guzi ayre	Catfish	*Aorichthys seenghala*
Kani pabda	Butter catfish	*Ompok bimaculatus*
Magur	Walking catfish	*Clarias batrachus*
Pangus	River catfish	*Pangasius pangasius*
Rita	Long barbed catfish	*Rita rita*
Shillong	River catfish	*Silonia silondia*
Shol	Snakehead murrel	*Channa striata*

Other Medium-Large Fish

Baila	Goby	*Glossogobius giuris*
Bamosh	Freshwater eel, Indian mottled eel	*Anguilla bengalensis*
Bara baim	Spiny eel	*Mastacembelus armatus*
Bata	Reba carp	*Cirrhinus reba*
Bhangon	Carp	*Labeo bata*
Bhol		*Barilius bola*
Choika		*Pellona ditchela*
Churi	Ribbon fish	*Lepturacanthus savala*
Churi		*Eupleurogrammus muticus*
Fesha	Anchovy	*Setipinna phasa*
Ghora maach		*Labeo pangusia*
Goinna	Carp	*Labeo gonius*
Kakila	Garfish	*Xenentodon cancila*
Khalla	Mullet	*Rhinomugil corsula*
Kuicha baim	Mud eel	*Monopterus cuchia*
Lal chewa	Goby	*Taenioides rubicundus*
Loittya maach	Bombay duck	*Harpadon nehereus*
Mohashoil	Carp	*Tor tor*
Nandil	Carp	*Labeo nandina*
Poa	Croaker	*Otolithoides pama*
Rupchanda	Chinese pomfret	*Pampus chinensis*
Sada chewa	Pouched goby	*Trypauchen vagina*
Shankar	Stingray	*Himantura uarnak*
Sharputi	Carp	*Puntius sarana*
Tapasi	Paradise threadfin	*Polynemus paradiseus*
Tatkini	Gangetic latia	*Crossocheilus latius*
Teli phasa	Anchovy	*Setipinna taty*
Tular danti	Whiting	*Sillaginopsis panijus*

Note: In alphabetical order of species by common Bangla name for ease of reference with the text where local names are used. The names may not be the same all over Bangladesh.

APPENDIX B. Locations mentioned in the text

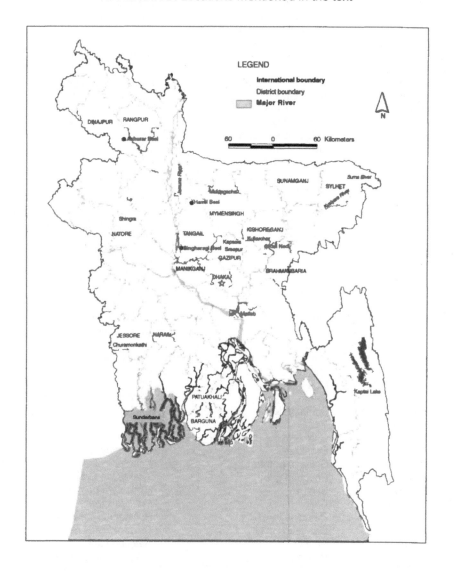

APPENDIX C

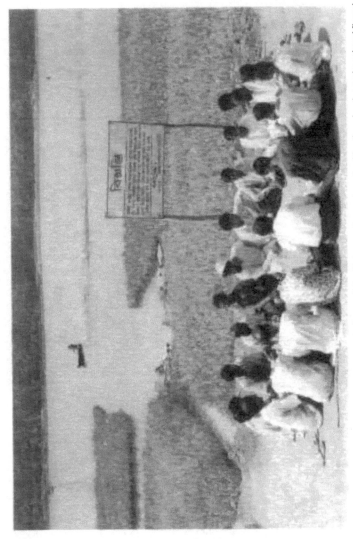

Beel Management Committee meeting in front of the fish sanctuary (marked by the sign board and red flags) in Ashurar Beel, northwest Bangladesh (photo: FermCom)

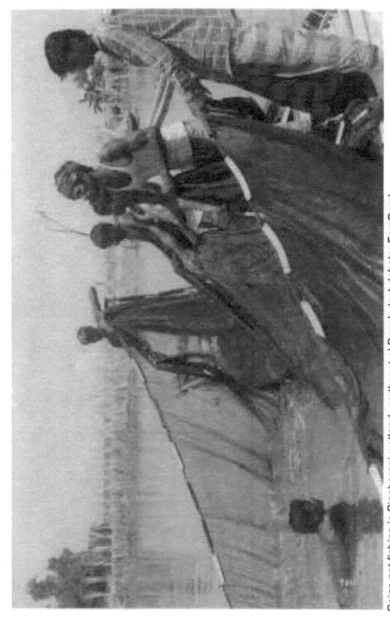

Seine net fishing in Singharagi wetland, northcentral Bangladesh (photo: FemCom)

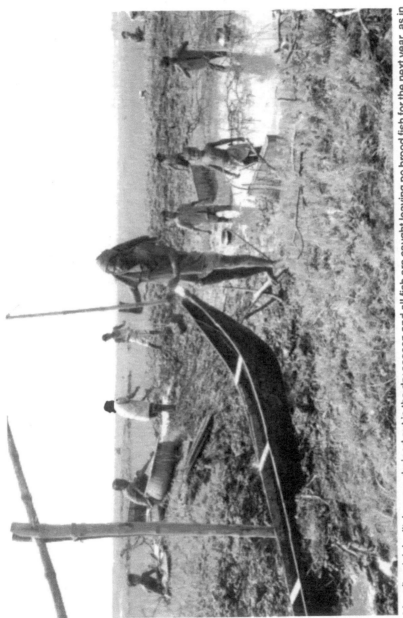

Most floodplain ditches are drained out in the dry season and all fish are caught leaving no brood fish for the next year, as in this floodplain in northwest Bangladesh (photo: FemCom)

APPENDIX C (continued)

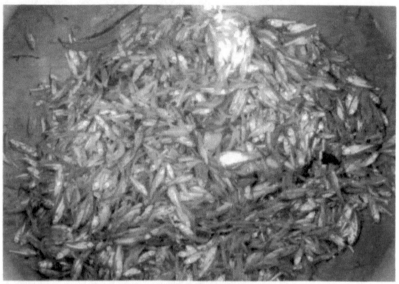

A catch of small indigenous fish species (SIS)—mostly mola (*Amblypharyngodon mola*)—and small shrimps (icha) from a floodplain in Kishorganij, Bangladesh (photo: Paul Thomson)

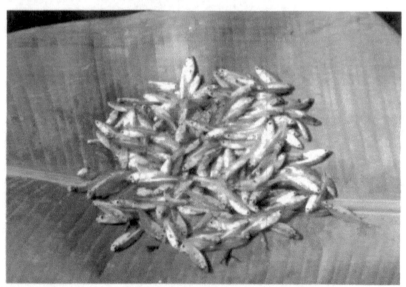

Mola (*Amblypharyngodon mola*)—a popular small indigenous fish species with a very high vitamin A content (photo: Paul Thompson)

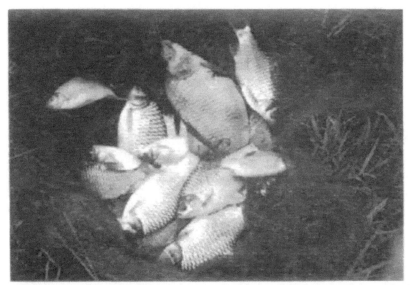

Puti (*Puntius* sp.)–the most commonly eaten groups of small indigenous fish species in Bangladesh (photo: Paul Thompson)

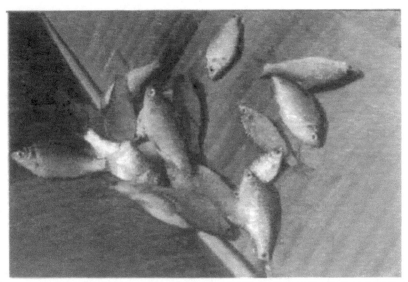

A catch of cultured fishes including Thai sharputi (*Barbodes gonionotus*) and common carp (*Cyprinus carpio*) from a pond in Kapasia, central Bangladesh (photo: Parvin Sultana)

Adoption of Crossbred Cow Technologies and Increased Food Security Among Smallholder Dairy Farmers in the East African Highlands

M. Ahmed
S. Ehui
M. Saleem

SUMMARY. This study investigates the household-level impacts of market-oriented dairy technologies (crossbred cows and complementary feed and management technologies) on incomes, food and non-food expenditures, nutrient intakes, and health of pre-school children. A recursive econometric model was employed using detailed household level survey data of production, income and consumption, nutrition, and health. Results show that market-oriented technologies are significant determinants of income. The size of the cultivated area, herd size, and purchased inputs are positively and strongly associated with the level of per capita income. Predicted income has a positive and significant influence on expenditures of food and non-food items. Price of food, however, has a negative and significant impact on expenditures. Results also indicate that womens' knowledge, expenditure on food, and price of nu-

M. Ahmed and S. Ehui are Economists and M. Saleem is Agronomist, International Livestock Research Institute, P.O. Box 5689, Addis Ababa, Ethiopia.
Adddress correspondence to: S. Ehui at the above address (E-mail: s.ehui@cgiar.org).

[Haworth co-indexing entry note]: "Adoption of Crossbred Cow Technologies and Increased Food Security Among Smallholder Dairy Farmers in the East African Highlands." Ahmed, M., S. Ehui, and M. Saleem. Co-published simultaneously in *Journal of Crop Production* (Food Products Press, an imprint of The Haworth Press, Inc.) Vol. 6, No. 1/2 (#11/12), 2002, pp. 319-337; and: *Food Systems for Improved Human Nutrition: Linking Agriculture, Nutrition, and Productivity* (ed: Palit K. Kataki, and Suresh Chandra Babu) Food Products Press, an imprint of The Haworth Press, Inc., 2002, pp. 319-337. Single or multiple copies of this article are available for a fee from The Haworth Document Delivery Service [1-800-HAWORTH, 9:00 a.m. - 5:00 p.m. (EST). E-mail address: getinfo@haworthpressinc.com].

trients are important determinants of nutrient intakes. The analysis of the factors affecting the health status revealed that womens' practice and knowledge, and age of the mother and female headship are important determinants of the weight-for-age and weight for height scores. Also, participation in village level health programs has a significant effect (at 10% level) on the weight for height. The policy implications resulting from this study clearly indicate that strategies that promote market-oriented smallholder dairy can improve food security as it contributes to an increased per capita income, thereby increasing per capita expenditure on food and non-food items. This increase in turn, positively affects the intake of nutrients. Therefore, to improve health, it is useful to focus on the role of woman in the household. *[Article copies available for a fee from The Haworth Document Delivery Service: 1-800-HAWORTH. E-mail address: <getinfo@haworthpressinc.com> Website: <http://www.HaworthPress.com> © 2002 by The Haworth Press, Inc. All rights reserved.]*

KEYWORDS. Dairy technology, food expenditures, food security income, nutrition

INTRODUCTION

Improving human nutrition, including their micronutrient status, is a critical element for achieving food security in East African Highlands. In contrast to the developed world where a lot of people eat too many animal products, most people throughout sub-Saharan Africa eat too few animal products for good nutrition. Thus, interest is mounting for food-based approaches (dietary change) to combat nutrient and micronutrient deficiencies (Ehui et al., 1998). Increased consumption of livestock and dairy products can make a unique and critical contribution to human nutrition because low levels of animal and fish consumption among the poor and the relatively high bioavailability of minerals and vitamins contained in animal products. Neumann, Bwibo, and Sigman (1993) have shown that consumption of animal products increases the bioavailability of minerals and vitamins in plant foods consumed at the same meal.

Animal products, especially dairy, also contribute to improving food security because they are a critical source of income for many smallholders in the East African Highlands. For many countries in the region, dairy production is the most important income generator (Ehui et al., 1998, p. 83). The introduction of market-oriented dairy technologies (e.g., crossbred cows and complementary feed and management technologies) can result in increased commercialization of dairy products by smallholder farmers when marketable surpluses exist. The increased income from sales of dairy products may also be spent on more and better quality food and result in improved nutrition and health. Consumption of more dairy products usually results in a positive effect on human nutrition and health (Neumann, Bwibo, and Sigman, 1993).

The objective of this paper is to determine the linkages between adoption of market-oriented dairy technologies, and household income, expenditures on food and non-food, and improved human nutrition as measured by calorie, protein, carotene, and iron intake, and preschooler's health indicators in Ethiopia. The above relationships are estimated using econometric recursive models to identify the determinants of these linkages. The dairy technologies being assessed are the results of a long-term research program between the International Livestock Research Institute (ILRI) and the Ethiopian Research Organization (EARO) that aimed at increasing milk and meat production, household income, use of dairy cows for traction, and nutritional status of household members.

The results of this study are particularly relevant for nutrition and food security policies in the East African region in general, and Ethiopia in particular, where there are several on-going programs to combat malnutrition. Examples of programs in Ethiopia include: community school and health-based nutrition education; regular provision of micronutrients to high risk (targeted) groups through supplementation programs; and ensured access at the household level to an adequate supply of nutrition through promotion of horticulture and livestock activities.

The paper is organized as follows: The next section expounds the theoretical household model; Section 3 outlines the empirical data used in estimation; The study area and the model are presented in section 4; The results are discussed in section 4 and the paper concludes in section 5.

THEORETICAL FRAMEWORK OF THE HOUSEHOLD MODEL

The farm household maximizes a utility function of the form:

$$U = U(X_a, X_m, X_l) \tag{1}$$

Subject to a cash income constraint:

$$p_m X_m = p_a(Q - X_a) - w(L - F) \tag{2}$$

Where X_a, X_m, and X_l are agricultural commodity (staple), a market purchased good and leisure, respectively. P_m and p_a are the prices of the market-purchased commodity and the staple, respectively, Q is the household's production of the staple, w is the market wage, L is total labor input, and F is family labor input. The quantity $Q - X_a$ is the household's marketed surplus, if positive. If $(L - F)$ is positive, the household hires labor, if it is negative, there is off-farm labor supply from the household.

A household also faces a time constraint:

$$X_l + F = T \tag{3}$$

Where, T is the total stock of household time. The other constraint the farm household faces is related to production technology that depicts the relation between inputs and outputs.

$$Q = Q(L,A) \tag{4}$$

Where, A is the household's fixed quantity of land.

The underlying assumptions for the above formulations are:

- In spite of the relevance of capital inputs such as fertilizer, pesticide, etc., they are not included in this illustration;
- The possibility that more than one crop can be produced is not included;
- Family labor and hired labor are perfect substitutes; and
- The three prices, namely p_m, p_a, and w are not affected by actions of the household, (i.e., the household is a price-taker in the three markets). This last assumption, if it holds, guarantees a recursive model.

Then, the three constraints (i.e., Equations 2, 3, and 4) can be combined as follows:

Substituting Equation 4 into Equation 2 for Q and the time constraint into the cash income constraint for F, yields a single constraint:

$$p_m X_m = p_a[Q(L,A) - X_a] - w(L - F) \tag{5}$$

Since $F = T - X_l$, Equation 5 becomes,

$$p_m X_m = p_a[Q(L,A) - X_a] - w(L - T + X_l) \tag{6}$$

Rearranging Equation 6 yields,

$$p_m X_m + p_a X_a + w X_l = p_a Q(L,A) - w(L - T) \tag{7}$$

Further rearrangement of Equation 7 gives,

$$p_m X_m + p_a X_a + w X_l = wT + p_a Q(L,A) - wL \qquad (8)$$

Finally from Equation 8, we get

$$p_m X_m + p_a X_a + w X_l = wT + \pi \qquad (9)$$

Where $\pi = p_a Q(L,A) - wL$ is a measure of farm profits. The left-hand side of Equation (9) represents the household's total expenditure on three items: market-purchased commodity, household's purchase of its own output, and household's purchase of its own time in the form of leisure. The right-hand side of the equation is the farm household's full income in which the value of the stock of time (wT) owned by the household is explicitly recorded.

In these equations, the household can choose the level of consumption for the three commodities and total labor input into agricultural production. The first order conditions for maximizing each of labor is:

$$\frac{p_a \partial Q}{\partial L} = W \qquad (10)$$

The household will equate the marginal revenue product of labor to the market wage. Since the other endogenous variables do not appear, and therefore, do not influence the household's choice of L, production decisions can be made independently of consumption and labor-supply (or leisure) decisions. Let the solution for L be

$$L^* = L^*(W, p_a, A) \qquad (11)$$

This solution can then be substituted into the right-hand side of the constraint to obtain the value of full income when farm profits have been maximized through an appropriate choice of labor input. The full income constraint can be rewritten as,

$$Y^* = p_m X_m + p_a X_a + w X_l \qquad (12)$$

Where Y^* is the value of full income associated with profit-maximizing behavior. Maximizing utility subject to this new version of the constraint yields the following first-order conditions:

The Lagrangian multipliers method for solving the above constrained optimization problem can be formulated as:

$$L(X_a, X_m, X_l, \lambda) = U(X_a, X_m, X_l) + \lambda(Y^* - p_m X_m - p_a X_a - w X_l) \qquad (13)$$

The first order conditions for maximization are:

$$\frac{\partial L(.)}{\partial X_a} = \frac{\partial U}{\partial X_a} - \lambda p_a = 0$$

$$\frac{\partial L(.)}{\partial X_m} = \frac{\partial U}{\partial X_m} - \lambda p_m = 0$$

$$\frac{\partial L(.)}{\partial X_l} = \frac{\partial U}{\partial X_l} - \lambda w = 0 \qquad (14a)$$

$$\frac{\partial L(.)}{\partial \lambda} = Y^* - p_m X_m - p_a X_a - w X_l = 0$$

From Equation 14a we get,

$$\frac{\partial U(.)}{\partial X_a} = \lambda p_a$$

$$\frac{\partial U(.)}{\partial X_m} = \lambda p_m \qquad (14b)$$

$$\frac{\partial U(.)}{\partial X_l} = \lambda w$$

$$p_m X_m + p_a X_a + w X_l = Y^*$$

Equation 14b holds the standard conditions from consumer-demand theory. For $i = m, a, l$, the solution of Equation 13 yields standard demand curves of the form:

$$X_i = X_i(p_m, p_a, w, Y^*) \qquad (15)$$

Equation 15 shows that demand depends on prices and income, where in the case of farm households, income is determined by the household's production activities. It therefore follows that changes in factors influencing production will also change Y^*, and hence, consumption behavior.

The nutrient intake including calorie, protein, iron and β-carotene can be derived directly from the demand equation for food in Equation 15 and can be represented as:

$$C = C(p_a, p_m, w, Y, Z) \tag{16}$$

Where the arguments are as defined above and Z is a vector of other household characteristics.

EMPIRICAL SPECIFICATION OF THE RECURSIVE MODEL

Based on the above description, the following issues are addressed recursively in assessing the impact of market-oriented dairy technologies:

- The impact of the dairy innovation on household incomes.
- The impact of incremental increases in income on food expenditure, and non-food expenditure.
- The impact of incremental increases in food expenditure on calorie, protein, iron, and carotene intake indicating better access to food and improved nutrition.
- The impact of incremental increases in nutrient intake on health indicators of preschoolers.

These issues and outcomes are modeled as part of the farm household's utility function, following Bouis and Haddad (1990) and Kumar (1994). The empirical recursive econometric model consists of income, expenditure, nutrients, and health relations. The explanatory variables can, generally, be disaggregated into resources such as labor, land, livestock holding size and composition, capital inputs and socio-economic variables describing household and farm characteristics that influence income, expenditure, and consumption decisions. Household socio-economic characteristics include family size, age, education, and sex of the household head, dependency ratio, ratio of women in the household and mothers' knowledge, attitude, and performance. Among farm characteristics are its proximity to the market. The following system of recursive equations is used in the empirical estimation.

1. Income equation:

$$Y = f(LAND, INPUT, TRACT, FLBOR, NFLBOR, LIVES, STRAW, \\ GROUP, EDUC, AGE, SEX, DRATIO, FRATIO, MKT) \tag{17}$$

2. Seasonal expenditure equations:

$$EXP_j = f(Y, PRICE, MKT, OFFSH, FS, DRATIO, FRATIO, AGE, \\ SEX, EDUC, d_t) \tag{18}$$

where j = food (f) or non-food (nf)

3. Seasonal nutrient intake equations:

$$C_i = f(EXP_f, NVPRICE_i, KAP, CEREAL, PULSES, DRATIO,$$
$$FRATIO, FS, EDU, SEX, AGE, AGEM, EDUM, d_t) \qquad (19)$$

where i = protein (p), calorie (cal), iron (ir) or β-carotene (car)

4. Health indicator equations:

$$WAZ = f(Ci, KAP, SEXC, EDUM, AGEM, PRVILH, KNBAL,$$
$$PRVAC) \qquad (20)$$

where:

- Y is the per capita income, which includes sales of farm products and off-farm income (Birr[1]);
- EXP_f and EXP_{nf} are per capita expenditure on food and non-food, respectively;
- C_i includes C_{cal}, C_p, C_{ir}, and C_{car} which are, respectively, per capita intake of calorie, protein, iron, and β-carotene;
- WAZ, WHZ, and HAZ are, respectively, the weight for age, weight for height and height for age Z-scores of the indexed child in the household;
- LAND is the area of land cultivated by the household (ha);
- INPUT is the value of purchased inputs including seed, fertilizer and other chemicals (Birr);
- TRACT is number of hours of animal traction applied to crop production (hrs);
- FLBOR is the number of family labor hours used in crop and livestock (hrs);
- NFLBOR is the number of non-family labor hours used in crop and livestock (hrs);
- STRAW is amount of straw produced during 1996 cropping year;
- LIVES is the livestock herd size expressed as tropical livestock units (TLU);
- PRICE is unit price of food;
- NVPRICE is the weighted average price per unit of nutrient (Birr);
- CEREAL is the area allocated to cereal (ha);
- PULSES is the area allocated to pulses (ha);
- GROUP is a dummy variable indicating if the household owns (CBC = 1 and 0 otherwise);
- EDUC is the highest education attained by the head of the household,
- AGE is the age of the head of the household (years);
- EDUCM is the highest education attained by the mother;
- AGEM is the age of the mother (years);

- SEX is the sex of the head of the household (male = 0; female = 1);
- SEXC is the sex of the indexed child (male = 0; female = 1);
- FS is the family size expressed in adult equivalent;
- DRATIO is the dependency ratio defined as the number of dependents to number of independent adults;
- FRATIO is the ratio of women in the household;
- MKT is the distance to the nearest market expressed in walking time to and from the market center;
- OFFSH is the share of off-farm employment in total income of the household;
- KAP is an index measuring mother's knowledge, attitude and practice;
- KNBAL is knowledge, specifically, of balanced diet (yes = 1; 0 otherwise);
- PRVILH is participation in village health program (yes = 1; 0 otherwise);
- PRVAC is participation in vaccination during pregnancy (yes = 1; 0 otherwise); and
- d_t is seasonal dummy variables.

Expenditure on food does not include the value of food produced on the farm, but only for that which is purchased. However, calorie intakes do include food from all sources, purchased and non-purchased. Because of the likelihood of the simultaneity problem, variables on the right hand side of each individual equation may be tested for simultaneity using Hausman's test (Hausman, 1978) at each stage in the system. If the test rejects the null hypothesis of no simultaneity, an instrumental variable technique is used. Also, multicollinearity may be detected using variance inflation factor (VIF) test. VIF is the diagonal element of the inverse of correlation matrix, which is $(1-R^2i)-1$, where R^2i is the R^2 obtained from regressing the ith independent variable on all other independent variables (Kennedy, 1985:153). Therefore, a high VIF indicates an R^2i near unity and hence suggests collinearity. According to Kennedy (1985), VIF of more than 10 indicates a harmful collinearity. This approach was used to exclude collinearity problems in the estimation process. The ependiture equations and nutrient intake equations were estimated each as a system using seemingly unrelated regression while the income equation and health indicator equations are estimated as single equations using OLS.

STUDY AREA AND SOURCES OF DATA

The study site is located in the Ethiopian highlands, about 40 km west of Addis Ababa in the vicinity of a small town called Holetta. The altitude of the research area is about 2600 meters above sea level. The average annual rainfall is 1100 mm with mean daily temperature of less than 20 degree centigrade. The main rainy period, known as the *Meher* season, starts in mid-June and continues up to September. The short rains or *Belg* are from February to April and are mainly used to break the soil. Farmers in Holetta depend on the *Meher* rains to plant crops. The farming system in the study area is classified as a mixed crop-livestock system with livestock playing an important role for provision of food (milk and meat), draft power, and dung, which is used for soil fertility enhancement as well as fuel.

The Holetta area is characterized by variable soils with a predominance of red brown soils, low water holding capacity on the slopes, and poorly drained heavy dark clay soils (vertisols) mostly in the valleys. Three types of soils can be identified on farm plots: vertisols, light and mixed upland soils, and heavy upland soils with vertisol properties. Farmers produce a wide range of cereal and legume crops on small parcels of land. The production is geared towards satisfying the household food requirements as well as a provision for feeding livestock in the form of straw and hay. The major crops are barley in the *belg* season, and wheat, teff, oats, and horse beans in the *mehr* season. Other minor crops include field peas, chickpeas, linseed, sorghum, and rapeseed. Farmers usually use manure, urea, and diammoium phosphate for soil fertility management. These inputs are either used individually or in combination, depending on availability, type of soil of the plot, and crops grown.

Beside crops, the household keeps a herd of animals, mainly consisting of dairy cows, at least two oxen for ploughing, heifers, bulls, goats, sheep, and chicken. Because of the dependency on animal traction for crop production, keeping at least a pair of oxen and a follower herd (heifers and bulls) for replacement is necessary despite the feed shortage. To ease the feed shortage, dairy-draft crossbred cows (CBC) and adoptions of on-farm forage production are encouraged. This technology allows the farmer to reduce the herd size while maintaining the capacity for both animal traction and milk production. However, farmers are reluctant to use crossbred cows for traction.

Holetta is one of the areas where crossbred cows were introduced to increase dairy production to meet the increasing demand of the neighboring urban areas and to improve farmers' incomes and nutrition. The area is considered to have a high dairy potential due to its adequate agro-ecological conditions and market access to Addis Ababa. Farm households are organized into peasant associations through which they are allocated usufruct rights to farmland. Individual farm households on small plots averaging about 1.5 hectares carry out crop production. They also have grazing areas of about 0.5-1.0 hectares. Because of the high population pressure and small farm sizes, intensification through the introduction of new technology is a distinct possibility. However, the practice of growing fodder crops for animals is rare, and there is an acute shortage of high quality feed, necessary for maintaining crossbred cows. Some of the newly introduced feeds intended to alleviate this problem include fodder beet, oat-vetch inter crop, and leguminous trees.

The data used for this study was generated by a collaborative dairy technology project involving the Ethiopian Agricultural Research Organization (EARO), and the International Livestock Research Institute (ILRI). One major objective of the project was to develop technologies to enable resource poor smallholder mixed crop-livestock farmers to participate in market-oriented dairying. Another objective was testing the use of crossbred dairy cows for traction, as well as milk production.

Pairs of crossbred dairy cows were introduced on 14 farms in Holetta in 1993, half for only milk production, and half for traction, as well as milk production. On-farm mean milk yield and average lactation days were not as such affected by traction, given adequate feeding (Stall, Steven, and Shapiro, 1994). Thus, the use of the crossbred cows for traction by households, in addition to dairy production, is not considered of relevance for the purposes of this study.

During 1995 and early 1996, 120 more crossbred cows were introduced into the community and an additional 60 households could use the cows for traction, in addition to milk production and reproduction. Another 60 control households using traditional practices of local Zebu cows for milk production and oxen for traction have been monitored starting mid-1996. In total, 134 households were surveyed for one year from October 1996 through September 1997. This enabled comparison of the income and nutritional status of the two groups of households, namely 65 households with crossbred cows (CBC participants) and 60 without crossbred cows (non-participants).

Data collection included land use, labor allocation to different operations, draught power use and source, input use, output disposal, income, expenditure, and price data. Food availability and food intake by household member were also collected. In addition, data on demographic, resources endowment, cropping and livestock activities were carried out. Food intake of 84 farm households was monitored for one day per month from March to December 1997. Special attention was given to the nutrition and health effects on children and women since they are the most vulnerable social group to food insecurity. The target population of the study thus included all members of households with preschool children of 6 months to 6 years. The nutritional records included both the CBC participants and non-participants.

The Ethiopian Health and Nutrition Research Institute (EHNRI) measured anthropometric indicators (weight for height, weight for age and height for age) on preschool children in all the households. Anthropometric measurements were focused on preschool children of 6 months to 6 years since they have relatively high risks of being affected by nutrient-deficiency resulting in health problems. Furthermore, due to their key positions in ensuring food availability for all household members, child health care measures and the nutritional knowledge of mothers were assessed. Environmental health factors, childcare and health care measures, child morbidity, and mothers' nutritional knowledge were also covered.

RESULTS

In the recursive analysis, the determinants of per capita income were estimated using the variables shown in Equation (17). Then the expenditure functions (Equation 18) were estimated after testing for simultaneity between the expenditure and income functions based on Hausman test (Hausman, 1978). The test rejected the hypothesis of no simultaneity between the two. Hence, the instrumental approach was used in the simultaneous estimation of the expenditure functions. A similar procedure was followed in the estimation of the parameters of the consumption functions, which were estimated simultaneously.

Impacts on Income

Test for multicollinearity among the independent variables was made using variance inflating factor (VIF). The higher the value of the VIF, the higher is the degree of multicollinearity, and hence, the lesser is the efficiency of parameter estimation. Usually, VIF of more than 10 is associated with a high degree of multicollinearity. Such a test was conducted for all variables in each of the models estimated.

A log-linear function was used to estimate the coefficients of the per capita income function determinants. Results are summarized in Table 1. As expected, adoption of the improved dairy cows significantly increases the per capita income of households. The results show that factor inputs such as land, and seeds and chemical fertilizer (*INPUT*), and straw production contribute significantly to per capita income. The signs of these variables are also as expected. As crop production is the most important source of household income, it is apparent that as the size of cultivated area increases, per capita income also increases. On the other hand, family size is found to have a negative impact on the level of per capita income. This impact is generally true when there is a high dependency ratio, which holds true also in the study area. Therefore, although a large family may provide a high reserve of labor for generating income, the children, elderly, and the disabled members of the household do not contribute to the income generation.

Family labor has a negative relationship with per capita income. But non-family labor is positively and significantly associated with per capita income. This relationship may be due to the fact that when a household earns

TABLE 1. Determinants of Income per Adult-Equivalent[1]

	β	t-value	Sig.	Collinearity Statistics	
				Tolerance	VIF
Constant term	3.4544	6.42	0.0000		
Cultivated area[*]	0.1952	4.03	0.0001	0.5339	1.8730
Input (seed, fertilizer, chemicals)[*]	0.0898	1.71	0.0891	0.2413	4.1445
Age of head of HH[*]	−0.3490	−4.54	0.0000	0.4782	2.0912
Straw produced in 1996[*]	0.3623	5.47	0.0000	0.1738	5.7549
Female ratio	0.0009	0.73	0.4652	0.7227	1.3836
Education of head (highest attained)	−0.0408	1.62	0.1063	0.4789	2.0883
Sex of head (Male = 1, Female = 2)	−0.2888	−3.27	0.0012	0.8525	1.1731
Traction hrs	0.0001	0.76	0.4462	0.7470	1.3387
TLU per adult-equivalent	0.0111	0.32	0.7511	0.4144	2.4131
Family labor[*]	−0.1276	−2.68	0.0079	0.3645	2.7437
Non-family labor[*]	0.1314	4.22	0.0000	0.3733	2.6789
Family size (adult-equivalent)	−0.0990	−8.26	0.0000	0.4252	2.3517
Dependency ratio	−0.0001	−0.29	0.7726	0.6991	1.4303
GROUP (CBC = 1, Non-CBC = 0)	0.2039	4.31	0.0000	0.6033	1.6575
Round trip travel time to nearest market	0.0002	0.50	0.6143	0.8121	1.2313
R square	0.70				
Adjusted R square	0.68				

[1] Natural log of the variable is used in the model.
[*] Sex: Male = 1; Female = 2.
Source: Unpublished data of ILRI, Dairy-draft project, 1997.

high income, it employs labor to operate on its farm and engages itself on other activities.

There are two unexpected signs in the estimated models: namely access to market and the level of education attained. The results further show that there is a negative relationship between the income level and the age of the head of the household. Although experience comes with age, it is possible that younger farmers are more able to acquire newer skills. The per capita income is negatively associated with female headship of the household. This result may be due to the poor resource basis of this group of farmers since the model depicted that the productive resources are important determinants of per capita income.

Impacts on Food and Non-Food Expenditures

Hausman (1978) provides a procedure to detect simultaneity between the predictor variable(s) and the dependent variable. Proceeding with the ordinary least squares (OLS) procedure without conducting this test would result in inconsistent estimates. Simultaneity implies that the predictor (explanatory) variable(s) will be endogenous, and therefore, correlate with the disturbance term.

For the determinants of food expenditure per capita, the relevant question is whether income (the predictor variable) is determined simultaneously with per capita expenditure (the dependent variable). The Hausman test is a two-step procedure. The first step involves OLS estimation of the income function by including all exogenous variables of the expenditure and the income functions (Bouis and Haddad, 1990; Pindyck and Rubinfeld, 1991).

The second step involves estimation of expenditure functions either on the predicted income or on the residuals of the income function estimated in step 1 and the other explanatory variables of the expenditure function. Finally, conducting a hypothesis test on the coefficient of either the predicted income or the residual term concludes the presence or absence of simultaneity (Bouis and Haddad, 1990; Pindyck and Rubinfeld, 1991). Following Pindyck and Rubinfeld (1991) the significance of the residual value in the step 2 of simultaneity test is used as an indicator of endogeneity.

Results of the test rejected the null hypothesis of no simultaneity indicating that simultaneity exists between the expenditure and income functions. Hence, the two expenditure functions shown in Equation (18) are simultaneously estimated using a three-stage OLS estimation procedure (White et al., 1990) with predicted income rather than observed income. The estimated parameters of the food and non-food expenditure functions are summarized in Table 2.

The result shows that (as expected) the instrumental variable explains the variation in the expenditure for non-food items rather than the expenditure on food. The result may be acceptable under the conditions of subsistence farmers who rely on their own food supply than on purchases of staples. However, with increased integration of improved dairy production and off-farm activities, the significance level of the influence may change. This result has also been evidenced by the fact that the share of off-farm income positively explains the expenditure on food.

As expected, the price of food has a negative and significant influence on the expenditure on food as well as non-food items. Moreover, the accessibility to markets has a negative and significant effect on expenditure. As hypothesized, the higher the proportion of female in the household, the more expenditure on food there will be. Moreover, the regression analysis shows that male-headed households tend to spend more showing perhaps the extent to which the male dominates the appropriation and disposal of the household income. The result is consistent with studies undertaken in Kenya (Kennedy, Peters, and Haddad, 1994).

Regarding the relationship between the ages of the heads of the household, the result shows that younger farmers tend to spend more on food and

TABLE 2. Determinants of Expenditure Functions

Variables	Expenditure on Food[1]		Expenditure on Non-Food[1]	
	β	t	β	t
Predicted per capita income'	0.0710	1.83[c]	0.0580	3.04[a]
Price of food'	−0.5057	−7.94[a]	−0.1480	−1.06
Access to off-farm work (share of income)	0.002	1.96[b]	0.0006	0.24
Distance to nearest market'	−0.1585	−5.16[a]	−0.2521	−3.79[a]
Female ratio in the household	0.0063	2.90[a]	0.0017	0.36
Dependency ratio	0.00002	0.03	−0.0013	−1.01
Family size	−0.0865	−6.47[a]	−0.0704	2.52[b]
Age of head of household'	−0.2682	−2.67[a]	−0.6369	−2.92[a]
Sex of head of household	−0.5516	−1.91[c]	−0.2471	0.39
Education of head of household	0.0415	1.45	0.0129	0.21
QUARTER1	0.2297	3.58[a]	1.4411	10.34[a]
QUARTER2	0.3872	5.96[a]	1.1856	8.41[a]
QUARTER3	0.3537	5.54[a]	0.8695	6.28[a]
Constant	4.7021	8.33[a]	6.6796	6.18[a]
R square	0.5594		0.4034	

[1] Natural log of the variable is used.
a, b, and c = sig. at 1%, 5%, and 10% level, respectively.
Source: Unpublished data of ILRI, Dairy-draft project, 1997.

non-food goods. Seasonality also plays a significant role in expenditure decisions. As the family size increases, the households tend to minimize the risk of food shortage by producing more of their subsistence requirement of their members. The result of the study proved this argument. The overall power of the models shows that about 56% of the variations in the expenditure for food is explained by the variables included in the model. The proportion is lower for the non-food expenditure model (40%).

Impacts on Consumptions of Nutrients

Recursive estimation procedure was adopted to estimate the consumption equations. Prior to the estimation of the consumption equation, Hausman test was performed to check if there was simultaneity between the consumption function and the expenditure function. Similar testing procedure was followed as described under previous section. In the first step, the expenditure function was defined including all exogenous variables of the expenditure and the consumption functions. In addition to the variables included in Equation (18), all variables exogenous to the consumption functions were included in the regression. The explanatory variables in the four consumption models are the same except for the prices of nutrition that depend on the type of nutrition under consideration.

In the second step, the residual of the model estimated in Step 1 is used together with variables in Equation (19). The result shows that the coefficient of the residual value in all the consumption models are found to be insignificant showing that there is no statistical evidence to accept the null hypothesis that there is no simultaneity. Hence, equations for calorie, protein, iron, and carotene and expenditure were estimated using the three-stage least squares method for simultaneously estimating the four systems of consumption function. The results shown in Table 3 show that there is a very strong and negative relationship between the unit prices of the nutritive value and their consumption. On the other hand, there is a positive and strong relationship between nutrient intake and expenditure on food, except in the case of calorie intake due to the reasons indicated above (i.e., reliance on own production). There is an inverse, but significant relationship between the age of mothers and per capita nutrient intake. Furthermore, there is a positive association between female-headed household and nutrient intake. Knowledge, attitude, and practices are more

TABLE 3. Determinants of Nutrient Intake

Variables	Calorie[1]		Protein[1]		Iron[1]		β-Carotene[1]	
	β	t	β	t	β	t	β	t
Food expenditure[1]	−0.0103	−0.41	0.0164	0.68	0.0742	2.17a	0.0982	2.16b
Nutrition value price[1]	−0.2054	−15.42a	−0.4140	−20.25a	−0.8462	−36.63a	−0.9905	−66.09a
KAP[1]	0.017	0.58	0.0693	2.49b	0.1666	4.23a	0.1461	2.79a
Family size	−0.0472	−6.62a	−0.0412	−6.05a	−0.0262	−2.72a	−0.029	−2.25b
Education of head of HH	−0.0582	−3.74a	−0.0407	2.76a	0.0278	−1.30	0.0296	−1.03
Education of mother	0.0132	2.45b	0.0059	1.15	−0.0059	−0.80	−0.010	−1.03
Age of mother	−0.0083	−3.87a	−0.0099	−4.83a	−0.0107	−3.67a	−0.0117	−3.03a
Age of head of HH	0.0054	3.39a	0.0063	4.15a	0.0082	3.81a	0.0091	3.18a
Sex of head of HH	0.3021	2.09b	0.1767	1.28	0.0568	0.29	0.1961	0.75
Dependency ratio	−0.0011	−3.61a	−0.0010	−3.25a	−0.0001	−0.32	0.0003	0.47
Female ratio in the HH	−0.0016	−1.46	−0.0003	−0.33	0.0011	0.79	0.0015	0.78
QUARTER1	0.0053	0.17	−0.001	−0.03	−0.0122	−0.29	0.0149	−0.26
QUARTER2	0.0081	0.24	−0.0054	−0.17	−0.0326	−0.72	−0.0420	−0.7
QUARTER3	0.0035	0.11	0.0076	−0.24	−0.0310	−0.70	−0.0400	−0.68
Cereals area	0.0001	2.78a	0.0001	3.97a	0.0001	4.63a	0.0001	2.95a
Pulse area[1]	0.0061	1.81c	0.008	2.49b	−0.0038	−0.83	−0.0056	−0.93
Constant	8.5542	43.25a	5.7025	29.18a	6.8402	25.48a	7.0228	19.78a
R square	0.493		0.473		0.753		0.946	

[1] Natural log of the variable is used.
a, b, and c sig. at 1%, 5%, and 10% level, respectively.

relevant determinants of micronutrients than of macronutrients. Family size and dependency ratio have negative and significant impact on nutrition intake per adult-equivalent. The R-square value shows that the estimated model captures most of the important determinants of nutrient intake.

Impacts on Health Indicators

The determinants of the nutritional status were estimated by regressing potential explanatory variables on the anthropometric measurements. There are difficulties in capturing essential variables explaining the health status of an individual. According to Shils et al. (1994), these variables may be physical, social, and emotional problems, which may interfere with appetite or may affect the ability to purchase, prepare, and consume adequate diet. Equitable access to consumption among the members of the household is an important factor, which is hardly captured in the model, due to the lack of data. Due to such difficulties, the econometric models of health and nutritional status are generally weak and R-squares ranging between 10% to 15% are supposed to be good estimates (Von Braun, Haen, and Blanken, 1991).

In this study, the values of the Z-scores (Height-for-age, weight-for-age, weight-for-height) computed from the anthropometrics measurements were used as a dependent variable and the nutrition intake discussed above, the KAP (mother's knowledge, attitude and practice) sex of the index child, age and education of the mother, participation of the mothers in village health program, vaccination during pregnancy, and specific knowledge of the role of balanced diet were used as explanatory variables. The estimated model shows that the weight-for-age (WAZ) and weight-for-height (WHZ) Z-scores, which reflects the current nutritional status, resulted in more efficient estimates of the model parameters (Table 4).

The result shows that KAP (mother's knowledge, attitude, and practice), age of the mother and female headship are important determinants of the WAZ and WHZ scores. Participation in the village health program has a significant effect (at 10% level) on the WHZ score. Unexpected sign of coefficients on protein and on β-carotene intakes were observed in the two models. In addition to targeting the income side to improve the nutritional status of the members of a household, intervention strategies should take the gender and the health aspects into consideration.

CONCLUSION

This paper assesses the impact of adopting market-oriented dairy technologies (cross bred cows and associated feed and management packages) on food

TABLE 4. Determinants of Nutritional Status of Children Under 6 Years

Variables	HAZ-Score		WAZ-Score		WHZ-Score	
	β	t	β	t	β	t
Constant term	−3.823	−2.85ᵃ	−2.688	−2.73ᵃ	−0.679	−0.73
Sex (male =1; female = 2)	−0.148	0.51	−0.399	−1.87ᶜ	−0.420	−2.07ᵇ
Age of mother	0.033	2.19ᵇ	0.028	2.50ᵇ	0.010	0.98
Education level of mother	0.024	0.33	0.035	0.65	0.016	0.33
KAP	0.046	0.39	0.191	2.20ᵇ	0.221	2.70ᵃ
Per capita protein intake	0.023	1.94ᶜ	0.001	0.12	−0.013	−1.60
Per capita iron intake	−0.007	1.33	0.002	0.48	0.008	2.09ᵇ
Per capita β-carotene intake	0.002	0.47	−0.003	−1.08	−0.006	2.12ᵇ
Knowledge of advantage of balanced diet (know = 1; 0 otherwise)	0.008	0.02	0.341	1.11	0.427	1.47
Participation in village health (yes = 1; no = 0)	−0.195	−0.44	0.298	0.91	0.572	1.84ᶜ
Vaccination during pregnancy (yes = 1; 0 = no)	0.451	1.37	0.016	0.07	−0.257	−1.12
R square	0.19		0.22		0.29	

a, b, and c indicate statistical significance at 1%, 5%, and 10%, respectively.

security. Food security is measured in terms of increased income, increased expenditures on food and non-food products, increased nutrient intakes, and better health status.

Results of econometric estimations using a recursive estimation procedure indicate that the proportion of crossbred cows owned, is an important determinant of income. Also resource bases like cultivated areas and purchased inputs, which are mainly obtained through the cash generated from dairy products, are important determinants of per capita income. Access to market is also an important factor determining the level of per capita income. Access to crossbred cows via income changes significantly and positively influences expenditures on food and non-food items and nutrient intakes. The higher the income level, the higher the expenditure on food and non-food items. Except for calorie intakes, higher expenditure on foods has had positive effects on other nutrients intakes. However, increased prices of food have had negative impacts on nutrient intakes. Finally, mother's knowledge, attitude and practice, age of mother, and gender of the household heads are important determinants of health status.

NOTE

1. Birr is the legal Ethiopian currency. At this time, 1 US dollar is about 8.3 Ethiopian Birr.

REFERENCES

Bouis, H.E. and L.J. Haddad. 1990. *Agricultural Commercialization, Nutrition and the Rural Poor: A Study of Philippine Farm Households*. IFPRI, Washington, DC, USA.

Ehui, S., H. Li-Pun, V. Mares, and B. Shapiro. 1998. The role of livestock in food security and environmental protection. *Outlook on Agriculture*, 27(2): 81-87

Hausman, J.A. 1978. Specification tests in econometrics. *Econometrica*, 46: 1251-1271.

Kennedy, P. 1985. *A Guide to Econometrics*, 2nd ed. The MIT Press, Cambridge.

Kennedy, E., P. Peters, and L. Haddad. 1994. Effects of gender of head of household on women's and children's nutritional status. In: Biswas, M.R. and M. Gabr (eds.), *Nutrition in the Nineties: Policy Issues*, Oxford University Press.

Kumar, S.K. 1994. *Adoption of Hybrid Maize in Zambia: Effects on Gender Roles, Food Consumption, and Nutrition*. IFPRI Research Report No. 100. IFPRI, Washington, DC, USA. 126p.

Neumann, C, N.O. Bwibo, and M. Sigman. 1993. *Diet Quantity and Quality: Functional Effects on Rural Kenyan Families*, Kenya Project Final Report, Phase II–1989-1992, Human Nutrition Collaborative Program Support Program, Office of Nutrition, USAID, Washington, DC.

Pindyck, R.S., and D.L. Rubinfeld. 1991. *Econometric Models and Economic Forecasts*. McGraw-Hill Book Company, New York.

Shils, M.E., J.M. Olson, and M. Sheke, 1994. *Modern Nutrition in Health and Disease*. 8th ed. Vol. 1, Williams & Wilkins, Baltimore, London.

Singh, M., P. Kumar. 1994. Natural induction of lactation–a report. *Indian Veterinary Journal*. 71(4): 405.

Staal, S.J., and B.I. Shapiro. 1994. The effects of price de-control on Kenyan Peri-Urban Dairy: A case study using the policy analysis matrix approach. *Food Policy*, 19 (6): 533-549.

Von Braun, J., H. de Haen, and J. Blanken, 1991. *Commercialization of Agriculture under Population Pressure: Effects on Production, Consumption and Nutrition in Rwanda*. IFPRI Research Report No. 85.

White, K.J., S.D. Wong, D. Whistler, and S.A. Haun. 1990. *SHAZAM Econometric Computer Program: User's Reference Manual*, Version 6.2. Ronalds Printing, Canada.

Delivering Micronutrients
via Food Fortification

M. G. Venkatesh Mannar

SUMMARY. Fortification of foods has been a successful strategy for the delivery of micronutrients in developed countries. Fortification requires modest investments, is cost effective, can build on existing technologies facilitated by the globalization of the food industry, supports other public health strategies to combat micronutrient deficiency induced malnutrition, and enhances sustainability. In developing countries, the success of food fortification has been encouraging, but varied, due to the decentralized food processing process and issues of quality control. Food fortification is an integral part of any food systems strategy and the choice of the appropriate food vehicle and its fortificant can be tailored to meet the local needs. This article discusses various aspects of food fortification: existing and future opportunities for food fortification, cost effectiveness, food fortification success stories with examples from different regions, and impact on nutritional status of humans. *[Article copies available for a fee from The Haworth Document Delivery Service: 1-800-HAWORTH. E-mail address: <getinfo@haworthpressinc.com> Website: <http://www.HaworthPress.com> © 2002 by The Haworth Press, Inc. All rights reserved.]*

KEYWORDS. Food fortification, food systems, iodine, iron, nutrition, vitamin A

M. G. Venkatesh Mannar is Executive Director, The Micronutrient Initiative, 250 Albert Street, P.O. Box 56127, Ottawa, Canada K1R 7Z1 (E-mail: vmannar@idrc.ca).

[Haworth co-indexing entry note]: "Delivering Micronutrients via Food Fortification." Mannar, M. G. Venkatesh. Co-published simultaneously in *Journal of Crop Production* (Food Products Press, an imprint of The Haworth Press, Inc.) Vol. 6, No. 1/2 (#11/12), 2002, pp. 339-363; and: *Food Systems for Improved Human Nutrition: Linking Agriculture, Nutrition, and Productivity* (ed: Palit K. Kataki, and Suresh Chandra Babu) Food Products Press, an imprint of The Haworth Press, Inc., 2002, pp. 339-363. Single or multiple copies of this article are available for a fee from The Haworth Document Delivery Service [1-800-HAWORTH, 9:00 a.m. - 5:00 p.m. (EST). E-mail address: getinfo@haworthpressinc.com].

INTRODUCTION

Deficiencies in three micronutrients–iodine, iron, and vitamin A–are widespread affecting more than a third of the world's population (World Bank, 1994). In their absence, individuals and families suffer serious consequences including learning disabilities, impaired work capacity, illness, and death. These deficiencies can be prevented and even eliminated if populations on a continuous and ongoing basis consume small quantities of the micronutrients (Table 1). During rapid growth, micronutrient intake must increase or else growth failure or deficiency diseases develop. It is during these periods that deficiency symptoms are most prevalent. For this reason, preschool-aged children, adolescents, and reproductive age women are high priority groups.

Nearly one in three people living in the developing world are affected by one or more micronutrient deficiency. Iron and iodine deficiencies are the most common and widespread nutritional problems. About half the reproductive age women in most of the developing countries suffer from iron deficiency anemia (IDA). Other high-risk groups include preschool and school age children and adolescents. Iodine deficiency disorders strike from 20% to 60% of people in different areas. Vitamin A deficiency has been widely recognized though at a lower clinical prevalence (around 1% in preschool children). However, vitamin A deficiency at a sub-clinical level (based on serum retinol assays) is thought to be around 10% to 25%. This level of deficiency is associated with increased mortality and morbidity risk in children and pregnant women. There are other deficiencies that are certainly widespread, but far less well recognized, e.g., rickets in young children, associated with calcium and vitamin D deficiency. Dietary intake surveys and limited biochemical indicators show that zinc deficiency is likely to be as widespread as that of IDA. Selenium and other micronutrients such as folate and vitamin E may have major role in reducing risks of chronic disease (e.g., cancers, heart diseases).

The major cause of micronutrient deficiencies is lack of adequate intake of bioavailable minerals and vitamins from the diet. This deficiency is exacerbated by the fact that commonly consumed foods and beverages (such as rice, wheat, corn, legumes, tea, and coffee) are high in inhibitors and low in enhancers of micronutrient absorption. Several delivery mechanisms are available ranging from high-dose supplements to consumption of micronutrient-rich foods to public health measures.

Food fortification is the addition of nutrients to commonly eaten foods so as to meet a demonstrable need in the population apparent from dietary, biochemical, or clinical evidence (Lofti et al., 1995; Venkatesh Mannar, 1987, 1993). Fortification should be viewed as part of a range of measures that influence the quality of food that include improved agricultural practices, improved food processing and storage, and consumer education to adopt good food prepara-

TABLE 1. Recommended Dietary Allowances (RDAs) for Some Essential Micronutrients

Category	Age or Condition	Minerals							Fat-Soluble Vitamins				Water-Soluble Vitamins						
		Calcium (mg)	Phosphorus (mg)	Magnesium (mg)	Iron (mg)	Zinc (mg)	Iodine (µg)	Selenium (µg)	Vitamin A (µg RE)[1]	Vitamin D (µg)[2]	Vitamin E (mg α-TE)[3]	Vitamin K (µg)	Thiamin (mg)	Riboflavin (mg)	Niacin (mg NE)[4]	Vitamin B6 (mg)	Folate (µg)	Vitamin C (mg)	Vitamin B12 (µg)
Infants	0-6 months	400	300	40	6	5	40	10	375	7.5	3	5	0.3	0.4	5	0.3	25	30	0.3
	7-12 months	600	500	60	10	5	50	15	375	10	4	10	0.4	0.5	6	0.6	35	35	0.5
Children	1-3 years	800	800	80	10	10	70	20	400	10	6	15	0.7	0.8	9	1.0	50	40	0.7
	4-7 years	800	800	120	10	10	90	20	500	10	7	20	0.9	1.1	12	1.1	75	45	1.0
	8-11 years	800	800	170	10	10	120	30	700	10	7	30	1.0	1.2	13	1.4	100	45	1.4
Males	12-14 years	1,200	1,200	270	12	15	150	40	1,000	10	10	45	1.3	1.5	17	1.7	150	50	2.0
	15-18 years	1,200	1,200	400	12	15	150	50	1,000	10	10	65	1.5	1.8	20	2.0	200	60	2.0
	19-24 years	1,200	1,200	350	10	15	150	70	1,000	10	10	70	1.5	1.7	19	2.0	200	60	2.0
	25-50 years	800	800	350	10	15	150	70	1,000	5	10	80	1.5	1.7	19	2.0	200	60	2.0
	51 + years	800	800	350	10	15	150	70	1,000	5	10	80	1.2	1.4	15	2.0	200	60	2.0
Females	12-14 years	1,200	1,200	280	15	12	150	45	800	10	8	45	1.1	1.3	15	1.4	150	50	2.0
	15-18 years	1,200	1,200	300	15	12	150	50	800	10	8	55	1.1	1.3	15	1.5	180	60	2.0
	19-24 years	1,200	1,200	280	15	12	150	55	800	10	8	60	1.1	1.3	15	1.6	180	60	2.0
	25-50 years	800	800	280	15	12	150	55	800	5	8	65	1.1	1.3	15	1.6	180	60	2.0
	51 + years	800	800	280	10	12	150	55	800	5	8	65	1.0	1.2	13	1.6	180	60	2.0
Pregnancy		1,200	1,200	320	30	15	175	65	800	10	10	65	1.5	1.6	17	2.2	400	70	2.2
Lactation	0-6 months	1,200	1,200	355	15	19	200	75	1,300	10	12	65	1.6	1.8	20	2.1	280	95	2.6
	7-12 months	1,200	1,200	340	15	16	200	75	1,200	10	11	65	1.6	1.7	20	2.1	260	90	2.6

Adapted from National Research Council–Subcommittee on the Tenth Edition of the Recommended Dietary Allowances, National Academy Press. Washington, DC. 1989

1 Retinol equivalents. 1 retinol equivalent = 1 µg retinol or 6 µg β-carotene
2 As cholecalciferol. 10 mg cholecalciferol = 400 IU of vitamin D
3 1 mg d-α tocopherol = 1 α-TE
4 1 NE (niacin equivalent) = 1 mg of niacin or 60 mg of dietary tryptophan

tion practices. Improved agricultural practices include the breeding of mineral and vitamin dense varieties of staple foods such as rice, wheat, maize, beans, and cassava for release to farmers in developing countries. It should also be linked to supplementation strategies that cover vulnerable groups.

Fortification involves the identification of commonly eaten foods in a country or region that can act as vehicles for one or more micronutrients and lend them to centralized processing on an economical scale. Fortification when imposed on existing food patterns, may not necessitate changes in the customary diet of the population and does not call for individual compliance. It could often be dovetailed into existing food production and distribution systems. Fortification levels aim to provide a part (usually 30-50%) of the daily adult requirements of the nutrient at normal consumption levels of the food vehicle. The levels also need to take into account variation in consumption of the food to ensure safety to those at the higher end of the scale and impact for those at the lower end. They should also consider prorated intakes by young children to ensure efficacious and safe dosages. Fortification can often be implemented and yield results quickly and be sustained over a long period of time. The benefits of fortification can extend over the entire life cycle. It can, thus, be the most cost-effective means of overcoming micronutrient malnutrition.

The Codex Alimentarius provides definitions for terminology relating to the addition of nutrients to foods (Table 2). Fortification or enrichment means the addition of one or more essential nutrients to a food whether or not it is normally contained in the food for the purpose of preventing or correcting a demonstrated deficiency of one or more nutrients in the population or specific population groups. Restoration refers to compensation for unavoidable nutrient losses during the course of Good Manufacturing Practice in the preparation and preservation of food or during normal storage and handling procedures. In many countries, there are requirements for the compulsory addition of micronutrients such as iron, niacin, and thiamine to bread and flour.

The concept of nutrient fortification of staple foods was developed in the early part of this century as a means of dealing with mineral and vitamin deficiency diseases that were prevalent in Europe and North America. Salt was iodized in Switzerland in the early part of the century. Margarine fortified with vitamin A was introduced in Denmark in 1918. During the 30s and 40s, milk was fortified with vitamin A and flour was fortified with iron and B vitamins in a number of European countries and in North America. In developed countries, where there is a high dependence on processed foods and industries are streamlined and automated, food fortification has played a major role in the health of the populations at large over the last 40 years and several nutritional deficiencies have been eliminated.

Over the past decade the contribution of salt iodization towards the virtual elimination in several developing countries has been substantial. Bolivia and

TABLE 2. General Principles for the Addition of Nutrients to Foods. (Adapted from : Codex Alimentarius Vol 4. CAC/GL09-1987. Food and Agriculture Organization 1984.)

1. The essential nutrient should be present at a level that will not result in either an excessive or an insignificant intake of the added essential nutrient considering amounts from other sources in the diet.
2. The addition of an essential nutrient to a food should not result in an adverse effect on the metabolism of any other nutrient.
3. The essential nutrient should be sufficiently stable in the food under customary conditions of packaging, storage, distribution, and use.
4. The essential nutrient should be biologically available from the food.
5. The essential nutrient should not impart undesirable characteristics to the food (e.g., color, taste, flavor, texture, cooking properties) and should not unduly shorten shelf life.
6. Technology and processing facilities should be available to permit the addition of the essential nutrient in a satisfactory manner.
7. Addition of essential nutrients to foods should not be used to mislead or deceive the consumer as to the nutritional merit of the food.
8. The additional cost should be reasonable for the intended consumer.
9. Methods of measuring, controlling and/or enforcing the levels of added essential nutrients in foods should be available.
10. When provision is made in food standards, regulations or guidelines for the addition of essential nutrients to foods, specific provisions should included identifying the essential nutrients to be considered or to be required and the levels at which they should be present in the food to achieve their intended purpose.

Ecuador are now IDD free. In many African countries (Nigeria, Madagascar, Eritrea, Cameroon) salt iodization levels are above 80%. Food fortification has also played a major role in substantially reducing Vitamin A and iron deficiency anemia. A national sugar fortification program in Guatemala has virtually eliminated VAD as a public health problem in that country. Flour fortification in Chile and Venezuela are substantially improving iron status in all sectors of the population. Today in Latin America, Asia, and Africa consumers of fortified products are as varied as margarine, milk, noodles, and cornstarch, which substantially protects them from a range of micronutrient deficiencies.

Based on more than 50 years of experience, food fortification has been proven effective in the control and prevention of a number of micronutrient deficiencies including IDA. Some examples of successful programs are summarized below.

- In the United States, after the introduction of flour fortified with niacin in 1938, deaths from Niacin deficiencies dropped from more than 3000 per year to negligible levels in approximately a decade (Figure 1). The current low levels of IDA in the US are attributable to fortified sources. Almost 1/4 of iron intakes in the US diet comes from fortified sources, much of that from flour products.

- Flour fortification with B vitamins began in Newfoundland during 1944. Within four years, deficiencies, which were found in nearly 20% of the population, dropped to negligible levels (Figure 2). In fact, Newfoundland was so convinced of the benefits of mandatory fortification that it made continuation of flour fortification a condition of the charter when it joined the Canadian federation.
- In the past decades flour fortification has been implemented in a number of Latin American countries. Chile has an IDA rate of less than 1%, which most observers attribute to a strong flour fortification program. More recently, all corn and wheat flour in Venezuela were fortified with iron, vitamin A and B vitamins. Fortifying to a level of 20-30 ppm, flour products currently contribute about 48% of RDA for iron in the average Venezuelan. The impact of flour fortification in Venezuela has been both swift and dramatic. Studies of anemia in children living in Caracas slum areas during the years immediately before and after fortification indicate anemia rates cut by about a factor of 2.5. It is important to note that this dramatic improvement occurred during a period when no other nutrition interventions were taking place and more importantly, at a time when economic pressures were causing an overall decline in the quality of the diet among the poorer classes of the country.

FIGURE 1. Reduction in mortality rates due to fortification of flour with niacin in the USA.

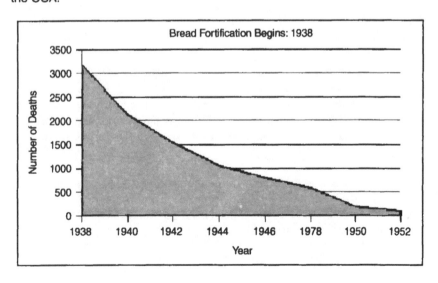

FIGURE 2. Reduction in vitamin B deficiencies in Newfoundland, due to fortification of flour with B vitamins.

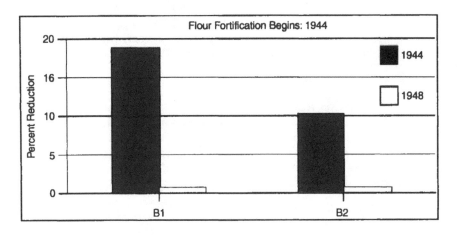

ADVANTAGES OF FOOD FORTIFICATION

Food fortification cannot expect to reach all populations deficient in essential micronutrients. When access to commercially or centrally processed food is limited, therefore, due to geography, poverty or cultural preference public health and welfare approaches to deliver supplements or dietary education are often the only viable options. However, for the large and expanding populations of all socio-economic classes that regularly purchase and consume commercially processed foods, fortification can make an enormous difference. Fortification offers a number of strategic advantages.

• Harnesses New Resources

By building on the existing food production and distribution infrastructure, fortification engages the market system and the private food sector. Industry provides much of the initial investment and the ultimate financing is borne by consumers. The private sector also offers technical expertise in production and marketing, and most importantly, a business-like approach to solving problems.

• Requires Modest Investment

Capital investment in fortification technology is minimal and easily absorbed by the producer. On the costs of fortificant, marketing and quality assurances are usually absorbed in the normal market fluctuations for most foods. Incremental costs often as low as 1-2% are either passed along to the consumer or simply absorbed by the producer. In Thailand, fortification added 0.05% to the cost of a pack of noodles. This hihger price was not discernable to the consumer, who experienced a price increase of 15-20% on account of inflation.

- Cost Effectiveness

   Fortification reaches broad populations at minimal cost. In Guatemala, sugar fortification protects the entire population for less than one-fourth the cost of supplementation. In Peru, a fortified school breakfast program offers protection against micronutrient deficiencies at a cost of $0.98 for fortification as against $1.52 for supplementation and $3.63 for dietary promotion.

- Builds on Existing Technology

   For many industries all over the world, the addition of conditioners, preservatives, vitamins, and minerals is not new. The additive equipment are already integrated into the process flow.

- Facilitated by the Globalization of the Food Industry

   Technology is rapidly becoming global with the expansion of trade and investments. Fortificants, premixes, and process know-how are now available internationally.

- Supports Other Public Health Strategies

   With fortification serving a bulk of the population, government can focus supplement delivery and dietary education on remote and disadvantaged populations that have limited access to fortified foods.

- Enhances Sustainability

   Fortification when integrated into the food processing and distribution system becomes a permanent feature and can be sustained with little external support or investment.

CONSIDERATIONS FOR PLANNING
A FOOD FORTIFICATION INTERVENTION

Food fortification involves the identification of commonly eaten foods in a country or region that can act as vehicles for one or more micronutrients and lend themselves to centralized processing on an economical scale. In developed countries, a range of cereals and cereal products, dairy products, processed foods, and beverages are fortified. In most developing countries, staple foods and condiments are the obvious choice for fortification given their consistent consumption by large sections of the population. In such situations, the choice of vehicles at the present time is limited to a handful of foods and condiments: cereals, oils and fats, sugar, salt, and sauces.

Fortification of foods is aimed to provide meaningful levels of the nutrient at normal consumption of the food vehicle. Variations in food consumption may affect the safety of those at the higher end of the scale and the level of impact for those at the lower end. They should also consider prorated intakes by young children to ensure efficacious and safe dosages. Food fortification also requires careful attention to food regulations and labeling and a careful assessment of the technical and analytical limitations for compliance with label declarations. The Codex Alimentarius has adopted a number of basic principles set out in Table 2 for the addition of nutrients to foods.

The selection of a suitable vehicle and a fortificant that meets all these conditions is often difficult. Salt iodization is one example of the successful large-scale fortification in the developing world–the primary reason being the simple and low cost technology and the narrow band of salt consumption quantities within a given region or population. There exist several other opportunities for single and multiple fortification of several commonly eaten foods like wheat and wheat products, rice, milk and milk products, cooking oils, salt, sugar, cereals, and condiments. As processed foods gain popularity in the developing world with an increasing market outreach, they offer new channels for micronutrient delivery. Table 3 indicates the feasibility of fortification of food vehicles with vitamins and minerals.

Depending on the food processing technologies, different addition methods have been developed.

- DRY MIXING for cereal flours and their products, powder milk, and powder beverages.
- DISSOLUTION IN WATER for liquid milk, drinks, fruit juices and in the water to be used for making bread pastas and cookies.
- SPRAYING as in iodization of salt and corn flakes where the vitamins do not support the cooking or extrusion step.
- DISSOLUTION IN OIL for the liposoluble vitamins for enrichment of oily products like margarine.
- ADHESION for sugar fortification where the vitamin A in powder form is adhered to the crystals surface by a vegetable oil.
- COATING of rice where the vitamins sprayed over the grain must be coated in order to avoid the losses when washing the grains before cooking.

- EXTRUSION of a blend of rice flour with micronutrients and stabilizers to provide a premix grains that can be blended with rice after milling.

Research and development efforts have enhanced the effectiveness of fortification technology. Better refining procedures and packaging have significantly improved the stability of iodine compounds in salt. In the case of iron, stabilizers and absorption enhancers are added along with the fortificant to retain it in an absorbable form or to improve its absorption. The structure of the iron or iron compounds has been modified to improve absorption. In the case of Vitamin A, work is ongoing to retard the loss of potency on storage. In all these cases, there is scope for further improvement and refinement for better product stability, absorption, lower cost, as well as development efforts need to continue.

Over the past decade, considerable experience has also been gained in the planning and implementation of fortification programs in the context of developing countries through support measures like advocacy and social communication, legislation and enforcement, monitoring and evaluation, and training. Given this background, it would be useful to review the global experience in food fortification with micronutrients–both successful and unsuccessful experiences–to assess the quality of available technologies and to identify the opportunities and challenges in their application. In addition, we need to understand the programmatic considerations that have a bearing on the large-scale application of the technologies.

Iodine

Over the past decade, there has been a remarkable growth in salt iodization programs. A significant proportion of the populations in over 110 countries are already having access to iodized salt and many countries are progressing towards the goal of Universal Salt Iodization. Once established in the country, salt iodization is a permanent and long-term solution to the problem. Iodine dosages range from 20 to 100 mg/kg of salt depending upon per capita salt consumption and the anticipated iodine losses between production and consumption. These losses are dependent upon the quality of salt and its packaging. Toxicity issues are negligible and cost considerations are fairly small.

While considerable progress in streamlining control programs of salt iodization have been achieved in several countries, producer compliance, quality assurance, logistic problems and bottlenecks do remain. The challenge is to systematically identify and tackle these constraints through effective advocacy, social communications, monitoring of salt iodine levels, regulation and enforcement.

TABLE 3. Opportunities for Food Fortification.

FOOD	VITAMINS											MINERALS	
	β-Carotene	A	D	E	B_1	B_2	B_6	C	PP	Folic	B_{12}	Fe	Ca
MILK:													
LIQUID	+	+	+	+	+	+	+	+	+	+	+	o	+
POWDER	+	+	+	+	+	+	+	+	+	+	+	+	+
WITH CEREAL	+	+	+	+	+	+	+	+	+	+	+	+	+
FLOURS:													
WHEAT	o	+	+	+	+	+	+	x	+	+	+	+	+
CORN	o	+	+	+	+	+	+	o	+	+	+	+	+
CASSAVA	o	o	o	o	o	o	o	o	o	o	o	o	o
RICE	o	+	+	+	+	+	+	+	+	+	+	+	+
RICE	o	+	+	+	+	+	+	+	+	+	+	+	+
SNACKS	o	+	+	+	+	+	+	+	+	+	+	+	+
CORN FLAKES	o	+	+	+	+	+	+	+	+	+	+	+	+
OIL			+		+		+	+					
MARGARINE	+	+	+	+	o	o	o	o	o	o	o	x	o
MAYONNAISE	+	+	+	+	o	o	o	o	o	o	o	x	o
JUICES	+	o	o	+	+	+	+	+	+	+	+	+	+
SUGAR							+						
POWDER BEVERAGES	o	+	+	+	+	+	+	+	+	+	+	+	+

+ : Possible   o : Trials needed   x : Not possible

Salt iodization is the first large-scale experience in national fortification of a commodity. It has provided valuable lessons in collaboration between government, industry, NGOs, the media, and other sectors. It has also given insights into building and sustaining an intervention program politically, technically, financially, and culturally.

Iron

While iron has potential for use in more food vehicles than iodine or Vitamin A, fortification with iron is technically more difficult than with other nutrients since iron reacts with several food ingredients. In the case of iodine and vitamin A, the problem is more of stability of the added compound under different storage and cooking conditions. The biggest challenge with iron is to identify a form that is adequately absorbed and yet does not alter the appearance or taste of the food vehicle. The buff colored insoluble iron phosphate compounds are stable under a variety of storage conditions but are poorly absorbed. The soluble iron salts like ferrous sulphate are well absorbed but easily discolor by reacting with food ingredients.

In addition to the general fortification criteria, iron fortification needs to take into account certain specific considerations.

- The vehicle should be a component of all meals because absorption varies inversely with the iron content of the meal.
- It should not require prolonged storage particularly under hot and humid climatic conditions since this could cause organoleptic problems.
- Vehicles that are dark in color or have a strong taste or odor, permit the use of more reactive iron compounds.
- Segregation of iron should not occur during mixing or storage.

While salt is clearly the mainstay for long term iodine deficiency prophylaxis, reducing the global prevalence of iron deficiency anemia will require the use of several alternative fortification compounds and food vehicles depending upon the local dietary patterns. Some promising possibilities are:

Wheat Flour and Bakery Products

In developed countries like the USA, Sweden, and Canada, these foods have had significant success as vehicles for iron (MI, 1995a; MI, 1995b; Popkin, Siega-Riz, and Haines, 1995). Stability problems have been largely overcome by using certain forms of reduced elemental iron. The bioavailability of iron added to wheat flour is several times greater than that added to other staple foods such as maize and rice. Further, it ensures even meal distribution of the added iron and provides a reasonably constant iron supply to each individual. More recently Venezuela, Ecuador, Brazil, and several other Latin American countries are implementing universal fortification programs for wheat and corn flour with iron, vitamin A, thiamine, riboflavin, and niacin.

Rice

Rice is a logical choice since it is a staple food for more than half the world's population and the main component of the diet in many countries where nutritional anemia is highly prevalent. Efforts in iron fortification of rice began in 1949 in the Philippines. In Papua New Guinea, a formulation that includes iron with vitamin B is used. It is noteworthy that in spite of these attempts there is still no large-scale program in operation. The Micronutrient Initiative (MI) has been working in Indonesia to integrate iron and/or vitamin A into the 'matrix' of broken rice grains that are powdered and reconstituted into full grains to produce a premix. The premix is then mixed with the rice in a certain proportion. Rice fortification is certainly an area that needs further work to develop a product that would be acceptable, and in which the iron would resist both washing and cooking, and yet, rapidly disintegrate in the intestinal tract. From the point of view of large scale application, it will be necessary to examine patterns of rice processing, availability of centralized milling points, and feasibility of large-scale fortification.

Salt

The technical requirements for iron fortification of salt are much more stringent than for iodine. Development efforts in India over the past 22 years have produced some positive results. During the mid seventies, a combination using ferrous sulphate with stabilizers like sodium acid pyrophosphate and a pH controller like sodium acid sulphate was tested extensively both in the laboratory and in field trials. The fortified salt showed good bioavailability and stability. This product is now commercially produced in limited quantities by a few companies in South India, but needs extensive promotion and governmental support.

In 1984, when the policy of universal iodization of salt was announced in India, the focus of work shifted to developing a formulation that would permit the addition of both iodine and iron. This formulation is needed because the acidic medium in which the iron compound is stable causes the rapid oxidation of iodide/iodate to free iodine, which vaporizes and is lost. In order to overcome this problem two approaches showed promise:

- The National Institute of Nutrition, Hyderabad has reported a formula using ferrous sulphate, a polyphosphate chelating agent (as stabilizer) and potassium iodate/iodide. This formulation is reported to be stable even in impure grades of salt.

- Recent work at the University of Toronto supported by MI has shown the feasibility of producing a dextrin encapsulation technique that provides a barrier between the iron and iodine compounds and improves stability. The salt is currently being field tested in Ghana for efficacy and consumer acceptability.

The successful testing and large-scale application of available technology for the double fortification of salt could represent a major breakthrough for combined iron and iodine delivery.

Condiments

In Thailand, fish sauce, which is consumed in many parts of the country, has been tested as a vehicle for iron. Fish sauce fortified with NaFeEDTA has shown good hemoglobin response. Fish sauce and fish paste have also been used as vehicles in the Philippines. Curry Powder used by an Indian population in South Africa has been fortified with NaFeEDTA with successful results. In China, the feasibility of using soy sauce as a carrier for iron is being examined. However, all these studies have been only pilot trials, and the constraints that retard their large-scale application have not been identified.

Processed Foods

There is a growing trend in several developing countries to increase the use of processed foods such as noodles, cereals, and soup cubes. Weaning foods for children are also becoming popular. Elemental iron of small particle size is being used for the fortification of processed cereals in several developed countries. In Chile, chocolate cookies have been fortified with dried hemoglobin for distribution as part of a school lunch program for good improvement in hemoglobin. In Mexico, chocolate milk powder is fortified with iron. In Tanzania a fortified orange beverage drink has been effective in improving iron and vitamin A status among school children. Barring such programs with a limited target population, it is not expected that processed foods or beverages could serve as a mainstay for food fortification programs in the developing countries. While fortifying foods that are not widely consumed by the population as part of the daily diet, it is virtually impossible to ascertain the effect of any one product on iron balance in the population and it is also difficult to regulate the level of iron supplied to the population.

Vitamin A

A variety of options are available for combating vitamin A deficiency including distribution of capsules, nutrition education, and introduction of farming techniques to grow carotene-rich foods in home gardens. However, given the magnitude and severity of vitamin A deficiency in some parts of the world, programs that can have an immediate impact are needed, while simultaneously dealing with the long term nature of the problem.

Recognizing this need, several countries in Central America like Costa Rica, Guatemala, Panama and Honduras passed laws in the 1970s stipulating that all sugar for home consumption had to be fortified. However, a combination of political and administrative constraints prevented this goal from being realized even though the technical feasibility of the process had been well established. The programs have had several ups and downs. Since the early 1990s, programs have been renewed with full cooperation from the sugar industry. Recent impact studies among Guatemalan school children have shown a sharp reduction in vitamin A deficiency.

In India, it is mandatory for Vanaspati to be fortified with vitamin A. However the efficacy of this measure and its benefits reaching low-income groups is still in question, especially since it is diverting scarce vitamin A from Maternal & Child Health supplementation programmes. In the Philippines, vitamin A fortification of margarine is mandatory. Shelf stable margarine containing 375 RE vitamin A per 15 g serving has been in the market since 1993. Studies showed that within 6 months of consumption, there was a 6% decrease in low serum retinol. Monosodium glutamate (MSG), a widely consumed condiment of daily use in several southeast Asian countries has been seriously considered as a vehicle for vitamin A, but still faces problems of stability and advisability of using MSG whose long-term health effects are still unknown. In Tanzania, and more recently in India, tea is being considered as a possible vehicle for vitamin A.

SELECTION OF FOOD VEHICLES

Potential food vehicles could be visualized as a three-tiered pyramid (Figure 3). Staple foods such as sugar, cereals and, grains, fats and oils form the base; basic foods such as breads and biscuits, packaged cereals and flours, and dairy products are in the middle; and value-added foods such as condiments, snacks, candies, and convenience and ready-to-eat foods are at the top. Fortifying less expensive staple foods at the base of the pyramid results in broader dissemination of micronutrients throughout the population, particularly the poor. Also, since basic and value-added foods are processed from staple commodities, fortifying foods at the base of the pyramid results in fortifying products throughout the food chain.

There are important differences in food consumption patterns between urban and rural areas. The urban population is more likely to consume many of

FIGURE 3. Food product pyramid showing examples for different categories of foods.

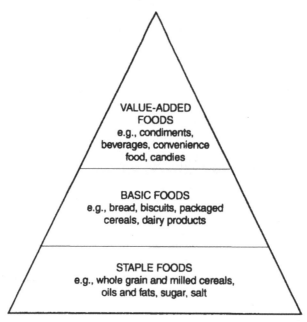

the potential fortified foods. They are more likely to consume rice and wheat products, tofu, dairy products, edible oils, and other condiments such as sugar, vinegar, sauces, and MSG. Moreover, it is highly likely that the products consumed in urban areas are centrally milled and processed, thus they are more readily fortifiable. It is clear that it will be harder to reach the rural population and most foods that can be fortified to reach the rural population will also reach the urban populations.

Infants and children under the age of 24 months consume a different dietary pattern than do older individuals. There are no major differences in consumption among children aged two years and older. Where there are few centrally processed complementary foods and consumption of such foods is infrequent and rare, careful research is needed on the best ways to address micronutrient problems of infants.

Condiments and cooking oils are best measured as total quantities consumed by each household, and then allocated among family members who consume foods that typically are the ones that contain these items. It also relates to the family size. Smaller families tend to be more likely to consume these oils and condiments, and this leads to some difference for individual statistics.

There are important differences in the dietary intake of different income groups, as we know from other research. For instance, wheat and rice consumption is less likely among lower income individuals. Consumption of dairy products, tofu products, canned vegetables and many condiments increase by income. One of the larger shifts is the increased likelihood that higher income families consume edible oils, soy sauce, MSG, and vinegar.

In a country where a universally consumed vehicle is not available, fortification of a number of foods offers several key strategic advantages. When a variety of food sectors are engaged, no single industry can resist on the grounds that it is being unfairly singled out. When multiple foods are fortified, each with less than the RDI per single serving, the possibility of consuming toxic levels of a micronutrient through excess consumption of a single food becomes more remote. For example, in Philippines, a variety of vehicles including margarine, flour, noodles, and sugar will offer protection from micronutrient deficiencies for specific consumer segments. When considering a multi-faceted approach, each food vehicle offers specific opportunities and constraints.

Staple Cereals

Inexpensive staples like rice corn and wheat flour reach the broadest population. However, these foods are often eaten where they are grown and processed at the community level. This limits opportunities to ensure quality and safety.

Cooking Media

Fats and oils may offer an option to meet a portion of the RDA. They are often centrally refined and packed.

Dairy Products

Milk may offer an option where centralized dairy processing exists. However, cost, distribution, and other factors may limit accessibility among vulnerable populations.

Condiments

Sugar, spices, starches, and sauces are attractive carriers. Some are processed centrally and consumed in regular quantities.

Value-Added Products

The most vulnerable populations may consume these higher priced products only sporadically. However, consumer awareness, technical breakthroughs, and marketing innovations often emerge from the development of fortified value-added products.

When no universally consumed vehicle is available in a country, the fortification of a number of foods offers several key strategic advantages. When a variety of food sectors are engaged, no single industry can resist on the grounds that it is being unfairly singled out. When a variety of foods are fortified, each with a lesser proportion of RDI, the theoretical possibility of consuming dangerous levels of a micronutrient through excess consumption of a single food becomes more remote.

FORTIFICATION OF COMPLEMENTARY FOODS

Child nutrition is an essential element in human development and is best improved in the context of coordinated investments in primary health care and early and basic education. Countries risk a "lost" generation unless they improve nutrition for children under age two, the stage of life when the body and brain experience maximum growth and development potential. The benefits of improving early childhood nutrition are multiple and tremendous. Synergistic benefits include:

- Nutrition impacts on health through immuno-competence and stronger resistance to life threatening infection.
- Health impacts on nutrition because reduced illness leads to weight and height gain.
- Nutrition and health improve psychosocial development and learning ability through better psychomotor skills and socialized vitality.
- Preschoolers who are well nourished are better socialized, less likely to drop out when they move to primary school, adjust better to the social and academic environment of school, and do better in the early grades.

Important as these findings are, the potential of the food industry to create nutritious foods for young infants has yet to be tapped and developed. For the food industry in the developing world, fortified complementary foods are at the cutting edge of product development and social marketing strategy for a huge untapped market. From the food technology perspective, the challenge is to increase both the energy density of complementary foods and levels of multiple vitamins and minerals at an affordable price. From the public health perspective, combination of proper regulation that protects infant health yet supports industrial innovation and strong public education on appropriate infant feeding practices and psychosocial care of the infant.

Industrially produced fortified complementary foods are recommended by pediatricians worldwide as an essential part of a nutritionally adequate infant diet and as a complement to breast milk and home-prepared foods. This combination is essential in order to meet the micronutrient requirements of infants, especially for iron and zinc. Beyond the superior micronutrient content of industrially fortified complementary foods over home-prepared rice porridge and other traditional infant foods, they have also the advantages of delivering higher bioavailability of micronutrients, higher energy density, and protein quality, not to mention the safety and convenience.

BUILDING A PUBLIC PRIVATE PARTNERSHIP

Food fortification calls for a multi-sectoral partnership between industry, national governments, international agencies, expert groups, and other players, to work closely on specific issues relating to technology development, food processing and marketing, free-market approaches with minimum price support mechanisms, standards, quality assurance, product certification, social communications, demand creation, monitoring, and evaluation. This coalition will benefit private sector partners, not just as a lever to improve performance in the marketplace, but also to show that the private sector has social as well as economic interests. It will benefit the government, which has a mandate to improve people's lives. And it will allow national and international development agencies to provide the technical support and seed money in an efficient, economic way.

Key areas where there is need for a clear understanding between the sectors include:

- Agreement on the common goal of eradication of micronutrient malnutrition via food fortification.
- What each partner is bringing to the table? What are their roles?
- Understanding each partners need? How they will be met?
- Establishing criteria/standards for partnership.
- Establishing a model and testing it in one or two countries.

SUPPORT MEASURES

To date, much of the focus in micronutrient fortification has been in the development and evaluation of fortified products. Needless to say, the success of any fortification program only occurs when the fortified product becomes available and, subsequently, consumed by the target groups.

Finally, the production of the fortified product has to be scaled up, packaged and distributed through normal trade channels and public institutions. This step, which is the production and distribution of the fortified product, is the least recognized bottleneck in the implementation of a fortification program. Here, industry plays a critical role in the production and distribution of these products. The private sector has the experience and the know-how to produce, distribute, and market the fortified product. It is the private sector that can make the fortification program sustainable.

Hence, the role that can be played by governments in the developing countries, international agencies, and non-government organizations is to make the environment conducive for to the private sector to produce and market fortified products.

This can be accomplished through:

- Communicating to the private sector that micronutrient malnutrition is an unmet consumer need;
- Establishing pragmatic fortification standards and regulations to foster level playing field and protect the consumer who purchases and consumes the product; and
- Increasing demand for the fortified product by raising profession and public awareness on the prevalence and consequences of micronutrient deficiencies and the benefits and values of fortified foods.

COST OF FORTIFICATION PROGRAMS AND FINANCING

Table 4 shows the vitamin and iron forms most commonly used for fortification and the corresponding annual cost per capita when supplementing the diet with 100% of the RDA (USRDA 1989). The costs indicated are only ap-

TABLE 4. Enrichment Cost of Foods.

VITAMIN	COMMERCIAL FORM	RDA	STANDARD OVERDOSES	FORTIFICATION/COST US$/PERSON/YEAR FOR 100% RDA
A	A Palm.250 CWS	1000 mcg RE	30	0.253
D	D3 100 CWS	400 UI	30	0.051
E	E Acet.50% CWS	10 mgTE	10	0.285
B_1	B_1 Mono	1.5 mg	30	0.032
B_2	B_2 USP	1.7 mg	20	0.053
B_6	B_6 HCl	2 mg	30	0.064
C	C	60 mg	50	0.558
Niacin	Nicotinamide	19 mg	10	0.067
Folate	Folic Acid	200 mcg	30	0.016
B_{12}	B_{12} 0.1% WS	3 mcg	30	0.053
Iron	Ferrous Sulphate	15 mg	-	0.040
TOTAL				1.470

proximate and indicate order of magnitude figures for actual processing and chemical cost at source only. They exclude program management, product promotion/marketing, and monitoring costs. In most cases, this additional cost works out to be between 5% to 10% of the micronutrient cost. Table 5 shows the impact of fortification of some commonly used foods on vitamin A intake using cost and consumption figures in Brazil. Table 6 shows the cost of fortification based on recent country experiences.

Often, the extra cost at source when passed on to the consumer, tends to get magnified at the various stages of distribution because the margins at every level will also increase proportionately. Therefore, the ultimate cost to the consumer will be progressively inflated as the food passes from producer to retailer. This cost increase is an economic question, which may need investigation on a case-to-case basis.

RECOMMENDATIONS FOR DEVELOPING A FOOD FORTIFICATION STRATEGY

Food fortification is an important component of the overall strategy to eliminate micronutrient malnutrition. A country's investment in an efficient program for food fortification can be very cost-effective. In addition, the food industry and trade can develop systems to derive economic and social benefits for themselves while simultaneously providing a social benefit to the community by fortifying the foods they produce and sell. However, for food fortification to be effective and well coordinated several issues need to be addressed.

- Food fortification is a unique example where industry and trade (who normally work in a largely commercial environment) are required to participate and play a leading role in a health intervention endeavor. In order to have an effective and sustainable fortification program, it is vital that the public and private sectors work in close collaboration, explicitly understanding and recognizing each other's viewpoints, concerns, and interests.
- The fortification strategy should be linked with other intervention strategies like supplementation, dietary approaches, and nutrition education
- An exercise in solviong a detailed technical problem should be carried out to confirm that the fortification process is feasible and does not alter the vehicle in any way and nutrient losses on storage and cooking are within tolerable limits. Industry could be involved in technology development, production, and quality control. Multinational companies with R&D facilities could be a source of technical expertise.

- Technology development will have to be followed up with field and pilot commercial trials to evaluate the techno-economic feasibility and consumer acceptability of the product.
- Food fortification programs should be planned to dovetail into existing food production and distribution systems within the country or region with minimum disruption and cost.
- Food quality should be monitored through regulation and effectively enforced.
- The importance of social communication cannot be over-stressed. All available media should be used to educate the population on the problems of micronutrient deficiencies and on the importance and safety of fortified foods. Consumers should be educated to demand a better product and accept a slightly higher price for that product.
- Whatever the external input, nothing can succeed without an adequate nucleus of well-trained nationals. Specialized training is especially called for in the assessment, fortification, quality control, and monitoring and evaluation procedures.
- As programs get under way, effective monitoring of process and outcome variables is critical. Measurement of food quality and fortificant levels in the foods at different levels from production to consumption is an essential step to ensure that adequate quantities of the nutrient are reaching the population. This must be combined with periodic estimation of clinical and biochemical indicators to evaluate the impact of the intervention. Programs should be envisioned as long lasting with evaluation as an essential component to identify progress, problems and needs.
- Inter-sectoral and international mechanisms of cooperation and coordination should be established for control of the distribution and marketing of fortified food products.

TABLE 5. Impact of Typical Vitamin A Fortification Levels on the Selling Price for Some Selected Foods.*

	IU/KG	% SELLING PRICE	PER CAPITA CONSUMPTION G/Day	NUTRITIONAL IMPACT IU/PERSON/DAY
LIQUID MILK	5000	0.16	74	500
MARGARINE	30000	0.10	5	150
WHEAT	10000	0.52	99	990
SUGAR	20000	0.55	31	3900

*Processing cost and customs duties are not included.

TABLE 6. Examples of Dosage and Cost of Food Fortification.

VEHICLE	FORTIFICANT	DOSAGE	COST (RANGE PER CAPITA/YEAR) (U.S.CENTS)	COUNTRY
Salt	Potassium iodate	50-80 PPM I_2	2-6 (1999)	Several
Salt	Ferrous sulphate Sodium hexametaphosphate Potassium iodate	1000 PPM FE 1000 PPM 50 PPM	12-18 (1994)	India
Sugar	Vitamin A	15 G/G	37 (1999)	Guatemala, Honduras, El Salvador
Corn flour/ Wheat flour	Iron, vitamin A, niacin, thiamine, riboflavin	20-50 MG/100 G	12 (2000)	Venezuela
Cookies	Haemoglobin	1.8 G HB/30	108 (1981)	Chile
Cooking fat	Vitamin A	50 IU/G	30-40 (1998)	India
Edible oils	Vitamin A	20 IU/G	N.A.	Pakistan
Margarine	Vitamin A	375 RE/15G	20 (1997)	Philippines
Breakfast meal	Multivitamins	-	175 (1998)	Peru

The control of micronutrient deficiencies is a realizable goal notwithstanding the magnitude of the task and the manny challenges and constraints that remain to be resolved. Food fortification could be an important strategy to help realize this goal. Effective fortification would require active collaboration between several sectors: scientific community, government, private industry, consumer groups, and international agencies.

The scientific community has identified the problems of micronutrient malnutrition and the possible solutions through enrichment of a variety of foods. During the past decade, considerable expertise has also been built up in the development of programs with in-built support measures like advocacy and social communication, legislation and enforcement, monitoring and evaluation, and training.

National governments must provide the administrative support and prescribe the framework within which the solutions can be implemented and regulated

The food industry has the technology, the capacity to mobilize resources, and the marketing capability to translate these needs into economically viable products that will be affordable and nutritious.

The consumer needs to be educated regarding the benefits and low cost of food fortification in order to create a 'demand pull' to which industry would have to respond.

International and bilateral aid agencies could provide initial advocacy and seed technical/funding support for development of strategies and interventions.

CONCLUSION

The control of micronutrient deficiencies is a realizable goal notwithstanding the magnitude of the task and many challenges and constraints that remain to be resolved. Food fortification could be an important strategy to help realize this goal. Effective fortification would require active collaboration between several sectors: the scientific community, the government, private industry, consumer groups, and international agencies.

REFERENCES

Arroyave, G. 1979. *Evaluation of sugar fortification with vitamin A at the national level.* Pan American Health Organization, Scientific Publication No. 384, Washington, DC, USA.

Bauernfeind, J.C., and P.A. Lachance, eds. 1991. *Nutrient additions to foods, nutritional, technological and regulatory aspects.* Food and Nutrition Press, Inc. Trumbull.

Codex Alimentarius. 1984. *Codex Alimentarius Volume 4, CAC/GL09-1987.* Food and Agriculture Organization.

Lofti, M., M.G. Venkatesh Mannar, R.J.H.M. Merx, and P. Naber-van den Heuvel. 1995. *Micronutrient fortification of foods: Current practices, research and opportunities.* Micronutrient Initiative and the International Agricultural Centre, Ottawa, 190 p.

MI (Micronutrient Initiative). 1995a. *Food fortification in Canada: Experiences and issues.* MI, Ottawa, 50 p.

MI (Micronutrient Initiative). 1995b. *Vitamin A deficiency: key resources in its prevention and control.* MI, Ottawa, 47 p.

National Research Council. 1989. *National Research Council–Subcommittee on the tenth edition of the Recommended Dietary Allowances,* National Academy Press, Washington, DC.

Popkin, B.M., A.M. Siega-Riz, and P.S. Haines. 1995. *The nutritional impact of fortification in the United States during the 1970's.* Department of Nutrition, University of North Carolina at Chapel Hill, Chapel Hill, NC 27514.

Venkatesh Mannar, M.G. 1987. Control of iodine deficiency disorders by iodination of salt: Strategy for developing countries. In B.S. Hetzel, J.T. Dunn, and J.B. Stanbury, eds. *The prevention and control of iodine deficiency disorders.* New York: Elsevier.

Venkatesh Mannar, M.G. 1987. *Complementarities: Fortification.* Paper presented at the United Nations ACC/SCN Micronutrient Forum, WHO, Geneva, February 15-16.

World Bank. 1994. *Enriching lives: Overcoming vitamin and mineral malnutrition in developing countries.* The World Bank, Washington, DC.

Designing Nutrition Interventions with Food Systems: Planning, Communication, Monitoring and Evaluation

S. C. Babu
V. Rhoe

SUMMARY. Household food security and nutrition are top priorities in many developing countries. In order to increase food and nutrition security, alternative policies and programs aimed at improving nutrition need to be formulated, implemented, and evaluated. There are three sets of strategies necessary for the successful implementation of a food and nutrition intervention program: planning strategy, communication strategy, and monitoring and evaluation strategy. In the process of explaining these three strategies, a conceptual framework for designing food and nutrition interventions using food systems approaches is developed as well as a model that illustrates the process is given along with specific activities, coordinating units, and personnel responsibilities. Finally, challenges and constraints facing developing countries are also discussed. *[Article copies available for a fee from The Haworth Document Delivery Service: 1-800-HAWORTH. E-mail address: <getinfo@haworthpressinc. com> Website: <http://www.HaworthPress.com> © 2002 by The Haworth Press, Inc. All rights reserved.]*

S. C. Babu is Senior Research Fellow and Senior Training Advisor, and V. Rhoe is Senior Research Assistant, IFPRI, 2033 K Street, N.W., Washington, DC 20006 (E-mail: s.babu@cgiar.org or v.rhoe@cgiar.org).

[Haworth co-indexing entry note]: "Designing Nutrition Interventions with Food Systems: Planning, Communication, Monitoring and Evaluation." Babu, S. C., and V. Rhoe. Co-published simultaneously in *Journal of Crop Production* (Food Products Press, an imprint of The Haworth Press, Inc.) Vol. 6, No. 1/2 (#11/12), 2002, pp. 365-373; and: *Food Systems for Improved Human Nutrition: Linking Agriculture, Nutrition, and Productivity* (ed: Palit K. Kataki. and Suresh Chandra Babu) Food Products Press, an imprint of The Haworth Press, Inc., 2002, pp. 365-373. Single or multiple copies of this article are available for a fee from The Haworth Document Delivery Service [1-800-HAWORTH, 9:00 a.m. - 5:00 p.m. (EST). E-mail address: getinfo@haworthpressinc.com].

KEYWORDS. Communications, food security, nutrition, planning

INTRODUCTION

Household food security and nutrition are top priorities in many developing countries. Low adoption rates of improved technologies, inadequate rainfall, and soil degradation have resulted in decreased food availability, and therefore, food and nutrition insecurity. In order to increase food and nutrition security, alternative policies and programs aimed at improving nutrition need to be formulated, implemented, and evaluated. Three sets of strategies are necessary for successful implementation of food and nutrition interventions: planning, communication, and monitoring, surveillance and evaluation strategy. This article first discusses the three processes of the planning strategy, followed by the communication, and monitoring and evaluation strategy. The concluding section stresses the challenges that developing countries face in implementing these three strategies when establishing food and nutrition intervention programs.

PLANNING STRATEGY

The planning strategy requires three basic steps: first, a situation analysis of the food and nutrition problems needs to be undertaken; second, past attempts to correct the existing problems need to be reviewed; and third, the costs and benefits of a new food systems intervention program should be explained. The situation analysis involves assessing the extent of the micronutrient malnourishment problem, analyzing the causes of this problem, and reviewing available resources. To assist in answering these three questions, the researcher should seek out the assistance of relevant local experts in the health, agriculture, food industry, and education sector. Gaining assistance from these local experts will help in the better understanding of the existing problem. Finally, the suggested food and nutrition intervention program needs to be directly linked to the existing national policy or the national policy needs to encourage the program in order to provide incentives to adopt it.

COMMUNICATION STRATEGY

Methods of food-related nutrition interventions in rural areas can be classified into six major groups, namely, food subsidies, growing of commercial crops, development of home gardens, supplementary feeding, food rations, and cropping systems changes (Kennedy and Pinstrup-Andersen, 1983). The components of the food systems approach are described in this volume, each of which include a system of collecting, documenting, and using existing information for incorporation into each of the above methods.

This section describes a conceptual framework and an organizational procedure for designing food and nutrition interventions using food systems approach. This framework is intended to provide guidelines to institutions involved in food and nutrition-related activities, such as ministries of agriculture and health as well as other non-government agencies in developing countries. It will assist them in developing a system of designing nutritional interventions using food systems approach. The conceptual framework, adopted from Babu and Mthindi (1994), for relating food security of rural households and food systems approach in nutrition and health is given in Figure 1. The availability of land and labor along with the improved technology and the use of modern inputs such as hybrid seeds and chemical fertilizers determine the food systems strategy that is adopted: crop diversification, new technology, commercial production of nutritive crops, post-harvest storage, home gardening, and animal production. The availability of markets for crops produced, the level of prices for outputs, and the ratio between self-consumption and market-oriented production determine the income from crop production through the food systems approach of these households. The non-farm income is determined by the nature and availability of employment and wages in the rural areas.

Household food security, while largely dependent on household income, is also determined by the food acquisition behavior of households. Furthermore, increased food availability and income of households do not automatically guarantee improved nutritional and health status. For example, due to the prevailing cropping and food consumption patterns, some essential vitamins may not enter the food system. This cropping or consumption pattern may result in nutritional deficiency in one or more nutrients among a group of households in a region or sub-regions of a country. It is in this stage that the identification and utilization of food systems approach will be beneficial to supplement essential nutrients and contribute to better health.

A model of the process of utilizing food systems approach in rural nutrition intervention programs with specific activities and the coordinating units and personnel responsible is shown in Figure 2. This framework is necessary to identify various steps and players involved in the process of implementing interventions. This framework is also necessary to develop consensus among those involved and to ensure their commitment for follow-up activities.

Problem Identification

In general, specific nutritional problems are identified through two major sources of information in developing countries. The most common are the na-

FIGURE 1. Conceptual framework relating to rural household food security through food systems approach to health and nutrition (adopted from Babu and Mthindi, 1994).

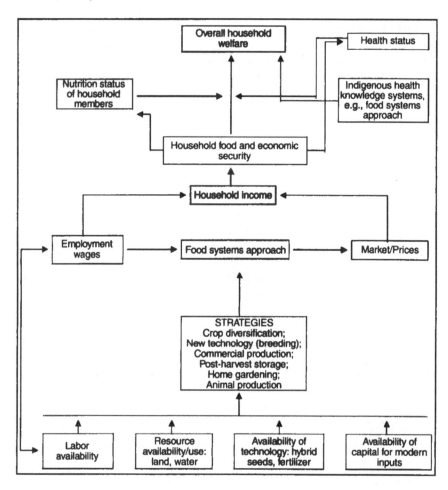

tional nutrition surveys, which identify various nutritional problems in different parts of the country. Ad hoc nutritional surveys can also be conducted based on reports from local hospitals so that the nature and the extent of the problem can be quantified. The Ministry of Agriculture or the Ministry of Health with the support of national statistical organizations usually carries out these types of surveys. In the case of deficiency disorders, once the problem is identified in a particular area, it has to be traced for deficiencies of one or more

FIGURE 2. A model of the process of utilizing food systems approach in rural nutrition intervention.

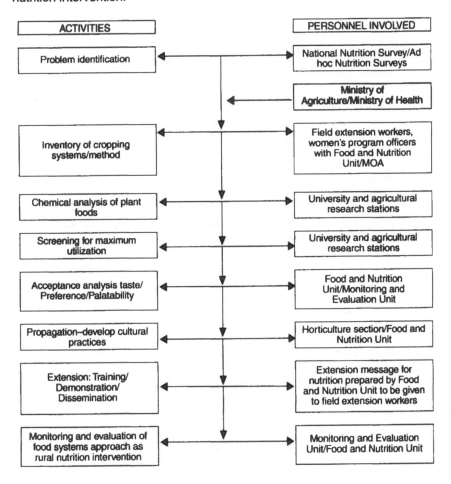

nutrients. One of the sectoral ministries such as Ministry of Agriculture or the Ministry of Health take the lead and alerts other sectoral ministries and organizations to identify solutions to the problem. This process is made easier in countries where a multi-sectoral nutrition committee, chaired by a President or Prime Minister's office, takes the lead role (Quinn, 1994). In what follows are the stages and activities for implementing rural nutrition interventions.

Making an Inventory

Having identified the problem and evaluated potential existing alternatives for intervention, there is a need to take an inventory of the food systems approaches used by households in different parts of the country. This survey would allow the planners to choose a cost-effective and the most acceptable food systems approach for further development and dissemination. In places where such information is not readily available, the existing agricultural extension system can be used for information gathering. The village level extension worker would be useful in developing the inventory by working with rural households that are familiar with the food systems approaches used in a particular area. In addition, the timing of making the inventory is also important.

Analysis and Screening

Once this inventory is prepared, the next step is to carry out a chemical analysis of the foods grown through the food systems approach for essential nutrients and vitamins. This analysis can be carried out in the laboratories of the universities and agricultural research stations. The chemical analysis of the food will help food technologists, nutritionists, and other agricultural scientists choose food that will have the maximum nutrient content.

Acceptance Analysis

The importance of taste in food acceptance has recently been recognized to play a crucial role in determining the success of food and nutrition intervention programs (Babu and Rajasekaran, 1991). It is well known that the quality of food taken is the major factor determining its nutritional impact (Kennedy and Alderman, 1987). Variations exist in the quality of food intake among subgroups of the population (Horton, 1985). It has also been suggested that increasing incomes could be a direct way of improving nutrition as the quality and variety of foods increases with income (Pitt, 1985). These considerations point to the need for assessing the acceptance of foods grown through various food systems approaches. An acceptance analysis should be conducted in order to determine the impact of tastes and preferences on the dietary intake pattern of different groups of households. Information based on the analysis could then be effectively used in targeting households for nutritional interventions using these foods and improving the success of the acceptance of these recently introduced foods.

Developing Cropping Practices

A common problem in the introduction of new plant foods into a community besides the issue of acceptance is the timely availability of propagation materials. The cultivation of annual varieties reduces the time between the planting and harvesting. Ensuring the local availability of planting materials is important in the case of annual varieties. This availability will enable better adoption of the newly introduced crops. Equally important is developing cropping practices for the new crops.

Extension and Training

Most of the efforts of the agricultural extension systems in developing countries are focused on increasing food production. Therefore, most of the technical messages delivered by extension agents are production-oriented. Given that traditional crops are grown year after year with the same agronomic practices, there are few new messages to be disseminated to the farmers. In the off-season, extension agents are relatively free to undertake additional activities such as nutrition education. One way of engaging extension workers in development-related activities is by utilizing and delivering messages on different food systems approaches. Feedback information from the field can also be sent to research units through the same channel. It is also important to document and disseminate the information on the success of food systems approaches in nutrition interventions.

MONITORING AND EVALUATION STRATEGY

The introduction of a food systems approach could be tried out as a pilot project in a small area to determine its success. Food systems approaches introduced should be monitored and evaluated for improvements of the nutritional status of the population in relation to particular nutritional problems for which they are recommended. The evaluation of the food systems approach as a method of rural nutritional intervention may provide useful insights and lessons. The evaluation studies should be carried out by the evaluation sections of the local agricultural divisions with the help of subject matter specialists for food and nutrition. Although capacity for such activities are severely lacking in many countries, one such evaluation is available for consultation (Babu and Chale, 1994). The results of the evaluations should be used in modifying and redesigning intervention programs. They are also useful in identifying operational, administrative, and technical problems in implementation. Thus, the cyclical process of identifying new food systems approaches and their evaluation for their effectiveness in improving nutritional status should be an integral part of on-going work of institutions involved in rural nutrition activities (Babu and Pinstrup-Andersen, 1994).

In order to scale-up nutrition intervention program, monitoring system must be established within the sectoral ministry that is implementing the intervention program. The information collected from the monitoring system should be processed into data that is useful for analysis of the progress made by the intervention. Both the process and outcome indicators should be monitored. Based on the analysis of the data, information should be generated that will be useful in redesigning intervention programs. An important element of the monitoring and evaluation activity, however, is the capacity for undertaking these activities. Emphasis should be given in strengthening this capacity at all levels (Babu and Chapasuka, 1997).

CONCLUDING REMARKS

Designing food and nutrition interventions through food systems approach requires careful planning and design of interventions. Ideally, the intervention should be implemented on a pilot scale and be evaluated for its benefits. Based on the lessons learned from the evaluation, it may be expanded to a large-scale project. A major challenge in developing countries is the capacity for designing, implementing, monitoring and evaluation of food and nutrition interventions. Institutional capacity for organizing large-scale interventions is also severely lacking. While it is important to build and strengthen such capacity, the design of intervention programs through food systems approach should be cognizant of the nature and extent of the existing capacity to absorb, assimilate, and adopt new strategies to address locality specific food and nutrition problems. The role of multidisciplinary approach where nutritionists, agriculturists, social scientists, and policymakers can work together can hardly be overemphasized.

REFERENCES

Babu, S.C., B. Rajasekaran. 1991. Biotechnology for rural nutrition: An economic evaluation of algal protein supplements in south India. *Food Policy.* 16: 405-414.

Babu, S.C., G.B. Mthindi. 1994. Household food security and nutrition monitoring: The Malawi approach to development planning and policy interventions. *Food Policy.* 19(3): 272-284.

Babu, S.C., B. Chale. 1994. *Indigenous Vegetables for Rural Nutrition: An Evaluation of Moringa in Salima.* BUNDA/IFPRI Working Paper No. 6. Bunda College of Agriculture, Lilongwe, Malawi.

Babu, S.C., P. Pinstrup-Andersen. 1994. Food security and nutrition monitoring–a conceptual framework, issues and challenges. *Food Policy.* 19 (3): 218-233.

Babu, S.C., E. Chapasura. 1997. Mitigating the effects of drought through food security and nutrition monitoring: lessons from Malawi. *Food and Nutrition Bulletin.* 18(1):71-83.

Horton, S. 1985. The determinants of nutrient intake–results from western India. *Journal of Development Economics.* 19:147-162.

Kennedy E.T., H. Alderman. 1987. *Comparative analysis of nutritional effectiveness of food subsides and other food related interventions.* Occasional Paper No. 7. International Food Policy Research Institute, Washington, DC.

Kennedy, E.T., P. Pinstrup-Andersen. 1983. *Nutrition-related policies and programs: Past performances and research needs.* International Food Policy Research Institute, Washington, DC.

Pitt, M.N. 1985. Food preference and nutrition in rural Bangladesh. *Review of Economic Statistic.* 67: 726-732.

Quinn, V. 1994. A history of the politics of food and nutrition in Malawi–the context of food and nutrition al surveillance. *Food Policy.* 19(3): 255-271.

Food Systems Approach
for Sustainable Nutrition Security:
A Synthesis and Way Forward

S. C. Babu

P. K. Kataki

SUMMARY. The problem of malnutrition in developing countries continues to be disquieting. Increasing the population's nutritional level through well-designed food and nutrition strategies and programs will contribute to the enhancement of human capital. Enhanced human capital is fundamental for increasing the productivity of society, which ignites economic growth. The articles of this volume form the components of, and addresses specific sets of food and nutrition interventions that are known as the food systems approach. In this chapter, an attempt is being made to synthesize the findings from these chapters in order to assist in operationalizing and mobilizing action towards implementing these strategies. *[Article copies available for a fee from The Haworth Document Delivery Service: 1-800-HAWORTH. E-mail address: <getinfo@haworthpressinc. com> Website: <http://www.HaworthPress.com> © 2002 by The Haworth Press, Inc. All rights reserved.]*

KEYWORDS. Agroforestry, animal production, cropping system, fish, food system, iodine, iron, nutrition, vitamin A

S. C. Babu is Senior Research Fellow and Senior Training Advisor, IFPRI, 2033 K Street, N.W., Washington, DC 20006 USA (E-mail: s.babu@cgiar.org).

P. K. Kataki is currently at the Department of Plant Agiculture, Crop Science Building, University of Guelph, Guelph, Ontario, Canada N1G 2W1 (E-mail: pkataki@uoguelph.ca).

[Haworth co-indexing entry note]: "Food Systems Approach for Sustainable Nutrition Security: A Synthesis and Way Forward." Babu, S. C., and P. K. Kataki. Co-published simultaneously in *Journal of Crop Production* (Food Products Press, an imprint of The Haworth Press, Inc.) Vol. 6, No. 1/2 (#11/12), 2002, pp. 375-381; and: *Food Systems for Improved Human Nutrition: Linking Agriculture, Nutrition, and Productivity* (ed: Palit K. Kataki, and Suresh Chandra Babu) Food Products Press, an imprint of The Haworth Press, Inc., 2002, pp. 375-381. Single or multiple copies of this article are available for a fee from The Haworth Document Delivery Service [1-800-HAWORTH, 9:00 a.m. - 5:00 p.m. (EST). E-mail address: getinfo@haworthpressinc.com].

WHY FOOD SYSTEMS APPROACH?

Any food systems approach will involve designing and implementing strategies for increasing the availability, accessibility, and utilization of macro- and micronutrients through increased food production, increased availability of nutrients in the food that is produced, and designing appropriate communications strategy that enhances the utilization of the foods produced.

Within the last three decades, cereal grain production has increased in several countries, directly and indirectly at the expense of crop and dietary diversification, respectively. The rate of malnutrition decline in humans has, therefore, been slow in recent years. Development of strategic linkages between agriculture and nutrition to combat both micro- and macronutrient deficiency related malnutrition is imperative. The food systems approach has evolved due to the partial successes and unsustainable nature of the supplementation and food fortification programs in developing countries. It includes programs and strategies that focus on increasing diversification of crops through changes in the farming systems; breeding staple food grains for increased micronutrient contents; producing and distributing vegetables, fruits, milk, fish, and other animal products; improving food processing methods and post-harvest storage processes; and providing appropriate planning, nutrition education, and monitoring and evaluation of these programs and strategies. Past strategies towards combating malnutrition have been mutually exclusive, and they have had limited successes. Food systems approach seeks to develop strategies that are specific to a region and have a long-term, sustainable impact in reducing malnutrition.

FOOD-BASED STRATEGIES

The potential of food-based strategies to reduce micronutrient malnutrition has been recently recognized (Ruel and Levin, 2001 in this volume). Food-based interventions aim at (1) increasing the production, availability, and access to vitamin A and iron-rich foods through the promotion of home production; (2) increasing the intake of vitamin A and iron-rich foods through nutrition education, communication, social marketing, and behavior change programs to improve dietary quality among vulnerable groups; and (3) increasing the bioavailability of vitamin A and iron in the diet either through home preservation or processing techniques.

Home gardening combined with promotional and education interventions have high potential to reduce vitamin A deficiency; however, very few studies have studied the impact of home gardens on household income, intra-household allocation, and micronutrient status.

Reducing iron deficiency through home gardens has been less popular, and hence, studies on this topic have been limited. Nevertheless, it is generally agreed that the bio-availability of iron from plant foods continue to be a challenge and it is not clear whether increased animal production at the household level results in improved iron intake due to the trade-off between income generation and consumption of animal products. Therefore, further nutrition education is needed to translate the local production into nutritional intake.

Clearly, food-based technologies and strategies have the potential to address many of the concerns about the intake and bioavailability of vitamin A and iron among impoverished populations. However, critical information gaps still exist in relation to both its efficacy and its effectiveness. Home processing technologies such as cooking, preservation techniques, home processing techniques, and food-to-food fortification have the potential to address some of the concerns about the bioavailability of vitamin A and iron. Yet, further expansion of these traditional and non-traditional technologies has been thwarted by a limited effort to promote, implement, and evaluate such technologies in community trials.

Implementation of food-based approaches by integrating production, nutrition education, and behavior change strategies has shown significant progress in the last 10 years, but evaluation of their efficacy, effectiveness, feasibility, sustainability, and impact on the diets and nutritional status of at-risk populations remains limited. While food based approaches could be an essential part of the long-term global strategy to alleviate vitamin A and iron deficiencies, their real potential has to be explored through appropriate planning, monitoring, and evaluation.

SHIFTING CROPPING PATTERNS

In much of South Asia, the introduction of green revolution technology along with irrigation in the 1960s and 1970s resulted in multiple cropping systems of cereal crops. While this approach helped to meet the calorie needs of the growing population, the micronutrient malnutrition among the vulnerable groups remains very high. This high level of micronutrient malnutrition is partly due to the reduced availability and accessibility of pulses, fruits, vegetables, meat, and fish, which are necessary for increasing the intake of micronutrients. For example, while the real prices of cereals have declined over the past 30 years in Bangladesh, the real prices of pulses, fruits, vegetables, meat, and fish have increased (Bouis, 2001). A recent study has shown that dietary diversity is a good indicator of the food and nutrition security (Hoddinot and Yohannes, 2001). A long-term sustainable approach to enhance diversity of diets is to increase the production of diverse foods. This diversity will require another shift in the cropping pattern from cereal based multi-crop systems to cropping systems that incorporate pulses and vegetables in between the cereal crops. Therefore, this approach will require policies that encourage crop diversification and should be further supported by institutions that produce and supply quality seeds and other inputs. Agricultural policies of developing countries should explicitly recognize the crop diversification strategy to encourage farmers to produce crops that will increase the availability and accessibility of micronutrients.

VEGETABLE PRODUCTION

Nutritional and economic benefits of fruits and vegetable production could be substantial, however, the per capita vegetable consumption in many developing countries remains far below the required level to meet the micronutrient needs. In addition to contributing directly to the increased availability at lower prices, production of vegetables can increase the income and enhance the efficiency of resources used in a farming system. Vegetable production could also form an important part of the crop diversification strategy to meet the increasing demand due to urbanization. Appropriate credit and marketing policies with investment in infrastructure for storing and distribution of vegetables are essential for promoting vegetable production and consumption. Furthermore, investment in research for addressing biotic and abiotic constraints is necessary to mitigate the risk inherent in vegetable production.

AGROFORESTRY FOR RURAL NUTRITION

Designing appropriate agroforestry systems that incorporate trees, animals, and annual crops to meet the nutritional requirements of people is seen as an effective food systems approach. Agroforestry systems increase nutrient availability for human consumption directly through the supply of fruits, vegetables, and other foods, and indirectly through the provision of feed to livestock and green manures for annual crops. While the full potential of agroforestry for human nutrition is yet to be exploited, a better understanding is needed on the trade off between resources used for tree and annual crops and in its cost effectiveness of supplying nutrients through tree-crop farming systems as compared to annual cereal-vegetable cropping systems. Research is also needed in evaluating the introduction of tree components for its nutritional benefits.

IMPROVING NUTRITIONAL QUALITY OF STAPLE CROPS

One way to address the nutritional quality of a diet where cereal staple crops such as rice and maize are eaten with minimal or no diversity of food is to improve the nutrient content of the cereal crops. Efforts to increase the protein quality of maize over the past forty years show that it is possible to increase the nutritional values of crops through appropriate breeding strategies, and thereby, benefit a large population in a rapid and effective manner without changing their traditional food habits. Recent efforts to fortify rice with micronutrients such as iron, zinc, and vitamin A through breeding indicate two major advantages of this approach compared with standard micronutrient supplementation and fortification through food processing.

First, the investment in the plant breeding approach to fortify cereal crops is made only once with minimal annual cost whereas with micronutrient supplementation and fortification through processing, the costs repeat year after year. Second, the cost of micronutrient supplementation programs must be borne by every developing country and the benefits are limited to the geographical location in which the program is implemented whereas with fortification through plant breeding the benefits can spread all over the world through transfers of technology. Given that the fortification of cereal crops through breeding can be accomplished without reducing the yield potential of these crops, adoption of field-fortified varieties will have added advantage over the varieties with less micronutrient content. However, plant-breeding strategies are at an early stage and information on their potential efficacy and effectiveness is not available. Research is needed to evaluate the bio-absorption and nutritional status of the population adopting this technology. Concerted efforts to extend the technology to small-scale farmers through appropriate seed multiplication and delivery systems will be needed to harness the full benefits of this approach.

FISH AND ANIMAL PRODUCTION FOR NUTRITION

Any food systems strategy should be adapted to maximize the resources of the region it is being intended for. A good example is the Bangladesh case. Vitamin A deficiency has been a major health-related problem in Bangladesh and the country has made substantial progress in the reduction of this problem (article by Schaetzel and Shankar in this publication), largely through distribution of vitamin A capsules. The progress made has been commendable, however, the recurring costs of supplementation of vitamin A capsules requires that Bangladesh continue to get financial support from foreign sources to meet the program costs.

After rice and vegetables, consumption of fish is the third highest component of a Bangladeshi meal making up 53% of the animal food intake (chapter by Thompson et al. in this publication). The micronutrient content of fish, including that of vitamin A in some of the commonly preferred fish species for consumption in Bangladesh is very high. However, physical changes brought about by the drive to bring more land under rice cultivation have adversely affected fish production. The potential and efforts for increasing fish production for the livelihoods and nutrition in the plains of Bangladesh should, therefore, continue through organized programs.

Similarly, Ahmed, Ehui, and Saleem in this publication, have discussed the potential role of animals for improving nutritional and economic status of households in Ethiopia. Even for a largely vegetarian population of Northwestern India, increased milk production, often referred to as the "White Revolution" and forming of co-operatives, have increased the consumption of milk and milk products and nutritional status of people in this region.

THE WAY FORWARD

Based on past experiences in designing nutrition interventions, it is clear that there is no magic bullet to solve malnutrition problems and that a single-disciplinary approach may not be enough. There is a need for professionals from various fields such as nutritionists, agronomists, plant breeders, biologists, social scientists, and planners to come together to design and implement nutrition interventions. Planners and policymakers need to address several challenges and constraints in order to translate a potential solution into improved nutrition. For example, the practical challenges of adoptive research that take into account local culture, food habits, living conditions, and resource constraints remain.

Monitoring and evaluating the program's benefits and risks is essential for learning from the intervention. Furthermore, the scaling up of a potential intervention requires appropriate institutions for planning, implementation, and redesigning the intervention based on lessons learned through the monitoring and evaluation process. Adequate capacity to undertake all of the above activities remains a major challenge in developing countries.

In implementing a food systems approach for improving human nutrition, several issues needs to be addressed in the future:

- Agricultural technologies developed should have a nutritional objective and other desired characteristics. Changes in cropping systems and introduction of new crops in the existing cropping patterns should include the final objective of increasing nutrition availability at the local level.
- It is not enough to develop the technologies that will increase the intake of micronutrients; therefore, nutrition education and communication is essential both at the public level and at the individual level.
- Breeding for increased micronutrient density of staple and non-staple crops should consider consumer acceptance. Further institutional sup-

port at the international level to organize information sharing on the nutritional characteristics of different crop varieties is required.

- Further studies are needed to understand the impact of various food-based strategies on the nutritional status of the targeted population. In addition to the short-term impact of various nutritional interventions, long-term sustainability issues need to be considered in cost-effectiveness studies.
- In order to promote the food systems approach, a multidisciplinary collaborative research team needs to be developed and strengthened at the country level. Furthermore, nutritionists and their work should be linked to the policymaking systems of the country. This linkage will help place nutrition at the top of the planning agenda.

CONCLUSION

Improving the quality of one's diet by increasing the availability, accessibility, and utilization of foods is important for reducing malnutrition in developing countries. The food systems approaches proposed in this volume provide strategies for meeting this objective. It attempts to bring together a multidisciplinary group of professionals to address the problem of malnutrition in a holistic way. We sincerely hope the review and results presented in this volume is useful for the planners, policymakers, and students of food, agriculture, and nutrition to take the concepts and ideas further towards serving the most important development goal of eliminating malnutrition from the face of the earth.

REFERENCES

Bouis, H. E. 2000. Commercial Vegetable and Polyculture Fish Production in Bangladesh: Their Impacts on Household Income and Dietary Quality. *Food and Nutrition Bulletin.* 21(4): 482-487.

Hoddinot J. and Y. Yohannes. 2001. *Dietary diversity as a food security indicator.* Seminar at International Food Policy Research Institute, Washington, DC, June 27, 2001.

Index

T - #0360 - 101024 - C12 - 216/152/23 - PB - 9781560221036 - Gloss Lamination